CANCER CONTROL
IN THE COUNTRIES OF THE COUNCIL
OF MUTUAL ECONOMIC ASSISTANCE

CANCER CONTROL IN THE COUNTRIES OF THE COUNCIL OF MUTUAL ECONOMIC ASSISTANCE

Edited by

N. P. NAPALKOV

and

S. ECKHARDT

AKADÉMIAI KIADÓ, BUDAPEST 1982

Copyright © Akadémiai Kiadó, Budapest 1982

ISBN 963 05 3036 8

Printed in Hungary

LIST OF AUTHORS

People's Republic of Bulgaria

MANOILOV K., Cand. Sci. /Med./, senior scientific worker, the Institute of Oncology, Sofia; MONOV N., Cand. Sci. /Med./, senior scientific worker, the Institute of Oncology, Sofia; POPOV I., Cand. Sci. /Med./, senior scientific worker, the Institute of Oncology, Sofia; STOICHEV D., Cand. Sci. /Med./, senior scientific worker, the Institute of Oncology, Sofia.

Cuba

MARINELLO I., Prof., Minister of Health of Cuba; KOCHNEV V.A., the prof. N.N. Petrov Research Institute of Oncology of the USSR Ministry of Health.

Czechoslovak Socialist Republic

GODÁL A., Cand. Sci. /Med./, senior scientific worker, Institute of Clinical Oncology, Bratislava; DVOŘAK V., Cand. Sci. /Med./, senior scientific worker, Institute of Oncology, Prague; DOLEJŠÍ V., Cand. Sci. /Med./, senior scientific worker, Institute of Experimental Oncology, Bratislava; DŮRKOVSKÝ J., Cand. Sci. /Med./, senior scientific worker, Institute of Oncology, Prague; KOLÁŘ V., Cand. Sci. /Med./, senior scientific worker, Institute of Oncology, Prague; KUBEC V., Dr. Sci. /Med./, the chief specialist on radiology of the CzSSR Ministry of Health, Prague; MAKOVICKÁ L., Cand. Sci. /Med./, senior scientific worker, Institute of Oncology, Prague; MAŇKA I., Cand. Sci. /Med./, senior scientific worker, Institute of Oncology, Prague; MECHL Z., Cand. Sci. /Med./, senior scientific worker, Institute of Oncology, Prague;

PLEŠKO V., Cand. Sci. /Med./, senior scientific worker, Institute of Oncology, Prague; RUBEŠ R., Cand. Sci. /Med./, senior scientific worker, Institute of Experimental Oncology, Bratislava; STACH J., Cand. Sci. /Med./, Institute of Oncology, Prague; TAUFROVÁ M., Cand. Sci. /Med./, senior scientific worker, Institute of Oncology, Prague; THURZO V., academician, Director of the Institute of Experimental Oncology, Bratislava; FREMMER J., Cand. Sci. /Med./, senior scientific worker, Institute of Oncology, Prague; ČEPČEK P., Dr. Sci. /Med./, senior scientific worker, Institute of Experimental Oncology, Bratislava; ČERNÝ V., Cand. Sci. /Med./, senior scientific worker, Institute of Experimental Oncology, Bratislava; ŠOMODI J., Cand. Sci. /Med./, Institute of Experimental Oncology, Bratislava.

German Democratic Republic
HEROLD H., Prof. Cand. Med. Sci., the Head of the National Register of Cancer Diseases, the Central Institute of Oncological Diseases, Berlin.

Hungarian People's Republic
PÉTER Z., M. D., the Head of the Organizing and Methodics Department, the Institute of Oncology, Budapest; ECKHARDT S., Prof., Cand. Med. Sci., Director of the Institute of Oncology, Budapest.

Mongolian People's Republic
DORZHGOTOV B., Cand. Sci. /Med./, the head physician of the Republican Oncological Hospital, Ulan Bator; NYAMDAVAA N., the head of a department of the Republican Oncological Hospital, Ulan Bator; OCHIRBAY S., inspector of the Therapeutic and Prophylactic Department, the Republican Oncological Hospital, Ulan Bator.

Polish People's Republic
SOSINSKI IR., M. D., the Deputy Director, the Marie Sklodowska-
-Curie Institute of Oncology, Warsaw.

The USSR
ALEKSANDROV N.N., the corresponding member of the USSR Academy of Medical Sciences, Professor, Director of the Institute of

Oncology and Medical Radiology of the BSSR Ministry of Health, Minsk; ARTYUSHENKO Yu.V., Cand. Sci. /Med./, senior scientific worker, the Oncological Research Centre of the USSR AMS, Moscow; BEREZKIN D.P., Dr. Sci. /Med./, the Head of the Laboratory of studying the efficiency of treatment of patients with malignant tumours, professor of the N.N. Petrov Institute of Oncology of the USSR Ministry of Health, Leningrad; BUSLAEVA M.M., Cand. Sci. /Med./, senior scientific worker of the Scientific and Organizing Department of the N.N. Petrov Institute of Oncology of the USSR Ministry of Health, Leningrad; GERASIMENKO V.N., Dr. Sci. /Med./, the Head of the Department of Rehabilitation of the Oncological Research Centre of the USSR AMS, Moscow; GUTMAN Z.M., Cand. Sci. /Med./, the Head of the Scientific and Organizing Department, the Institute of Oncology and Medical Radiology of the BSSR Ministry of Health, Moscow; DEMIDOV V.P., Dr. Sci. /Med./, the Chief of the Board of Oncological Assistance of the USSR Ministry of Health, Moscow; YEGOROV P.I., Cand. Sci. /Med./, assistant professor of the N.N. Petrov Institute of Oncology of the USSR Ministry of Health, Leningrad; YEKIMOV V.I., physician of the Scientific and Organizing Department, N.N. Petrov Institute of Oncology of the USSR Ministry of Health, Leningrad; ZARUBOVA A.E., Cand. Sci. /Med./, senior scientific worker, the Oncological Research Centre of the USSR AMS, Moscow; KLIMENKOV A.A., Dr. Sci. /Med./, the Head of Department of the Oncological Research Centre of the USSR AMS, Moscow; LAZO V.V., Cand. Sci. /Med./, the Head of the Department of otorhinolaryngologic oncology of the N.N. Petrov Institute of Oncology of the USSR Ministry of Health, Leningrad; MERABISHVILI V.M., Cand. Sci. /Med./, senior scientific worker, the Scientific and Organizing Department of the N.N. Petrov Institute of Oncology of the USSR Ministry of Health, Leningrad; MIROTVORTSEVA K.S., Cand. Sci. /Med./, worker of the sector of coordination of the Scientific and Organizing Department, N.N. Petrov Institute of Oncology of the USSR, Ministry of Health, Leningrad; NAZARENKOV V.P., junior scientific worker, the Scientific and Organizing Department of the N.N. Petrov Institute of Oncology of the USSR

Ministry of Health, Leningrad; NAPALKOV N.P., the corresponding
member of the USSR AMS, Professor, Director of the Institute,
N.N. Petrov Institute of Oncology of the USSR Ministry of
Health, Leningrad; ORLOVSKY L.V., Dr. Sci. /Med./, Professor,
the Central Institute of Education, Moscow; PESTOVSKAYA G.N.,
Cand. Sci. /Biol./, senior scientific worker, the Oncological
Research Centre of the USSR AMS, Moscow; PETERSON B.E., Dr.
Sci. /Med./, Professor, Director of the Moscow P.A. Gertsen
Oncological Institute of the RSFSR Ministry of Health, Moscow;
SAVELJEV M.N., Cand. Sci. /Med./, the acting Chief of the
Department of Foreign Relations of the USSR Ministry of Health,
Moscow; STRELKOVA R.M., Cand. Sci. /Med./, senior scientific
worker of the Department of Medical Information of the Onco-
logical Research Centre of the USSR AMS, Moscow; SYAGAEV S.A.,
Cand. Sci. /Med./, the Chairman of the CMEA Health Service
Commission, Moscow; TIKHONOVA N.A., Cand. Sci. /Med./, senior
scientific worker, the Head of the Scientific and Organizing
Department of the Oncological Research Centre of the USSR AMS,
Moscow; FALILEYEV Yu.V., Dr. Sci. /Med./, Professor of the
Central Institute of Advanced Training of Physicians, Moscow;
CHAKLIN A.V., Dr. Sci. /Med./, Professor, the Head of the De-
partment of Epidemiology of Tumours of the Oncological Research
Centre of the USSR AMS, Moscow; SHABASHOVA N.Ya., Cand. Sci.
/Med./, senior scientific worker, the Scientific and Organizing
Department, N.N. Petrov Institute of Oncology of the USSR
Ministry of Health, Leningrad.

PREFACE

This volume is an English version of the book entitled "Cancer Control in the Countries of the Council of Mutual Economic Assistance" edited by N.P.Napalkov and S.Eckhardt in 1980, in Russian. The Editorial Board of this publication is composed of a group of experts from the CMEA countries such as Bulgaria, Cuba, Czechoslovakia,the German Democratic Republic, Hungary, Mongolia, Poland and the Soviet Union. The book enlists a series of geographical, socio-economic and demographic background information as well as data on the cancer incidence of these countries. It describes the structure, organization and cancer control activities including aspects of professional and public education at the given areas.

The reader will find various patterns of cancer incidence in the different countries, and the preventive, diagnostic and therapeutic measures taken against malignancies also vary within wide limits. Nevertheless in each country discussed there is an effort to organize the fight against cancer by creating a centralized plan which is a part of the national health care programmes. These programmes prescribe methods of prevention, early detection, diagnosis, treatment and follow-up of cancer. Although to a various degree, most of the CMEA countries have also educational programs directed to the medical personnel and to the community.

It is obvious that cancer as a number two killer in many countries deserves special attention. It is also quite clear that the fight against malignant diseases cannot be

successful without an international and interdisciplinary collaboration of all experts in this field. This was the reason
why the Editors and members of the Editorial Board of this
book felt it necessary to publish their experience in English.
It is their hope that by the aid of their present contribution a new bridge will be opened among various parts of the
world.

The Authors are fully aware of the fact that without the highly competent and effective assistance rendered by
the Publishing House: Akadémiai Kiadó to the Editors this book
could not have been published. Therefore, they wish to express
their gratitude to all who assisted in completing this work.
Special thanks have to be attributed to dr. Zoltán Péter whose
devoted assistance was of great value in the editorial work.

Sándor Eckhardt

X

CONTENTS

CANCER CONTROL IN THE USSR

INTRODUCTION

Whatever social systems and health care services can be, a majority of the countries in the world are faced today with the necessity to solve the problem of cancer the importance of which for national and international public health is only too obvious.

The representatives of the Soviet Union expressed the view in the Third Committee of the Fourteen Session of the UN general Assembly that the fight against malignant neoplasms called for joint efforts on the part of the UN member-states. This view was supported by the world public, and its support manifested itself in the development of wider international contacts of scientists working on various aspects of the "malignant neoplasms". This view was declared again in 1973 when the Twenty Sixth World Health Assembly proclaimed a resolution calling on all countries to coordinate their efforts within the framework of a long-term scientific programme aimed at controlling malignant neoplasms. Led by the Soviet Union, the CMEA member-states have taken an active part in the elaboration of this programme and have made, in this respect, a significant contribution.

The cooperation amongst the CMEA countries reveals a considerable development. It has to be pointed out here that from among the most important medical problems included in the programme of cooperation priority was given to the integrated problem of "malignant neoplasms". In December 1973, at the Eighteenth Session of CMEA in Moscow the competent organs of the CMEA member-states signed a protocol of an Agreement on scien-

tific cooperation on the problem of "malignant neoplasms".
Each participating country was assigned to elaborate some selected scientific topics in accordance with the programme provided for in the Agreement.

A large volume of organizational work that followed this
agreement made it possible to work out detailed programmes of
the proposed research and involve the scientific research institutes of the CMEA member-states in this effort which had
expressed their consent to participate and cooperate in this
work. The countries which had decided to take part on a joint
basis in this project entitled "The Scientific Foundations of
the Organization of Cancer Control" are as follows: Bulgaria,
Czechoslovakia, Hungary, the German Democratic Republic, Cuba,
Mongolia, Poland and the USSR.

It should be emphasized that the social nature of the
problem of "malignant neoplasms" has brought about considerably
greater interest and development of scientific research in the
field of organization of cancer control, which is only natural.

The necessity for early diagnosis, investigation, comprehensive treatment and follow-up of many people simultaneously
suffering from malignant neoplasms, the questions of their rehabilitation, social security and provision of assistance and
care in the course of progress of their primary disease have
brought about a situation when the questions of organization
have acquired a dominant significance in a system of assistance
to patients with malignant neoplasms.

In countries where the type of pathology is non-epidemic
the work aimed at improving oncological assistance has been
going on rather intensively in recent years. It is obvious that
directions in the development of oncological assistance are
determined, to a considerable extent, not only by the level of
medical services in the given country, but also by the latter's
state system, geographic, ethnic and "way of life" pecularities,
by the composition of its population, and so on.

The study of this question reveals that the premises on
which the organization of oncological assistance is built in
various countries of the world are extremely diverse and the
great efforts by a number of countries to reorganize and

2

modernize their oncological services show that they are not
quite satisfied with the forms and results in this field of activity.

In this respect, the experience of the countries of the socialist world in the field of organization of oncological assistance to the population has been attracting a great deal of attention all over the world in recent years. It should be noted
that this interest is quite natural for it is precisely in the
countries of socialism where a harmonious and logically substantiated system of oncological assistance has been built which
comprises a functioning network of oncological institutions providing prevention, diagnostic, treatment and dispensary services
for patients with malignant neoplasms. This work which is vast
in scope is conducted on a planned basis and in accordance with
the existing oncological doctrines and conceptions and in a close
connection with other treatment institutions of the country, as
their natural integral part; at the same time, this system possesses also a certain amount of autonomy, it has certain features which are specific to its activities only and, lastly, it
is intended exclusively to meet the needs of patients with malignancies and preblastomatoses. All this cannot but lay a
special imprint on its functions. The concentration of efforts
on the elaboration of this single problem has made it possible
to create a harmonious system of measures in a comparatively
short period of time definite results has been achieved by its
improvement in the fight against malignant neoplasms. In organizing their own systems of cancer control, the countries of the
socialist world relied on the Soviet Union's rich experience in
the field of organization of oncological assistance the beginnings of which go back in that country to the 20's of this century. At the same time, the forms of oncological assistance
created in these countries do not follow entirely the system
adopted in the Soviet Union, they bear an imprint of individual-
ity in which the state, national, geographic and other pecularities of these countries are reflected. It should be noted that
these methods of fight against malignant tumours which are
unique in nature and are organized and implemented on a nation-
-wide scale are not known to an adequate extent in the world.

3

This monograph entitled "Cancer Control in the CMEA member--countries" is a first publication of this kind and contains a description of all aspects of organization of oncological assistance to the population in the CMEA member-states. The monograph is intended to fill, to some extent, the gap existing in this field and to give organizers in the field of public health, oncologists and physicians interested in the problems of cancer control and opportunity to get to know the state system of organization of oncological assistance in the socialist countries more or less fully.

At the same time, the monograph represents, to a certain extent, a summing up of the process of integration of scientific research by the CMEA member-states, which, following the agreement of 1973 on the technic-scientific cooperation within the framework of the problem of "Public Health" has become especially fruitful.

It is intended to give a thorough description of the system of organization of oncological assistance in the CMEA member--states in the monograph. It has been considered advisable to give information on the organization of oncological assistance to the population in each country in accordance with a uniform plan so that one could adequately assess the distinctions and peculiarities characteristic of individual countries. But with all the differences of approach to the question of prevention, diagnosis and treatment of patients with malignant neoplasms, the existence of a strictly regulated organization of curative and social assistance to persons afflicted with malignant neoplasms deserves attention and studies for this may prove extremely useful for the further work in this field.

N. P. Napalkov

S. Eckhardt

CANCER CONTROL IN BULGARIA

THE COUNTRY'S GEOGRAPHIC, ECONOMIC AND DEMOGRAPHIC PROFILE
AND THE DEVELOPMENT OF CANCER CONTROL FROM A HISTORICAL ASPECT

I. Popov

Bulgaria lies in the south-eastern part of the Balkan
Peninsula between north latitudes of $41^{\circ}14'$ and $44^{\circ}13'$ and between longitudes of $22^{\circ}21'$ and $28^{\circ}36'$ east. On the south it is
bordered by Turkey and Greece, while on the west by Yugoslavia.
With Rumania to the north, the border is mainly the line of the
river Danube while there is an eastern frontage on the Black Sea.

Bulgaria occupies an area of 110,911 square km. The terrain
is characterized by a variety of relief and its frequent change.
The mean height above sea level is 470 m. Lowlands /31.5 per
cent of the territory/ and low hills /41 per cent of the terri-
tory/ occupy a predominant area; elevations 600 m high and even
higher occupy 27.5 per cent of the entire territory of the
country.

Water resources are not abundant in Bulgaria. To make up
for this deficiency, many artifical lakes have been constructed
during the last decades and subsurface waters are tapped on a
great scale. A great source of the country's wealth are mineral
springs /140 fields with more than 500 springs the total flow
of which exceeds 2,000 litres/sec/. Among them cold springs are
predominant the temperature of which is $20^{\circ}C$. Hot springs are
to be found in several regions - the Srednegorskaya region
where the mineral water has a temperature from 25 to $60^{\circ}C$, the
Marishka, where the temperature of mineral water reaches 50 to
$70^{\circ}C$, the Rilo-Rodopskaya region where water temperature reaches
$100^{\circ}C$. Together with the extensive beaches on the Black Sea
coast, mineral springs immensely enhance the importance of the

5

Republic as a balneological and health resort centre.

Bulgaria possesses various ore and non-metalliferous mineral deposits /iron, manganese, lead, zinc, copper, chromium, fireclay, kaolin, limestone, barite, salt and other/. Oil and gas extraction has been started on a limited scale, though.

During the last two to three decades Bulgaria has undergone great changes in the course of its economic development. Formerly a country of fragmented agriculture in which a predominant part of the population was engeged /77 per cent in 1939/ Bulgaria has, in a historically short period of time after the World War II and the Liberation, become an industrial-agrarian state. In 1972, industry accounted for 65 per cent of the total social production and for 56 per cent of the national income.

In 1939, 3,349 small industrial enterprises employed altogether 92,164 workers; the nationalization of industry was followed by the latter's considerable development so that in 1970 the number of workers employed in the industry reached 1,186,284. A considerable growth has been recorded in the production of electricity and fuel, in ferrous and non-ferrous metallurgy, mechanical engineering, chemical, light and food industries.

Significant structural changes have taken place also in the Bulgarian agriculture. Small peasant holdings have now been amalgamated into 696 cooperative farms distributed between agrarian-industrial and industrial-agrarian complexes, 170 in total. They are all equipped with modern implements for the cultivation of land. This enables the leaders to make large--scale plans of mechanization, fertilizing, irrigation and other land reclamation measures which, involve annual increases in agricultural production. The living and working conditions of the agricultural population are also undergoing vast changes and resemble more and more those of the urban population.

The climate in Bulgaria is determined by a number of factors, of which the most significant one is abundant solar radiation, characteristic for the latitudes where the country lies and the latter's geographical position.

The mean annual temperature for the 1915-1955 period was

6

10.5°C. As we go from north to south the mean annual temperature rises in some southern areas to 12.2°-13.9°C.

A great variety of climatic conditions can be explained by the proximity to the Mediterranean and the Black Seas and the predominant western-eastern circulation of air masses. As we go from north to south and from west to east the continental nature of climate becomes milder and shows features which are transitional between continental and Mediterranean types of climate. The southern part of the country is characterized by a great number of clear sunny days, hot summers and comparatively mild winters while the northern part by longer and colder winters and more frequent north-western and north-eastern winds.

Rainfall is unevenly distributed among the seasons and months and depends on the mean height above sea level. Mean annual rainfall for the 1896-1945 period was 698 mm but is showed differences depending on the mean height above sea level.

The soils of the country show a great diversity of types. In North Bulgaria one can find black and brown soils which are rich in humus. In South Bulgaria brown loessial and dense chernozem-like soils and their varieties /"smolnitsi"/ are to be found. In mountainous areas brown loessial and mountain-meadow soils are wide-spread.

The soil composition is suitable for supporting rich vegetation - forests, natural meadows, wild medicinal plants and herbs, agricultural crops: grain, vegetables, oil plants, tobacco, hemp, cotton, fruit trees, grapes, etc.

Demographic Situation

The demographic processes that have been taking place in Bulgaria in the 20th century can be divided into three periods. The first period began in 1900 and ended in the years 1920-1925. A gradual decline of a previously high natality was characteristic for this period, which lasted till the end of the World War I. This was followed by a 7-to-8 year period of demographic compensation with both natality and the growth of population significantly on the rise. As a result of the hard conditions of life after the war, mortality and morbidity were also rising.

The second period /1925-1945/ was characterized by a steady trend towards a lower natality which reached its lowest level /21.4 per 1,000/ in 1939 and remained stabilized at that level till 1945.

The third period /after 1945/ was also characterized by a trend towards a lower natality /14.9 per 1,000 in 1966/. A number of measures introduced at the end of 1967, and at the beginning of 1968 by the Government on a countrywide scale in order to raise natality gave good results; at the present time, we encounte a certain rise in natality /17.2 in 1974/.

Mortality also showed an upward trend in the first period and a downward trend in the second and third periods and at the present time - from 23.8 per 1,000 for the 1900-1910 period down to 17.9 for the 1926-1930 period and from 12.3 for the 1946-1950 period down to 8.8 for the 1966-1970 period.

Infant mortality per 1,000 new-born children was 147.1 in 1926-1966 period and 30.5 for the year 1972. In 1974, infant mortality dropped to 25.4 per 1,000 newborns.

The general mortality for the country as a whole was 9.8 in 1972; for the urban population it was 7.4 and for the agricultural population - 12.8; among males mortality was 10.5 and among females - 9.1 per 1,000. A considerable proportion is due to diseases of circulatory organs and malignant neoplasms. Mortality from these disease in 1969 was 426.2 and 135.0 per 100,000 people, respectively. /see Fig. 1/.

In Bulgaria average life expectancy has increased from 53 years for males and 56 years for females at the end of the World War II to 69 years for males and 73 years for females in the 1969-1970 period. The structure of the Bulgarian population has considerably changed, too /see Fig. 2/.

In terms of its nationalities, the Bulgarian population can be considered homogeneous. As at December 1965, Bulgarians made up 87.9 per cent of the total population, Turks 9.5 per cent, gypsies 1.8 per cent, while Armenians, Jews, etc. the remaining almost 1 per cent.

The rate of employment in the population is 51.3 per cent /58.1 per cent for men and 45.7 per cent for women/.

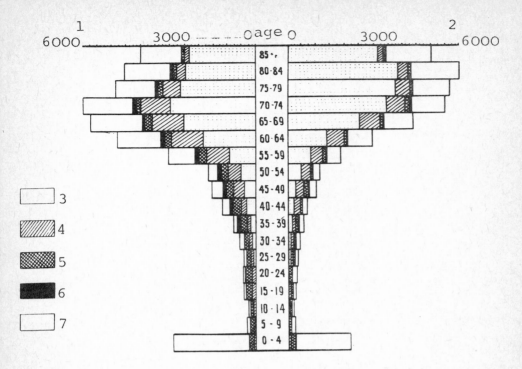

Fig. 1. Mortality in Bulgaria caused by major groups of diseases for the year 1969.

1. Males - 2. Females - 3. Cardiovascular diseases - 4. Malignant neoplasms - 5. Accidents, injuries, poisoning - 6. Tuberculosis - 7. Other diseases

In 1972, the average density of population for the entire territory of Bulgaria was 77.5 per cent sq. km with considerable differences between regions - from 48.5 to 118.7 in some regions and 979.1 people per sq. km in Sofia.

According to preliminary estimations, the population of Bulgaria has increased by December 1975 /the last population census/, by 12.4 per cent as compared with 1946, to reach the total of 8,729,720 of which 5,061,458 people live in towns and 3,608,285 in villages. The number of men /4,356,826/ is somewhat lower than that of woman /4,372,894/. The urban population has grown from 24.7 per cent in 1946 to 59.4 per cent in 1974 while the agricultural population has diminished from 75.8 per cent to 40.6 per cent mainly as a result of migration and urbanization. In 1946, there were 113 small towns in the country

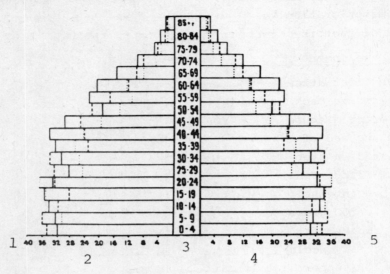

| I968 |
| I956 |
| I946 |

Fig. 2. The age-sex distribution of the population of Bulgaria
for 1946, 1956 and 1968
1. Years - 2. Males - 3. Age - 4. Females -
5. Years of age

/the capital Sofia had 366,800 inhabitants, there were three
towns with a population from 50 to 126 thousand inhabitants,
11 towns with a population from 30 to 50 thousand and 30 towns
with a population up to 5,000/. At the present time, the country's capital has a population of 965,728, together with the
population of the suburbs 1,064,712; there are 2 cities with
a population from 250,000 to 300,000, 4 with a population from
100,000 to 160,000 and 14 towns from 50,000 to 100,000 people.

During the last decades, industry has developed at an accelerated rate, which has contributed to the growth of a number of towns and villages with industrial areas and has changed
the number and composition of their population.

The geographic and demographic changes that have taken
place in Bulgaria are of great importance for the health of
its population. While playing a positive role in raising the

10

living standards of the population and its cultural level, the processes of growing industrialization and urbanization, of the development of the productive forces and the accelerating economic and social changes lead, at the same time, to environmental deterioration which occupies a distinct place in the complex of factors affecting the health of the population.

Development of Oncological Assistance in Bulgaria

The first attempts to make public the control of malignant neoplasms date back to 1928 when the problems of cancer were taken up for discussion at a congress of physicians of the country; at the end of the 30s, a Cancer Control Committee was established, a step which was soon followed by the opening of the Anti-Cancer Centre with the total of 20 cancer beds at the Chair of Roentgenology of the Medical Faculty in Sofia in 1937. There were 200 grams of radium obtained for treatment purposes. But the impact of these measures on meeting the needs of the population in oncological assistance was negligible because of the lack of support from the State. Thus, the physicians directed their efforts to solving, mainly, curative tasks while the questions of prevention of cancer and its early diagnosis remained outside their purposeful endeavours.

The social and economic changes that took place in Bulgaria after the World War II have made it possible to achieve a rapid improvement in the field of public health. It is now based on such socialist principles tested by the Soviet health service as prevention, humanism, provision of free medical care, general accessibility and planned nature. A wide network of medical services available to the entire population with specialized oncological institutions for monitoring patients with malignant neoplasms has been set up and is continually developing.

The great social importance of morbidity and mortality caused by malignant neoplasms has made it imperative to carry out organized cancer control. It is necessary to emphasize that among the causes of death, malignant tumours have taken the second place in Bulgaria and in a number of other economically developed countries.

Nevertheless, the high cancer mortality is not the only reason why the problem of malignant neoplasms has been the object of so much concern on the part of public health authorities and the medical profession. The advances made in the study of the etio-pathogenesis of cancer have demonstrated that cancer is preventable, while the complex methods of its treatment allow new approaches to be adopted in solving this intricate socio-biological problem. These complex methods provide the basis for organization and development of specialized oncological care as a part of the system of health service.

In Bulgaria, organized cancer control began in 1950-1951 when free medical care was decreed and the main principles of organization of cancer control - prevention, early detection, diagnosis, treatment, follow-up, reduction of invalidism and rehabilitation of patients with malignant neoplasms - were introduced. For the implementation of the above measures on a wide and co-ordinated basis within the system of health service a special organization for cancer control under the auspices of the Ministry of Health and District Departments of Health has been set up.

In accordance with the new tasks, a number of normative documents on organization and activities in the field of the health service have been elaborated. During the period of 1971-1974 the following documents were adopted: the Law on Health, the Law on a System of Prophylactic Mass Examinations and the stages of its realization, the Programmes for the development of individual branches of health service including that of cancer control. The general perspectives for the development of health service have been laid down and contributed to an improved oncological assistance for the population.

The Research Institute of Oncology set up in 1950 under the Ministry of Health has become a scientifico-methodological centre for prevention and treatment of malignant tumours in the country while the thirteen District Oncological Dispensaries have become the main links in the pattern of organization, guidance and implementation of cancer control measures within the boundaries of the areas they serve. This pattern of

administrative and scientifico-methodological guidance ensures
a successful participation of all the organs of the health
service in the cancer control of the entire population of the
country /see Fig. 3./

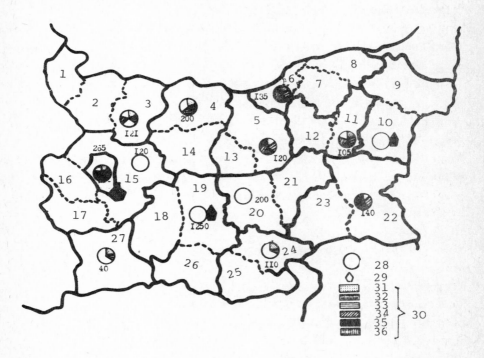

Fig. 3. The network of oncological institutions in Bulgaria

1 - Vidin	15 - Sofia	28 - Oncological
2 - Mikhaylov-	16 - Pernik	institutions
grad	17 - Kyustendil	29 - Medical
3 - Vratsa	18 - Pazardzhik	Academy
4 - Pleven	19 - Plovdiv	30 - Radiotheraphy
5 - V.Turnovo	20 - Stara	methods
6 - Ruse	Zagora	31 - Deep roentgen
7 - Razgrad	21 - Sliven	therapy
8 - Silistra	22 - Burgas	32 - Surface
9 - Tolbukhin	23 - Yambol	therapy
10 - Varna	24 - Khaskovo	33 - Closed
11 - Shumen	25 - Kurdzhali	isotopes
12 - Turgovishte	26 - Smolyan	34 - Open isotopes
13 - Gabrovo	27 - Blagoevgrad	35 - Gammatron
14 - Lovech		36 - Betatron

Before the specialized network of oncological institutions

was organized, the country's statistical data on cancer morbidity and mortality was incomplete. Use was made mainly of the information regarding the patients who had undergone treatment and those who had died in the medical institutions, and mortality was partly registered in some cities of the country.

The elaboration of statistics relating to the incidence of malignant neoplasms, which is necessary for planning, guidance and improvement of organization of cancer control, began on a countrywide scale in 1952. To meet the need in statistics for the above-mentioned purposes, a system of registration of each newly diagnosed patient, alive or dead, with a malignant neoplasm and permanent information on the registrations to the respective District Oncological Dispensary has been introduced and made compulsory. The postmortem examination and registration of patients with malignant neoplasms has also been made more efficient. It has become possible to identify the extent of the disease, specific features of, and trends in, the patterns of its incidence in the country and also to study the causes behind the appearance of malignant tumours under the influence of certain factors.

The public health organs study and analyse the statistical data on morbidity, incidence and mortality, in case of malignant neoplasms and the effectiveness of prophylactic activities. This provides the basis for the elaboration of perspective programs of step-by-step development of the oncological network, for the specialized training of medical personnel with a view to improve their qualification and knowledge in oncology, for strengthening the prophylactic character of cancer control, improving the care and management of patients, and for guiding research activities in the field of etiopathogenesis, prevention, clinical behaviour, and treatment of tumours, synthesis and testing of anti-cancer preparations.

In Bulgaria the leading role in the organization of cancer control is played by the specialized oncological institutions /see Fig. 4/.

The Institute of Oncology has sections, in-patient clinics /the total of 265 beds/ and laboratories for diagnostic,

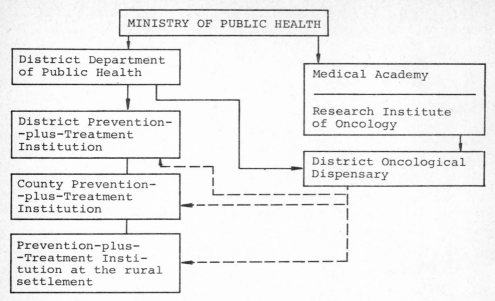

Fig. 4. The pattern of organization of oncological assistance
in Bulgaria

thrapeutic, experimental, organizational-methodological and
preventive activities. The Institute has studied, elaborated
and introduced new methods in the diagnosis, treatment and
prevention of cancer. It conducts experiments on carcinogenesis,
biology and immunology of tumours and investigates anti-tumour
substances. Besides, the Institute studies the extent of, and
trends in, the incidence of malignant neoplasms in certain
groups of population, carries on research aimed at the elucidation of certain features of these neoplasms from the point of
view of their epidemiology, and estimates the effectiveness of
monitoring the oncological patients, etc. The Institute offers
opportunities /through training courses and individually/ to
medical workers to receive a speciality in oncology and improve
their knowledge in this respect, publishes manuals, monographs,
etc. on the questions of theoretical and practical oncology,
sponsors congresses, symposia, workshops, and ten-day colloquies
on cancer. The workers of the Institute render, on a systematic
basis, scientific -methodological and consultative assistance
to oncological dispensaries and other treatment-plus-prophy-

lactic institutions in the question of prevention, diagnosis and treatment of malignant neoplasms and organization of cancer control. The comprehensive nature of its activities has made the Institute a leading scientific, consultative and therapeutic establishment and a methodological centre of oncology for the whole country.

The integration of the Institute with the Medical Academy in 1973 has opened up a prospect of improving the quality of undergraduate and postgraduate training in oncology. Thus the possibility was also created to involve not only oncologists in the scientific —methodological assistance in the questions of prophylaxis and treatment of pre-cancerous diseases and malignant neoplasms but also respective specialists from other highly qualified units of the Academy.

The District Oncological Dispensary belongs to the Department of Health of the local District Council. As for its activities in the district it is entrusted to serve, the Dispensary plans them after consultations with the local Department of Health and reports to the latter on the implementation of these activities.

In accordance with the standards relating to established posts in treatment institutions, the oncological dispensaries in Bulgaria fall into two categories: first category dispensaries serve areas with a population of over 500,000; second category dispensaries serve areas with a population under 500,000. The area to be served by each dispensary is determined and approved by the Ministry of Health.

At the end of 1951, when the oncological dispensaries were opened on the basis of district hospitals, they had to operate on a very small scale for they had no more than 5 to 10 beds for the hospitalization of patients with malignant neoplasms. Later a definite direction was set for the development of the dispensaries with a country-wide standard of 3 oncological beds per 10,000 inhabitants. The number of beds in the oncological institutions including those in the Institute of Oncology increased up to 315 at the end of 1953, 1,115 by 1965 and the present total of 1.681 /1.93 per 10,000 inhabitants/.

Now the majority of dispensaries have 100 to 200 hospital beds.

The specialized comprehensive treatment of patients with malignant tumours is ensured to a considerable extent by the organization of in-patient departments in the oncological institutions. A part of the oncological patients /mainly those needing surgical treatment and pharmacotherapy/ is admitted to the district or city treatment-plus-prophylactic institutions, or to the institutes and in-patient units of the Medical Academy.

As a result of the intensive activities of the oncological network, the number of patients receiving treatment in specialized institutions is increasing every year. An oncological dispensary has the following units: consulting rooms, laboratories, registration department with a card file, organizational and methodological department with a statistical section and also an administrative and financial division /see Fig.5/.

In accordance with the standard establishment and normatives concerning the established posts for medical personnel of treatment Institutions in Bulgaria, the availability of physicians, including those working in the oncological dispensaries and the diagnostic, treatment and prophylactic units of the Institute of Oncology, reached 3.62 per 100,000 inhabitants in 1974; among them surgeons - 0.77; gynaecologists - 0.41; radiologists - 0.47; therapists - 0.37; organizers and statisticians - 0.45; roentgenologists - 0.18; pathologists - 0.18, etc.

Out of the total number of physicians in the country which reached 209.4 per 100,000 inhabitants at the end of 1974, 91 per cent join the physicians of oncological institutions in carrying out diagnostic, therapeutic and prophylactic measures in the field of cancer control.

The supply of oncological institutions with diagnostic apparatus and facilities is getting improved each year.

The role of oncological dispensaries in the realization of the provisions of the normative documents approved by the Ministry of Health is determined by the documents themselves.

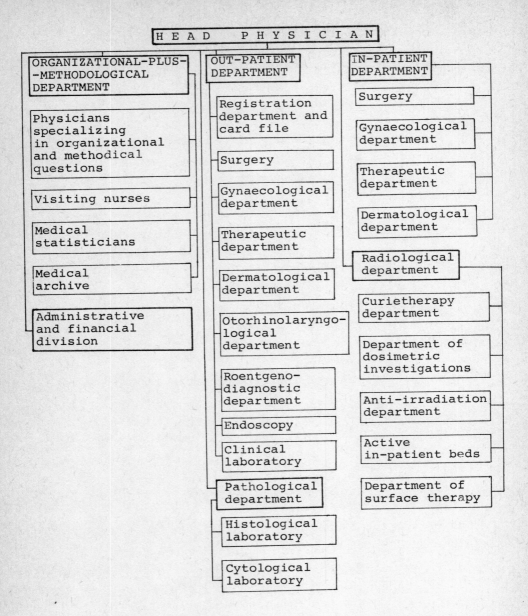

HEAD PHYSICIAN

ORGANIZATIONAL-PLUS--METHODOLOGICAL DEPARTMENT

- Physicians specializing in organizational and methodical questions
- Visiting nurses
- Medical statisticians
- Medical archive
- Administrative and financial division

OUT-PATIENT DEPARTMENT

- Registration department and card file
- Surgery
- Gynaecological department
- Therapeutic department
- Dermatological department
- Otorhinolaryngological department
- Roentgeno-diagnostic department
- Endoscopy
- Clinical laboratory
- Pathological department
- Histological laboratory
- Cytological laboratory

IN-PATIENT DEPARTMENT

- Surgery
- Gynaecological department
- Therapeutic department
- Dermatological department
- Radiological department
- Curietherapy department
- Department of dosimetric investigations
- Anti-irradiation department
- Active in-patient beds
- Department of surface therapy

Fig. 5. Structure of a District Oncological Dispensary

The main task of an oncological dispensary is cancer prevention. In accordance with this, the dispensary studies the extent of, and trends in, the incidence of malignant

18

tumours among the population in the area it serves, makes efforts to detect them, examines the effect of carcinogenic factors to which the population is exposed at work and at home and also studies pre neoplastic diseases

The responsibility of the dispensary in connection with the primary prevention of cancer is to notify the public and sanitary organs of air, water and soil pollution, to work for a strict observance of the standards and regulations related to the protection of natural and social environment from the effects of harmful substances, especially those of carcinogenic character.

The dispensary elaborates and proposes to the district health departments an exact plan of organization of prophylactic examinations of the population for the early detection of precancerous diseases and malignant neoplasms, exercises methodological guidance in the course of their performance and involves its physicians in this work; it also issues directions for out-patient and in-patient departments of the general treatment institutions with regard to strengthen to prophylactic aspect of daily check-ups and attention to cancer. Together with respective specialists of the district hospitals, the dispensary analyses the data obtained in the course of the prophylactic examinations of the population, directs and organizes measures aimed at the restoration of the health of detected oncological patients and, besides, organizes, directs and carries out monitoring of such patients.

The oncological dispensary's second main task consists in ensuring early diagnosis and specialized comprehensive treatment of malignant neoplasms and precancerous diseases. It renders systematic assistance to prevention and treatment institutions, on a systematic basis, in introducing new methods of diagnosis and treatment of the oncological diseases and also consultative assistance, if necessary. The dispensary keeps under its effective control and studies every case of malignant neoplasm in an advanced stage, every postmortem diagnosis, every case of malignant neoplasm first diagnosed only after death and organizes measures aimed at reducing their number. The participation of oncologists in the meetings of specialized consultative teams is also a contribution to this. These teams were established in 1972 in the district hospitals for the diagnosis of malignant tumours in sites less accessible for investigation. Consultative assistance and methodological guidance is rendered to the district hospitals by the Institute of Oncology.

The dispensary takes steps for a timely admittance of patients with malignant neoplasms to oncological and other treatment institutions.

The oncological dispensary's third main task consists in organizing, directing, supervising and ensuring registration and monitoring of patients with malignant neoplasms and precancerous diseases. In view of this treatment institutions are required to notify it promptly of every newly identified case of cancer, every suspected case of malignant tumour and every case of malignant tumour first identified after death, and lastly, all deaths from malignant neoplasms. A notification to this effect is sent within 24 hours to the local oncological dispensary in the area of which the case has been identified. Should the object of the notification be a person not residing in the area served by the oncological dispensary in question the latter verifies the diagnosis, if necessary, and promptly transmits to the dispensary in the area of which the person resides. At the beginning of each year, every dispensary transmits copies of prompt notifications to the Institute of Oncology after verifying them. This makes it possible to study the patterns of incidence of malignant neoplasms for the country as a whole and distribution of malignant tumours by districts, taking into account the influence of various factors causing them.

The oncological dispensary registers each patient with a newly diagnosed malignant neoplasms; it fills in his personal medical card on the basis of the examination or epicrisis performed by another treatment institution which made the diagnosis or carried out a treatment. Personal medical cards form the dispensary's file where they are arranged in alphabetical order as well as according to the address of the patients.

The method of monitoring ensures an active detection of persons with malignant tumours and their observation on a systematic basis. The observation is effected by the oncological dispensary with the aid of the control cards which are distributed according to the sites of cancer, with months and days set for carrying out examinations in the county hospital and rural curative services of each county.

The city and district treatment and prophylactic institutions enter the newly diagnosed cases of malignant tumours into the patients' personal medical cards on which they put a special sign of an oncological disease and place it in the general card file. The results of examinations performed to verify the diagnosis, epicrises about the treatment made or control examinations, instructions of the oncological dispensary regarding the care of patients in home conditions are attached to them. The documentation provided by these institutions contains the necessary evidence regarding the incidence of the malignant neoplasms in the given area; it is used by medical workers as an aid in treating the patients in accordance with the oncological requirements.

Registration of patients with malignant neoplasms which is done by the 13 oncological dispensaries countributes to the more expedient and up-to-date solution of the problem of diagnosis and treatment of malignant tumours. Information gathered by the dispensaries and systematic analysis of the results of oncological assistance ensure timely identification of shortcomings and measures for their elimination. The statistical analysis of morbidity and mortality from, as well as susceptibility of the population to, malignant tumours and the examination of the results of medical treatment provide the basis for studying the epidemiological pecularities of the incidence of malignant tumours and the level of prophylactic examinations in various districts of the country.

The oncological dispensaries compile annual reports about the number of newly diagnosed cancer cases and those to be found in their registration files /Form 61-zh/ and also about

their activities /Form 10/ and transmit them to the Central
Statistical Office administered by the Cabinet at the beginning
of each year where these reports are collected on a country-
-wide scale. Besides, the dispensaries present to the Organizational and Methodological Section of the Institute of Oncology yearly analyses of their activities accompanied by
their reports. The Section assesses the results of the oncological assistance in the country and the activities of individual dispensaries, and presents them for discussion at the
joint meeting of chief physicians and heads of the organizational and methodological departments of the oncological dispensaries. The generalized conclusions of these meetings provide a basis for elaborating the prospects of development of
oncological assistance for the current year and the beginning
of the next one.

The verified notifications of newly diagnosed patients
with malignant neoplasms and the reports of the oncological
dispensaries received by the Organizational and Methodological
Section make possible to enlarge the scope of the statistical
and scientific research regarding the results of cancer control
in the country. The extent, structure and trends of the morbidity of the population from malignant neoplasms are determined. Studies are made on the requirements of the population
in a specialized oncological assistance and of the measures
necessary to take for the further development of such assistance.

During the last five-year period the stabilized and relatively low level of mortality and the growing morbidity of the
population reflect the positive results achieved in the course
of improving oncological assistance.

The analysis of the dynamics of the statistical indicators average for the five-year period ending with 1972 shows
not only the extent of, and trends in the morbidity of the
population from malignant neoplasms but also characterizes
the level of cancer control for the country as a whole /see
Figs 6 and 7/.

Information collected and sorted annually makes possible

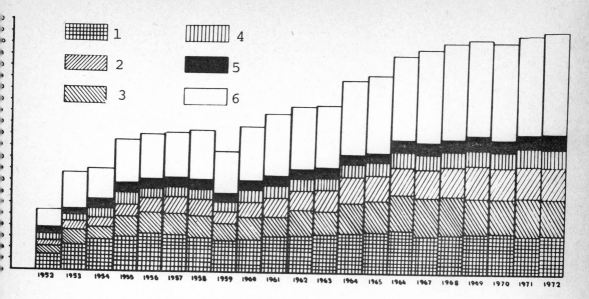

Fig. 6. Morbidity of the population in Bulgaria from malignant
neoplasms at some sites /per 100,000 inhabitants/
1. Skin - 2. Stomach - 3. Lung - 4. Breast -
5. Uterus - 6. Other sites

to carry out valuable epidemiological research on cancer and
to identify a number of socio-hygienic aspects of the oncological assistance necessary to determine the directions of its
further development and improvement.

THE SYSTEM OF REGISTRATION OF PATIENTS WITH NEWLY
DIAGNOSED MALIGNANT NEOPLASMS
N. Monov and I. Popov

The main sources of the information regarding the incidence of malignant neoplasms among the population in Bulgaria
are the compulsory registration of the cancer cases and deaths,
certificates of death and the annual reports of the oncological
dispensaries. On this basis, the Organizational and Methodological Section of the Institute of Oncology determines the

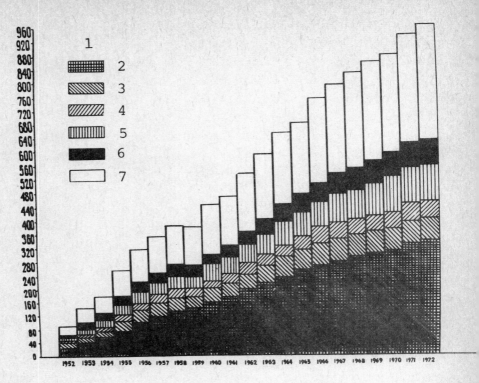

Fig. 7. The rate of patients with malignant neoplasms in Bulgaria from the 1952-1972 period

1. Sites per 100,000 inhabitants   - 2. Skin   - 3.Stom-
ach - 4. Lung - 5. Breast - 6. Uterus - 7. Other
sites

the rates of incidence of, morbidity and mortality from these
neoplasms for the country as a whole and by individual districts, for urban and rural population. Apart from that, the
therapeutic results in the district oncological dispensaries
and institutions of the general network are analysed, the
directions of the activities of these institutions in the organization of the oncological assistance to the population are
determined.

The tables of the incidence, mortality and morbidity of
malignant neoplasms for the five-year period have been calculated on the basis of data regarding the number and composition
of the population, which have been made available by the Central
Statistical Office.

24

In the middle of 1972, the population of Bulgaria totalled 8,576,200, of whom 4,285,708 /49.97 %/ were men and 4,290,492 /50.03 %/ women. The urban population numbered 4,721,847 /55.18 %/ while rural population 3,854,353 /44.82 %/. The relative proportion of the population aged 60 and over was 10.44 % in urban and 21.29 % in rural areas.

The registrations of patients with newly diagnosed malignant neoplasms for the 1970-1974 period averaged 18,371 per year, which means a rate of incidence of 214.21 per 100,000 inhabitants.

The number of newly diagnosed cases of malignant neoplasms in the period under review increased from 17,435 or 205.4 per 100,000 inhabitants in 1970 to 19,128 or 220.4 per 100,000 inhabitants in 1974. Thus, the rate of incidence increases annually by 3-3.5 per 100,000 inhabitants.

According to the standardization proposed by M. Segi, the average rate of incidence for the 1970-1974 period in Bulgaria equalled 196.04 per 100,000 inhabitants.

Although the morbidity of urban and rural population is examined separately in Bulgaria, the demographic and migratory processes of the last decades make it difficult, to a certain extent, to study the influence of certain factors on morbidity in the town and countryside.

The registrations of patients with newly diagnosed malignant neoplasms among the urban population for the 1970-1974 period averaged annually 9,003, or 190.26 per 100,000 inhabitants.

The rate of incidence among the urban population increased from 186.8 in 1970 to 196.6 in 1974. The increase was 2.3 per 100,000 inhabitants. The standardized rate of incidence for 1974 /population of Bulgaria in 1970 was taken as standard/ was 182.6; registrations of patients with newly diagnosed malignant neoplasms among the rural population averaged for the 1970-1974 period 9,368 or 218.34 per 100,000 inhabitants.

New cases of malignant neoplasms in the rural areas increased from 9,139 or 231.82 per 100,000 inhabitants in 1970 to 9,461 or 253.63 per 100,000 inhabitants in 1974. According to the M. Segi standard, the rate of incidence among the rural population in Bulgaria was 154.66 per 100,000 inhabitants.

The standardization of rates makes it obvious that the increase in their values is partly attributable to the increase in the percentage of people of older age groups.

The rate of increase is $V = 5.4$ per 100,000.

Registrations of male patients with newly diagnosed malignant neoplasms in Bulgaria for the 1970-1974 period averaged annually 9,916 per year or 231.4 per 100,000 inhabitants, while those of female patients 8,405 or 195.9 per 100,000 inhabitants.

According to the M. Segi standard, the male incidence rate equals 181.31 and the female incidence rate 145.97 per 100,000 inhabitants.

The male incidence rate of men shows less variation in some years as compared to that of women. In both sex groups, the highest incidence was recorded in 1974 /238.14 and 200.95, respectively/.

Men are more frequently affected by cancer of the lung, stomach, skin, lip, rectum, while women by cancer of the skin, stomach, cervix uteri, lung and so on.

In the average incidence for the 1970-1974 period, the first place occupied by the cancer of the skin - 16.2, followed by that of the stomach - 15.2, the lung - 13.7 and the breast - 7.8.

In men, the highest incidence was observed in older age groups while in women in the middle age groups in certain localizations /cervix uteri, breast/.

Concerning localization, cancer incidence in Bulgaria shows a considerable variation by districts and regions.

Administratively, the country is divided into 28 districts. The population of Sofia, the country's capital is over 1 million, while that of the Smolyan district, which is the smallest, is 162,296. There are differences between the districts not only in the number of their population but also in the ratio of urban and rural population, in the prevalence of some or other ethnic group and in the age distribution of population. People aged 60 and over comprise 22.02 per cent of the population in the Lovech District while in the Kurdzhali District

7.66 %. The differences in the incidence of malignant neoplasms depend to a similar extent also upon the climatic and geographic conditions, upon production and living conditions.

When characterizing the incidence of malignant neoplasms by individual districts it should be noted that it is the highest in the Trnovo District, 290.04, Vratsa District, 274.72, and Pleven District, 264.05 per 100,000, and it is considerably lower in the Smolyan District, 112.60, and Kurdzhali District, 121.19 per 100,000 inhabitants.

Among the urban population, the highest incidence was observed in Sofia, 241.33, in the towns of the Plovdiv District, 223.35, the V. Trnovo District, 221.94, while a lower incidence was observed in the Khaskovo District, 80.15 and Smolyan District, 90.96 per 100,000 inhabitants.

In the countryside, the highest incidence of malignant neoplasms has been observed in the Gabrovo District, 380.92, the Vratsa District, 350.80, the V. Trnovo District, 342.09, while the lowest incidence in the Kurdzhali District, 98.05 and the Smolyan District, 127.98 per 100,000 inhabitants.

Among men, the highest incidence was recorded in the V. Trnovo District, 304.75, the Vratsa District, 287.54, the Plovdiv District, 274.26, while the lowest in the Smolyan District, 126.94 and the Kurdzhali District, 140.46 per 100,000 inhabitants.

A high incidence of malignant neoplasms of each localization was observed among women in the V. Trnovo District, 273.91, the Vratsa District, 261.12, while a low incidence in the Kurdzhali District, 66.36 and the Smolyan District, 95.73 per 100,000 inhabitants.

The observed variation in the incidence of malignant neoplasms by districts can be explained by the different age distribution of the urban and rural population and by certain climatic and geographic, occupational and other conditions.

Some variations exist also in the levels of incidence of malignant neoplasms of different localization.

Cancer of the skin

In the structure of incidence, the cancer of skin occupies

the first place in Bulgaria. During the 1970-1974 period, its incidence averaged 34.63 per 100,000 inhabitants; it should be noted here that the highest incidence, 35.33, was observed in 1970 while the lowest, 33.79 in 1971. The annual variation in the incidence of cancer of the skin is insignificant; the rate of annual increase - V = 0.06 per 100,000 inhabitants. By the M. Segi standard, it is 25.27.

The incidence of cancer of the skin is higher than the national average in the Vratsa District, 61.43, the Khaskovo District, 49.61, the Plovdiv District, 46.25, while it is significantly lower in the Kurdzhali District, 14.48 and the Smolyan District, 18.07 per 100,000 inhabitants.

Among the urban population, the incidence of cancer of the skin is significantly higher in the Plovdiv District, 36.85, the Shumen District, 35.63, the Khaskovo District, 36.22 and it is lower in the Smolyan District, 9.96 and the Sliven District, 14.74 per 100,000 inhabitants.

Among the rural population, the incidence of cancer of the skin is significantly higher in the Vratsa District, 84.22, the Stara Zagora District, 74.60, while low incidence was recorded in the Kurdzhali District, 13.26 and the Silistra District, 21.85 per 100,000 inhabitants.

Apart from the factors mentioned above in connection with the differences in the incidence of cancer of the skin between the various districts of the country, it is of great importance, that a considerable proportion of the population is engaged in agriculture thus highly exposed to solar radiation.

The processes of migration and the changing conditions of agricultural labour have brought about an equalization in the incidence of the cancer of the skin among the rural and urban population.

Cancer of the stomach

Cancer of the stomach occupies the second place among malignant neoplasms in Bulgaria. Registrations of patients with cancer of the stomach for the 1970-1974 period averaged annually 2,787 or 32.49 per 100,000 inhabitants or 25.27 according to M. Segi.

The incidence of cancer of the stomach is high in the Gabrovo District, 51.50; in the V. Trnovo District, 49.55; it is significantly lower in the Smolyan District, 20.14 and the Vidin District, 20.57 per 100,000 inhabitants.

Among the urban population the highest incidence of cancer of the stomach is registered in the V. Trnovo District, 37.80, the Gabrovo District, 32.98, while in the Vidin District it is 10.25, the Mikhaylovgrad District 12.84 and the Smolyan District 13.10 per 100,000 inhabitants. These figures are considerably lower than the national average. To a certain extent, these differences are evidently due to the prevalence of certain trace elements in the soil and water.

A wide variation is observed in the incidence of cancer of the stomach between men and women.

Cancer of the stomach occurs more frequently in men than in women /39.34 and 25.48 per 100,000 inhabitants, respectively during the period under review/. The standardized rates of incidence according to M. Seg, 30.55 and 17.61, also confirm the existence of a considerable difference. It is possible that a higher consumption of alcohol and tobacco by men may be responsible for the higher incidence of the cancer of the stomach.

Cancer of the lung

In Bulgaria, cancer of the lung occupies the third place in the incidence structure. In the period under review, registrations of new patients averaged annually 2,511 or 29.27 per 100,000 inhabitants, or 20.14 according to M. Segi.

A high incidence of this cancer localization is connected with a high concentration of carcinogens in the atmosphere, especially in the large cities, with smoking and a number of occupational exposures.

The incidence of cancer of the lung in many district is close to the national average which equals 29.27; the highest incidence was recorded in the Mikhaylovgrad District, 40.26, while the lowest in the Smolyan District, 15.57 and the

Kurdzhali District, 18.33 per 100,000 inhabitants. The incidence of cancer of the lung in the period under review was 25.55 in the towns and 33.87 per 100,000 inhabitants in rural regions. According to the M. Segi method, the incidence was 25.07 for the urban population and 18.75 for the rural population. The high incidence of the cancer of the lung among the urban population can be explained, obviously, by the influence of a number of aetiological factors. The incidence among the urban population may be expected to be higher but the permanent migration of rural population into towns results in a somewhat lower figure. The highest incidence among the urban population was recorded in the Plovdiv District, 32.26, and the lowest in the Smolyan District, 13.36; in rural areas, the highest incidence was recorded in the Lovech District, 56.99 and the lowest in the Smolyan District, 17.13.

In its incidence,   cancer of the lung shows large differences according to sex.

In men, the incidence is 49.39, and in women 8.32. According to M. Segi, the incidence of cancer of the lung in Bulgaria as a whole is 20.14, in men 38.0 and in women 5.88 per 100,000 inhabitants. The incidence of cancer of the lung in men is 5.94 times higher than that of women, a fact which can, evidently, be explained by a higher consumption of tobacco and more frequent and prolonged stays in the environment polluted by carcinogens.

Cancer of the breast

Cancer of the breast occupies the fourth place in incidence with the value of 16.67 in the 1970-1974 period; the highest incidence, 18.19, was recorded in 1974, while the lowest, was 14.74 per 100,000 inhabitants in 1970. According to M. Segi, the incidence was 13.18. A comparatively high incidence of cancer of the breast in the period under review is associated with the reduction or absence of breast-feeding and frequently interrupted pregnancies, reduction in birth-rate, etc.

The incidence of cancer of the breast is considerably higher among the urban population than among rural population: 18.91 against 13.91, or 18.10 against 9.25 according to M. Segi.

Except for a shorter period of breast-feeding and a larger number of abortions in towns, an adequate explanation for this
difference has not yet been found.

The highest incidence was recorded in Sofia, 22.27, while
the lowest in the Kurdzhali District, 3.84, the Smolyan District, 7.29, the Blagoevgrad District, 9.50 and the Razgrad
District, 9.76 per 100,000 inhabitants.

Cancer of the cervix uteri

Registrations of new patients for the 1970-1974 period
averaged annually 556 or 6.49 per 100,000 inhabitants. The highest incidence of this period, 6.97, was recorded in 1974, and
the lowest in 1971 when it was 6.09 per 100,000 inhabitants. In
relation of women only, the incidence of cancer of the cervix
uteri is 12.78 per 100,000 inhabitants or 10.3 according to M.
Segi. The low incidence of cancer of the cervix uteri in Bulgaria can be attributed to the mass prophylactic examinations
carried out by the State.

There is a wide geographical variation in the incidence
of cancer of the cervix uteri.

Among the urban population, the incidence is 7.68, while
among the rural population it is 4.93 per 100,000 inhabitants,
or 7.19 and 3.46, respectively, according to M. Segi. The highest incidence was recorded in Sofia /the standardized rate according to M. Segi is 19.1/, and the lowest in the Smolyan District, 4.44.

Usually, the lower incidence of this cancer localization
is recorded in districts with a moslem population, where men
are circumcised.

Cancer of the lips

Cancer of the lips, especially that of the lower one,
is not rare in Bulgaria, which can be explained not only by
the geographical features of the country but also by the way
of living and the pursuits of the population in the past.

Registrations of new patients for the 1970-1974 period
averaged annually 523 or 6.10 per 100,000 inhabitants, and
4.61 according to M. Segi.

The highest incidence in the period under review was recorded in 1974 when it equaled 6.59, while the lowest in 1971
when it equaled 5.68 per 100,000 inhabitants.

The frequency of this cancer is greater in men than in
women /10.10 and 2.05 respectively per 100,000 inhabitants or
8.03 and 1.43, respectively, according to M. Segi/. This can be
attributed to a heavier alcohol consumption and smoking, less
care for the hygiene of the oral cavity, and a greater exposure
to unfavourable atmospheric conditions.

This cancer localization occurs more frequently among the
rural population. During the 1970-1974 period it was 3.75 for
the urban population and 8.99 per 100,000 inhabitants in the
rural population, or 3.64 and 5.45, respectively, according to
M. Segi. Its incidence is especially high in the Vratsa District, 11.59 while in Sofia it is the lowest, 2.69 per 100,000
inhabitants. The wide range of incidence points to the influence
of the way of living on the inception of tumour in this localization.

The higher incidence in the country can be explained by
a more frequent exposure to sun and wind; it is also obvious
that the conditions for the hygiene of the oral cavity are less
favourable in rural localities and this can also be a contributing factor.

Cancer of the rectum

The cancer of the rectum occurs rather frequently in
Bulgaria. Registrations of new patients in the period under
review averaged annually 661 per year or 7.7 per 100,000 inhabitants.

The highest incidence of cancer of the rectum, 8.95, was
recorded in 1974, and the lowest, 6.70 per 100,000 inhabitants,
in 1970.

Standardized incidence rates for 1974 /population in 1974
was taken as standard/ equaled 8.45 which clearly points to a
rise in the incidence of cancer of the rectum; the increased
percentage of persons of older age in the year under review
seems, in this respect, to be not the only contributing factor.

The incidence in men is somewhat higher than in women: the rates in the 1970-1974 period were 8.53 and 6.91, respectively, per 100,000 inhabitants, or 6.56 and 4.95 according to M. Segi.

The incidence of cancer of the rectum is somewhat higher in the town than in the country: 8.58 in the town against 7.04 per 100,000 inhabitants in the country /6.96 and 5.85, respectively, according to M. Segi/.

In Bulgaria registrations of all patients with malignant neoplasms /both newly diagnosed and surviving/ are made annually. On this basis, a coefficient of effectiveness /the relation between all oncological patients registered earlier and those registered for the first time/ is calculated.

In 1974, the incidence was calculated as an average of three preceeding years /1972, 1973 and 1974/.

The coefficient of effectiveness for all cancer localizations was 4.85 in 1974. For the most important cancer localizations, the coefficient shows a wide variation /cancer of the lip 12.60; cancer of the skin 10.37; cancer of the cervix uteri 7.6; cancer of the breast 6.84; cancer of the pharynx 5.36; cancer of the mouth 5.1; cancer of the stomach 2.09; cancer of the lung 1.8, and so on/.

The suggested method makes possible to assess the effectiveness of oncological assistance by years and by individual districts. While not supplanting the methods used for the study of perspective results of treatment of malignant neoplasms, it does give a certain idea of the possible results of diagnostic, therapeutic and preventive procedures and advances obtaining more accurate incidence rates.

Mortality from malignant neoplasms is studied in Bulgaria on the basis of the diagnoses registered in the death certificates. They are taken into account only when a malignant neoplasm has been the main cause of death.

For the 1970-1974 period mortality averaged 137.09; among the urban population it was 115.9, while among the rural population 162.6.

Considerable differences are found in the mortality rates by sex: thus in men the mortality rate is 162.35, while in women it is 111.86 per 100,000 inhabitants of respective age and sex; the standardized rate, according to M. Segi, equals 102.40 for the entire population, 114.93 for the urban population, 94.23 for the rural population, 26.04 for men and 81.06 for women.

The differences between these groups originate from a variation in both the age composition and the patterns of incidence of various cancer localizations in men and women. The lower mortality in women can be attributed to the fact that they show a high incidence of cancer in localizations which are more responsive to treatment /breast, cervix uteri, skin, etc./. Men are afflicted more often with cancer of the lung and stomach in which cases the therapeutic results are still unsatisfactory.

Among the above-mentioned localizations the highest mortality is caused by cancer of the stomach, 33.53, and of the lung, 27.27. Mortality from cancer of the breast is 7.31, leukemia 5.61, cancer of the rectum 5.42, of the cervix uteri 1.94 per 100,000 inhabitants of respective sex and aged.

According to M. Segi, the standardized mortality from cancer of the stomach is 24.19, cancer of the lung 20.01, cancer of the breast 5.65, leukemia 4.88, cancer of the rectum 3.88 and cancer of the cervix uteri 1.5.

Territorially, the highest mortality from all malignant neoplasms is observed in the Vratsa District, 183.7 while in the Smolyan and the Kurdzhali Districts it is 77.97 and 78.86, respectively, per 100,000 inhabitants.

Among the urban population, the highest mortality is observed in Sofia, 136.28, while in the Smolyan District 60.55 and the Kurdzhali District 76.30 per 100,000 inhabitants.

Among the rural population, mortality is considerably higher than the national average in the Vratsa District, 227.9; a low mortality, 80.14 per 100,000 inhabitants is observed in the Kurdzhali District.

In general, it can be concluded that the differences in mortality /both general and by localization in individual districts are determined by various of rates incidence and by the influence of the age composition of the population.

In recent years, mortality form all malignant neoplasms in Bulgaria has been fluctuating within very narrow limits. In 1968, it was 138.4, while in 1974 139.6, with a rate of increase of 0.57 per 100,000 inhabitants. This can be attributed to a constantly improving organization of cancer control /see Figs 8, 9, 10/.

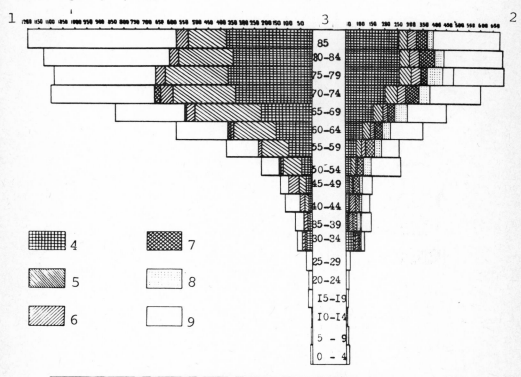

Mortality per 100,000 inhabitants 1972											
Sites	20-29		20-24		15-19		10-14		5-9		0-4	
	M	F	M	F	M	F	M	F	M	F	M	F
Stomach	0.6	1.3	0.3	0.3	-	0.3	0.3	-	0.3	-	-	0.3
Lung	-	0.6	0.6	0.3	0.9	-	0.6	0.6	-	-	-	-
Rectum	-	0.3	-	0.6	0.3	-	-	-	-	-	-	-
Breast	-	0.6	-	-	-	-	-	-	-	-	-	-
Uterus	-	1.0	-	0.3	-	-	-	-	-	-	-	-
Other	12.9	7.9	10.0	4.4	10.4	5.4	4.8	4.1	6.4	4.0	7.3	6.3

Fig. 8. Mortality in Bulgaria from malignant neoplasms of different localization in a distribution according to age and sex, for the year 1972.
  1. Males - 2. Females - 3. Age - 4. Stomach - 5. Lung - 6. Rectum - 7.Breast - 8.Uterus - 9. Other

35

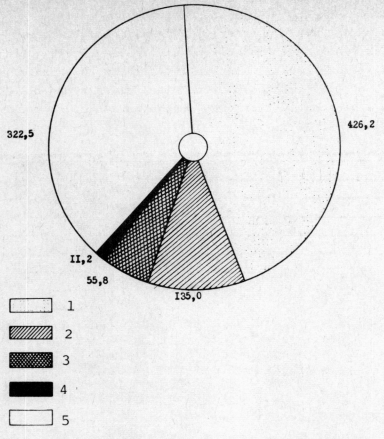

Fig. 9. Mortality in Bulgaria by main groups of diseases.
For the year 1969 /per 100,000 inhabitants/

1. Cardiovascular diseases - 2. Malignant tumours -
3. Accidents, injuries, poisonings - 4. Tuberculosis
- 5. Other

In 1974, out of the total number of patients, 23.1 per
cent were treated surgically, 29.3 per cent by radiotherapy,
and 47.6 per cent received a combined only chemotherapeutic
treatment.

A rather high percentage of those who receive radiotherapeutic treatment in Bulgaria can be explained by the high incidence of cancer of the skin and the lip.

On the basis of 1974 data survival of patients for five
years or longer after the treatment in the percentage of those
living at the end of the year of treatment is the following:

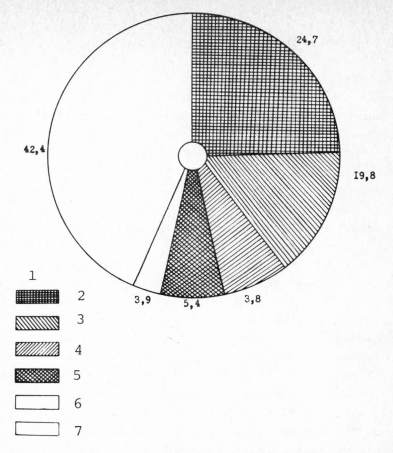

Fig.10. Mortality in Bulgaria from malignant neoplasms by different localizations for the year 1972.

1. Site - 2. Stomach - 3. Lung - 4. Rectum - 5. Breast - 6. Uterus - 7. Other

cancer of the stomach 22.8 per cent; lung 6.7, breast 40.2, cervix uteri 48.6, lip 58.4, skin 47.9 per cent,and so on.

ORGANIZATION OF DETECTION AND EXAMINATION
OF ONCOLOGICAL PATIENTS
I. Popov and K. Manoilov

In recent years, in Bulgaria a new, essentially prophylactic strategy was launched for the active preservation of health of the population, for the active early detection of persons with a high risk of the disease and for the applica-

tion of prophylactic measures to them, as well as for the early
detection of patients with malignant tumours and for their timely treatment.

This qualitative change in the system of public health
corresponds to the main directions in the development of oncological assistance because early detection of malignant neoplasms and cancer prevention depend, above all, on how intensively the general medical services conduct their activities.
It is there that the patient with more or less definite complaints regarding his health and also persons subject to prophylactic examination are seen for the first time. To ensure an
earlier detection of oncological diseases the Ministry of Health
has issued methodological instructions regarding the early diagnosis of malignant neoplasms and mass prophylactic examinations.
They contain a description of the duties for panel doctors and
factory medical consultants and also for those working in out-
-patient clinics, with regard to cancer control. Their oncological alertness can help a great deal in arriving at a correct
interpretation of anamnestic data, which is necessary for the
determination of the clinical status of patients under examination and also for a timely detection of persons already
afflicted with a malignant tumour, or suspected of being
afflicted. For the verification of the diagnosis, the physician
should refer the patient to a treatment institution possessing
facilities for conducting special investigations. Those cases
which are difficult to diagnose in out-patient conditions are
referred to in-patient hospitals and if the diagnosis is confirmed the report to that effect is promptly dispatched to an
oncological dispensary. If necessary, a consultation is sought
with an oncologist or the patient is admitted to an oncological
dispensary.

Apart from the clinical diagnosis, laboratory, roentgenological, endoscopic, radioisotope, morphological /cytological and
histological/ and other methods are used.

As for the laboratory methods, in recent years a wide use
has been made of radioisotope procedures, not only in confirm-
ing or excluding any doubts the clinicians may have regarding

the presence of a malignant neoplasm but also in determining
the extent of its spread.

X-ray procedure remains a main method of diagnosis of malignant neoplasms of the digestive tract, the lung, the uro-
genital system, the bone and a number of other anatomical sites.

Apart from fluorography and roentgenoscopy, cancer of the
lung is diagnosed also with the aid of bronchoscopical investigation; in case of special symptoms, angiographic methods can
also be resorted to.

In the primary detection of cancer of the breast in high-
-risk females, mammography have come into use, with the analysis of results and their assessment in connection with the
utilization of this method in mass prophylactic examinations.

Endoscopy has an important role in the diagnosis of malignant neoplasms. Thus, bronchoscopy, esophagogastroscopy, rec-
toscopy, cystoscopy, mediastinoscopy and laparoscopy have
been introduced. To improve the early diagnosis of cancer of
the stomach and the lung, use is also made, though to a limited
extent, of fibergastroscopy and flexible fiber optic bronchos-
copes.

The examination of a patient suspected of having a malignant tumour should be completed within 15 days. If the suspicion of a malignant neoplasm is not dispelled during this period of time and the diagnosis remains unclear, the patient
should be referred to an oncological dispensary for examination
but within a shorter period of time.

Consultation with a specialist is sought for the patient,
if necessary, or the latter is referred to a highly specialized
medical institution for additional examination and elucidation
of the nature of affliction.

An important requirement is to reduce to the minimum the
psychological trauma the patient with a malignant neoplasm may
suffer. Therefore the documentation where the diagnosis is
entered should not be accessible to the patient when he is referred to another institution for a consultation and investigation. The patient should be informed of his disease in a way
inspiring confidence in the favourable result of treatment
rather than fear of his fate. The diagnosis is made known not

to the patient but to his family; nevertheless, exceptions can be made if the patient refuses to undergo a prescribed treatment; in that case the patient and the persons accompanying him are explained all the seriousness of the affliction and the possibility of fatal outcome if the necessary steps are not taken, and examples of favourable therapeutic results in similar cases are also given.

In the course of comprehensive prophylactic examinations of organized groups of population which have been conducted since 1950 for the purpose of detecting chronic and occupational diseases including the oncological ones, the oncological institutions are required to render the institutions of general medical services methodological and consultative assistance.

The positive experience gained in the field of cancer control has made possible for the Ministry of Health to issue an order in 1956 to carry out annual prophylactic examinations of women aged 30 and over with the purpose of early detection of tumours and precancerous diseases of the female genital organs and the mammary gland. In the urban areas, the responsibility for the organization of the examinations has been entrusted to treatment institutions; examinations are made by obstetricians-gynaecologists. In rural areas, they are performed by panel doctors and obstetricians. The lists of women subject to prophylactic examination are preliminarily drawn up by women's consultation clinics and medical services at enterprises and these lists are annually revised. To educate the population on the importance and usefulness of such examinations, the latter are preceded by a wide variety of mass educational work. Women with alterations in the cervix uteri detected in the course of prophylactic examinations are subject to colposcopy which is performed by the gynaecologist of the district hospital; the surgeon examines the breast. After 1965, special examination rooms were opened in a number of out-patient clinics in towns where trained obstetricians conduct prophylactic examinations of women attending the out-patient clinic in connection with other complaints. Women with certain changes in their genitalia and breast are immediately referred to the gynaecologist or surgeon for the verification of the diagnosis.

From 1968 on, the entire adult population of the country is covered by roentgenofluorography which, apart from detection of tuberculosis and other chronic diseases, promotes a better diagnosis of cancer of the lung. The number of people examined so increases annually /from 1,527,000 in 1970 to 2,077,000 in 1974/.

To put the mass prophylactic examinations of women on a modern basis, in the oncological institutions cytologic laboratories staffed with physicians, biologists and laboratory assistants opened in 1970; these laboratories quickly became an integral part of the medical services and annually make as many as 2.300,000 cytologic tests. The positive effect of this work can be confirmed by the number of women examined with the aid of cytologic tests – 585,696 in 1973 and 888,115 in 1974. The detection rate per 1,000 women examined with the aid of the cytologic method was 3.6 and 2.8, respectively; the use of the histological method gave the detection rate of 0.51 and 0.42, which is quite satisfactory for the initial stage in the utilization of this method. The high effectiveness of this method is confirmed by the fact that out of the total number of 605 newly diagnosed patients with cancer of the cervix uteri in 1974 118 had cancer in situ, 39 microinvasive and 215 invasive cancer, i.e. early forms of the disease. Besides, there were registered 111 cases of dysplasia of which 76 were benign and 35 suspected of cancer.

The sputum of persons who in the course of roentgenofluorographic examinations were found to have pathological symptoms in the lung has begun to be tested cytologically.

Apart from improving the existing forms of prophylactic work on the basis of the achievements of the medical science, technological progress and rational organization and management of work of the medical personnel, in 1972 the Ministry of Health organized new units for mass prophylactic examinations of the population in polyclinics attached to district and some town hospitals. Their task is the timely detection of persons, who can be considered as belonging to high-risk groups and

requiring early diagnosis of a pathological alteration, thus
they bear a great medical, economic and social importance.
This new organizational form helps to organize mass prophylactic examinations consistently from time to time. These examinations are supplementing other kinds of existing prophylactic
health surveys.

Several oncological dispensaries, relying only on their
own staff, organize prophylactic examinations of high-risk
population groups where the rate of detection of pretumourous
diseases and primary forms of cancer is higher compared to the
examinations performed by the general medical services. In the
comprehensive health-improvement measures that are being implemented the dispensaries see the possibility for a sharp
reduction in the incidence of cancer of localizations accessible
to examination: the skin, the lip, the pharynx, the uterus,
the breast and also for working out methodological instructions
for the prophylactic work carried out by general medical services.

The cases of precancerous diseases are registered for monitoring by the district polyclinics and some of them are under
the observation by oncological dispensaries. Patients are treated and followed up till their final recovery and one year later
they are removed from the follow-up list.

The further development, improvement and coordination of
various kinds of prophylactic examinations and the introduction of personal control cards for the purpose of timely examination of various groups of population are tasks to be solved
in the nearest future. They will contribute to a sharp improvement of cancer control in our country and a favourable change
in morbidity and mortality from malignant neoplasms.

ORGANIZATION OF HOSPITALIZATION AND TREATMENT
OF PATIENTS WITH MALIGNANT NEOPLASMS
K. Manoilov

The indications for hospitalization of oncological patients are based on the uniform oncological doctrine adopted
in the country and on the existing methodological instructions

issued to ensure the timely diagnosis and treatment of patients with malignant neoplasms.

Referral for hospitalization is made by the physician of an out-patient clinic who is guided in his action by the need:

- to perform special diagnostic procedures in unclear cases and on patients with malignant neoplasms and pre-tumourous diseases, i.e. procedures which   should be carried out only under hospital conditions;

- to perform such forms of treatment of patients with malignant neoplasms and pre malignant diseases which are impossible under out-patient conditions;

- to give medical assistance to patients in advanced stages of the disease, which is done in accordance with special instructions.

The conditions for comprehensive treatment of patients are present in almost all oncological institutions, some district hospitals, clinics and the institutes of the Medical Academy located in the three largest cities of the country, which admit oncological patients most often.

The shortage of hospital beds in specialized oncological institutions and considerations of medical-social nature lead to a situation where a very considerable number of patients with malignant neoplasms needing of surgical treatment and also patients in advanced stages of the disease needing symptomatic and palliative treatment have as yet to be hospitalized in district, town and county hospitals. If the patients operated upon in the above-mentioned istitutions need radiotherapy, they undergo it in radiological departments of oncological institutions and of the Medical Academy.

The period within which oncological patients should be hospitalized is determined by the physicians of the out-patient clinics at the time of making the diagnosis and it depends on the indications for hospitalization, on the localization affected and the extent of the disease as well as on the number of beds available in those treatment institutions which possess all the facilities for a high quality treatment. If radical treatment is indicated for patients with malignant neoplasms, they are subject to hospitalization, in principle, within five days from the date of the diagnosis. Patients, who are suspected of having a malignant neoplasm and need to be examined under in-patient conditions, are also subject to hospitalization within a short period of time. Other patients are admitted by oncological institutions within 10 to 30 days or are referred to some institutions of the general medical services with a recommendation to carry out the necessary treatment according to their possibilities. This cooperation is contributed to by the close relations between oncological and other therapeutic institutions.

Since the oncological institutions possess only limited facilities for the treatment of malignant tumours of the nervous system, of the eye, of the urinary organs, of the bone, and acute leukemia, these have to be treated by respective specialized units of district hospitals and of the Medical Academy.

After a comprehensive clinical assessment of indications is made for the application of possible therapeutic methods to achieve an effective treatment and the general condition of the patient is determined, a plan of treatment is designed.

Surgery and radiotherapy are the main methods of treatment and, depending on the indications, they may be used independently or in combination. The surgery may be extended for the purpose of removing the tumour together with the affected lymphatic nodes or it may be palliative to relieve the suffering of the patient and it may be combined with radiotherapy or chemotherapy in order to obtain a maximum curative effect.

Radiotherapy is used separately or in combination with surgical and chemotherapeutic methods.

In order to improve the general condition of the patient with a malignant neoplasm and to counteract the changes that may set in as a result of the treatment, measures are taken to stimulate the organism's protective system. Immunotherapy of certain malignant tumours has begun to be developed.

The study of causes behind complications and in-patient lethality is the responsibility of heads of departments and clinics serving patients with malignant neoplasms and also of oncologists who render methodological assistance for them. The nature of the tumour, the general condition of the patient and his age, abnormalities resulting from one application of diagnostic and therapeutic precedures, the developed anatomo-functional loss and causes of death are assessed.

The detection of patients in advanced stages of tumour development even in localizations accessible to examination is a task which has not yet been solved completely. The study of causes of late detection of persons with the disease and the dead in whom the malignant neoplasm was diagnosed only post-mortem are the main requirements for achieving an improved organization of cancer control. This responsible work has been entrusted to oncological institutions since the time of their organization by an instruction on organization and methods of cancer control and the Ministry of Health has confirmed this provision in a special order. The oncological dispensaries involve their specialists in the work aimed at finding the causes which delayed the detection of patients with malignant neoplasms. A special questionnaire is filled in for such patients /Supplement 1/.

The oncological dispensaries analyse and generalize the data collected with the aid of the questionnaires, verify the causes leading to the development of advanced forms of tumours and assess the diagnostic possibilities of the therapeutic institutions which have identified the patient or caused the delay in referring him to another institution for carrying out the necessary examinations.

The generalizations and conclusions made as well as measures to be adopted with a view to remove the causes behind delays in detecting cancer patients, thus to avoid the development of the disease to advanced stages are discussed at meetings and conferences of physicians of county hospitals. To reduce cases of delayed detections of malignant tumours caused by the ignorance of the patient, public education is organized about cancer, while to avoid the same caused by the fault of medical workers postgraduate training courses are arranged for them and their alertness to cancer in their daily work is

QUESTIONNAIRE

for the patient with an advanced malignant neoplasm

1. Number of personal medical card, history of the disease
   _____

2. Institution where the card was filled in _____
   _____

3. Forename, middle name, and family name of the patient _____
   _____ age _____ years _____ sex ___
   place of residence _____ address _____
   _____ occupation _____

4. Diagnosis and stage of disease _____
   _____

5. Date of the diagnosis of the tumour in an advanced stage
   _____

6. Date of first symptoms of the disease _____

7. Date of first examination of the patient _____

8. Name and address of the institution _____

9. Date of the diagnosis of the malignant neoplasm and name
   and address of institution _____

10. If the patient treated, when _____
    where _____ in connection with what _____
    _____

11. Was the patient examined prophylactically _____
    when _____ where _____

12. Was the patient present at talks on cancer _____
    when _____ where _____
    how many times _____

13. Reasons for the late application for medical help /under-
    line/: repugnance, fear of the possibility of cancer, un-
    specified symptoms, etc. _____

14. In a chronological order state the visits of the patient
    to the physician in connection with this disease and indi-
    cate the date, method of examination in each particular
    institution, diagnoses made, treatment given and the
    results of the treatment _____
    _____
    _____
    _____
    _____
    _____

15. Analysis of causes behind the advanced state of the dis-
    ease: /underline the cause/ incomplete examination of the
    patient, diagnostic mistake /clinical, roentgenologic,
    pathological/ long examination of the patient, concealed
    nature of the disease, late attendance to a clinic to seek
    medical advice or other _____

16. Conclusion _____
    _____
    _____

                    Signature: _____

developed. Measures are adopted to improve the supply of diagnostic apparatus in the medical institutions and for the better
utilization of diagnostic possibilities to increase the number
of early detections of cancer.

MONITORING OF PATIENTS WITH MALIGNANT NEOPLASMS
I. Popov

Until 1968, monitoring of patients with malignant neoplasms was carried out by the physicians of oncological rooms
of the county hospitals and, partially, by the staff of the
oncological dispensaries.

In order to improve monitoring, the Ministry of Health
has entrusted observation of oncological patients to the oncological dispensaries. The latter have organizational and
-methodological departments where the staff includes the head
of the department, a staff-physician and two visiting nurses
per 150,000 population. The physicians working in this department are given the opportunity to acquire a specialty and improve their qualifications in the respective departments of
the dispensary or another medical institution in the given
town or city.

Periodic control examinations of patients with malignant
neoplasm under observation are organized by the physicians of
the organizational and methodological departments and are
carried out by oncologists in the dispensary either alone or
jointly with the physicians of the out-patient departments of
county hospitals. The results of the examinations are entered
in the personal medical card and the personal control card of
the patient in the card file of the dispensary; the medical
institution in the area of which the monitored patient resides
is notified of the epicrisis and, if necessary, of additional
medical procedures required to be carried out on an in-patient
basis, out-patient basis and at home. If a medical institution
follows up the patient with a malignant neoplasm for some time
after completing his treatment it should notify the oncological
dispensary of the general condition of the patient and agree
with it in the necessary prescriptions.

If a patient fails to appear at the control examination within the period of time set for it, it is the duty of the dispensary to find out the reasons for non-attendance, in which it relies on the assistance of local medical institutions or on its nurses and physicians who visit the patients. In the period of time before the date of the control examination, an oncologist may pay visits for certain patients who have completed their treatment for carrying out additional procedures, pharmacotherapy, settling questions of rehabilitation, job replacement, solving medical-social and other questions. This work is necessitated by the fact that the number of patients who need a prolonged chemo- or hormonotherapy after the completion of their hospital treatment is rather considerable and, besides, it is necessary for the assessment of the condition of patients who need of additional radiotherapy, either on out-patient or on in-patient basis.

An oncologist sets for each patient a different period of time before a control examination, which depends on his assessment of the patient's condition, methods of treatment that have been applied, the degree of tumour development, etc. Control examinations are frequent in the first year after treatment, then they become rarer and after 5 years are made only once a year. With respect to some cancer localizations the oncological dispensaries make enquiries with the local medical institutions.

The patients are under observation till they die. The question of discontinuing observation of certain groups of patients after completion of a certain well-substantiated follow-up period is now under discussion.

Data about the number and dynamics of monitored patients with malignant neoplasms are shown by the oncological dispensaries in their annual progress reports. These reports include also those patients who are put on register and those struck off the register by the end of the year, and the survival of patients during one, two, three, five and more years. Besides, on the basis of the collected information about the monitored patients the dispensaries analyse and evaluate distant results of treatment, prophylactic and therapeutic procedures for individual cancer localizations. Such concrete investigations on each cancer localization have not been made on a countrywide scale; but the incidence, morbidity and mortality of all kinds of malignant neoplasms and certain primary localizations have been forecast.

Organization and performance of monitoring work depend on a correct clinical assessment of the condition of oncological patients and an accurate reflection of its stages in the respective documentation. Therefore, a timely removal of mistakes and compensation of omissions made by other institutions forms part of the tasks of the oncological dispensaries. They follow the requirement to present the diagnosis in accordance with the International Classification of Diseases, with an accurate indication of the localization of tumour, stage of tumour development and its clinical group and with a histological result, if possible. Since the prognosis, therapeutic recommendations and methods of treatment depend on the size of the tumour, its structure and the degree of spread into neighbouring and distant organs and tissues, the correct assessment of the stage of the disease before treatment is an essential requirement. Oncological assistance can be effective only if patients are given an active care. This requirement can be fulfilled if the observation of certain clinical groups of patients is carried out on rational lines, if the diagnosis of persons suspected of having malignant neoplasms is timely verified, if patients with precancerous diseases are given an adequate treatment, if patients newly diagnosed with cancer are ensured a special or radical treatment, if patients are followed up regularly after their radical treatment so that possible recurrences and metastases could be detected early, if terminal patients are given systematic medical and social assistance. The existing system of registration of patients with malignant neoplasms by the oncological dispensaries and the introduction of the improved form of monitoring have made possible to bring the specialized oncological assistance closer to the population. Frequent contacts of oncologists with the physicians of the general medical services in the areas they serve contribute to the latters' oncological alertness in their everyday work with the patients and their active involvement in cancer control.

The fact that the oncological dispensaries solely bear the responsibility for registration and observation of patients with malignant neoplasms has been proved effective in the conditions of Bulgaria. The number of people they serve is not large, they are located quite closely to the institutions of general medical services, which gives the oncologists an opportunity to carry out systematic methodological, monitoring and consultative work in the areas they serve. In this respect it is also important that the patients referred to oncological and other treatment institutions for examination and treatment can use public transport free of charge.

The improvement and stabilization of the indices by which one can judge about the level of oncological assistance offered in recent years also confirm the positive assessment of the measures that have been implemented in this field of activity.

THE STUDY OF EFFECTIVENESS OF TREATMENT OF
ONCOLOGICAL PATIENTS
D. Stoichev

The assessment of treatment of patients with malignant neoplasms is based on the study of their survival.

The rate of survival for assessing the effectiveness of treatment is most often calculated for a control period of 3, 5 years or longer.

The method used in the study of survival of oncological patients in Bulgaria is that of Hill-Merkov; the method of calculation of five-year survival rates is also used, partially, and, recently, also that of the probability of survival.

In the absence of a single and generally accepted method for the calculation of survival and assessment of results of various treatment methods, the studies suffer the disadvantage of incompleteness, the conclusions made are incomparable and there are errors in interpreting the collected evidence. Therefore, with an eye to the introduction of a single method of calculation and analysis of results of treatment of patients

with malignant neoplasms, an experiment was carried out in
Bulgaria for the introduction and observance of the following
principles:

1. Calculation of survival of cancer patients is made at
the end of each year of the follow-up period and is based on
the total number of registered patients /whether treated or
not/.

2. Results of treatment of patients are assessed from the
start of the treatment. Survival of patients who have undergone no treatment is calculated from the date the experts make
their decision that the patient is not subject to treatment.

3. Survival of patients with multiple tumours is calculated for each localization separately.

4. If the patient had been treated in various out-patient
clinics, dispensaries and hospitals in the course of his treatment, the effectiveness of the latter is studied for each institution separately.

5. The diagnosis of a malignant tumour should be confirmed histologically. In the absence of morphological diagnosis, the results of treatment are calculated separately.

6. The control follow-up period may, by choice or according to the biological characteristics of the tumour, last
three, four, five, ten years or longer.

7. Since what is intended is to arrive at a single method
of assessing therapeutic results, the study should be accompanied by a general statistical analysis of treated patients.

8. A retrospective study of the medical documentation
regarding the patients under observation /indirect observation/
allows them to be grouped into the following categories:

Category "O" which includes those who died in the period
of control observation.

Category "A" which includes those lost to follow-up.

Category "W" which includes those alive at the time the
results of treatment are assessed.

As a measure to prove the reliability of assessment of
treatment, the representative error is calculated. If survival
calculations are made with the aid of the direct method, the

representative error is determined by the following formula
$m \sqrt{\dfrac{P/I-p/}{D + W}}$. If survival calculation is made with the aid of
the actuarial method, the representative error is determined by
the following Greenwood formula $P_n \sqrt{\sum \dfrac{q_i}{m_i + p_i}}$.

It should be noted that the study of survival has been
limited so far to individual oncological institutions and some
other institutions where malignant neoplasms are treated. The
introduction of new requirements in the practice and the proposed introduction of the automated system of management and
information in the field of monitoring oncological patients
should make possible the processing of data regarding the treatment of patients with malignant neoplasms and the assessment
of effectiveness of their treatment on a centralized basis.

ORGANIZATION OF MEDICAL DETERMINATION OF DISABILITY
AND REHABILITATION OF ONCOLOGICAL PATIENTS
I. Popov and K. Manoilov

The degree and duration of post-treatment disability to
work arising in patients with malignant neoplasm should be assessed in a responsible and competent manner. In arriving at
their decision, the experts who carry out the medical examination of the patient rely on the prognosis of his disease and
take into account the temporary or permanent malfunctions
exhibited by the patient and also the possibilities for his
rehabilition. In this respect, they are also guided by the
instructions, approved by the Ministry of Health, on the work
performed by experts in prevention and treatment institutions
in relation to temporaly disability to work and also on the
activities of the medical boards for industrial disability.
The medical boards dealing with cases of temporary disability
are authorized to extend the duration of the medical certificate
of temporary disability up to 6 months if there is a possibility
of rehabilitating the patient in question within one year after
his treatment is completed.

If the condition of the patient and the nature of his

occupation make possible to ease his conditions of work it can
be arranged so in the agreement with the management and the
trade union of the enterprise where the patient is employed. If
the enterprise finds it impossible to comply with the recommendation of the medical board, it recompensates the patient
for the damages. The result of examinations of the patients are
entered in a special "MB Decisions Book" and in the personal
medical cards.

The medical board refers patients for expert medical
labour   testimony in the following cases: 1/ every two months
after the expiration of the 6-month period of temporary disability; 2/ at any time in case of a prolonged period of disability to work /invalidity/; 3/ if, according to the medical
certificate temporary disability occurs, and it was stated not
later than two years before, every two months for a total period of 12 months, either because of a single disease or because
of different ones. The patient is referred to the medical board
for industrial disability with a medical protocol of the Medical Board in which the results of examinations and treatment
and also purpose of referring the patient to the court are
stated.

The medical board for industrial disability examines persons in connection with: 1/ the need to prolong their leave
because of a disease; 2/ granting of pensions; 3/ job replacement; 4/ provision of social assistance; 5/ the need for receiving a skill category or for retraining; 6/ the need to determine
the degree of loss of ability to work; 7/ a respective request
on the part of the patient; the board establishes a disablement
category for each person: persons who, due to the condition of
their health, will not be fit for work any longer are classified
as belonging to the first disablement category; persons who are
not fit any longer to pursue their usual occupation, but are
able to continue work provided that special conditions are
created for them are classified as belonging to the second
disablement category, while persons who have changed their occupation or who are in need of changing it and also in reducing their skill category are classified as belonging to the

third disablement category.

Such classification by disablement categories makes possible for a considerable number of persons to return to the labour after their treatment. In cases when the individuals are retrained and their new occupation entails a lower remuneration for work, they are classified as belonging to the third disablement category so that their remuneration could be brought up to the former level, i.e. to what it was before the onset of the disease. Persons working in special conditions are classified as belonging to the second disablement category. If the persons are classified as belonging to the first disablement category and are in need of special care they receive a pension allowance to enable them to hire someone for this purpose.

The chances of cure and rehabilitation can be considerably increased by improving the diagnosis and earlier detection of patients with malignant neoplasms. Besides, the extended surgery and the methods of treatment that are employed require the adoption of social and psychological measures in the field of rehabilitation but these have not yet been developed to an adequate extent. The social workers employed by the oncological institutions receive special training. There is a demand for psychologists and pedagogues for work with patients and their near relatives. The program worked out and launched by the Department of Therapeutic Physical Training of the Institute of Oncology is directed mainly towards the recovery of motor functions that may be impaired as a result of surgical treatment of cancer of the breast, the female genitalia and the lung. There has been successfully introduced a scientifically established baro stimulation method for the diagnostic investigation of neural reflectory mechanisms of the inferior margin of the colon in order to determine the causes of fecal incontinence and this is used for the repair of function for therapeutic and rehabilitation purposes. For breast restoration in women operated upon in connection with cancer of the breast prostheses are used to achieve aesthetic correction of the defect. The initial experience accumulated by the Institute of

Oncology is included in the training program for dispensary's physicians. With all the successes mentioned above, it should be noted that since rehabilitation has not been given in our country a necessary organizational form, the results in this field still fall short of the possibilities offered by modern medicine and public health.

The field of cancer control has achieved definite successes in terms of early detection, diagnosis and comprehensive treatment of malignant neoplasms, and the end-results of treatment of some cancers and labour prognosis of treated patients have improved. Nevertheless, with all the positive results in this field, there are still many questions regarding temporary and prolonged disability to work, disablement, job replacement and rehabilitation of oncological patients which need adequate elucidation and find no reflection whatever in the scientifically established methodological recommendations.

If the expert testimony obtained to determine temporary or prolonged post-treatment disability to work is expected to correspond to modern requirements, the elaboration of methodological instructions regarding some cancer localizations as an aid for the experts is absolutely indispensable.

The rehabilitation directed towards achieving a post--treatment decline or prevention of disablement amongst oncological patients calls for the elaboration of a special programme with the indication of measures, necessary manuals and specialists needed for its realization. No other approach will result in the perfect and definite satisfaction of the requirements of patients with malignant neoplasms.

ORGANIZATION OF MEDICAL ASSISTANCE TO PATIENTS WITH ADVANCED TUMOURS

I. Popov

In the organization of oncological assistance to the population, the most challenging questions are those pertaining to treatment and care of patients with malignant neoplasms in an advanced stage.

The decision that the patient has reached the terminal

stage should be based not only on the results of all out-patient and clinical investigations but, in some cases, also upon
the exhaustion of all diagnostic and treatment possibilities in
in-patient conditions, including surgical intervention for the
purpose of establishing the extent of tumour.

In cases where the determination of the extent of tumour
is made in hospitals of the general medical services and at
the clinics of the Medical Academy, advice of experienced oncologists must be sought. Patients with persistent tumours are
accepted for in-patient treatment if their condition calls for
an urgent intervention in connection with complications, such
as bleeding, ileus, constriction of the oesophagus, etc. and
also for palliative therapy. Since the number of beds available in the oncological institutions is not sufficient, instructions have been issued to admit patients with persistent malignant neoplasms into general hospitals for symptomatic and
palliative therapy. The organization of specialized institutions
for hospitalization of patients with persistent tumours is not
considered advisable in our country. In connection with the
organization of departments for completion of cure and for
long-lasting treatment of oncological patients in general hospitals it is expected that conditions will be created there for
medical and general care of patients with persistent tumours.

Medical care at home is made available for patients with
persistent forms of malignant neoplasms, in according with the
respective instructions of the oncological dispensary. The home
care consists of visits by nurses and physicians of the oncological dispensary who carry out certain treatment procedures
and prescriptions, but most of all by local physicians and
nurses for symptomatic therapy.

TEACHING OF ONCOLOGY, TRAINING OF PHYSICIANS SPECIALIZING
IN ONCOLOGY AND MIDDLE-LEVEL PERSONNEL FOR ONCOLOGICAL
INSTITUTIONS

I. Popov

With the organization of the Medical Academy in 1973 and
the incorporation of the scientific institutes of the Ministry

of Health into it, the conditions for training and postgraduate training of physicians in oncology have become more favourable.

The curriculum for undergraduates provides for optional lectures on the topic of malignant neoplasms presented at the respective chairs of the Medical Academy and also for a period of practical training in oncological institutions.

At the special and postgraduate training courses for physicians of general medical services which are organized by the Medical Academy, lectures on the diagnosis, treatment and prophylaxis of malignant neoplasms are given by specialists from the Institute of Oncology who have scientific degree.

The Institute of Oncology annually offers an opportunity to physicians of oncological dispensaries and general treatment institutions for specialization and advance in the form of specialized courses or on an individual basis. This is done in accordance with a special programme which covers the main parts of oncology - surgery, gynaecology, radiology, dermatology, chemotherapy, as well as the epidemiology and prophylaxis of malignant neoplasms, morphology of tumours and so on. The Institute organizes specialized courses for middle-level medical workers on radiology, histopathology and cytology, courses for visiting nurses, medical statisticians, etc.

A majority of oncological dispensaries train middle-level medical workers to treat patients with malignant neoplasms correctly. They organize seminars with a view to improve the knowledge of physicians and obstetricians of general medical institutions on prophylaxis, early detection and diagnosis of malignant neoplasms and monitoring of oncological patients.

HEALTH EDUCATION OF THE PUBLIC ON THE PROBLEMS OF CANCER
I. Popov

The work in the field of public education on cancer is guided by the National Institute of Medical Education. The departments of medical education of district hygienic-plus-
-epidemiologic institutes, the Bulgarian Red Cross and the "G. Kirkov" Society for Dissemination of Scientific Knowledge take part in the organization of this work.

Methodologically, the public education about oncology is carried out jointly by the Institute of Oncology and the Institute of Medical Education, by specialists of oncology, trained physicians and middle-level medical workers of other medical institutions.

The purposes and objectives of public education about cancer are determined by considerations about achieving definitive results in implementing prophylactic measures.

Public education on cancer should be oriented towards making people more cancer-conscious and alert to this disease, towards educating them to the need of seeking medical advice in good time, and also towards persuading certain groups of the population to participate in prophylactic examinations carried out to achieve early detection of cancer and precancerous diseases. Other objectives of public education about cancer include cultivation of medical and hygienic habits which would promote the health of both individuals and collectives of people, eradication of habits and customs harmful to health and also of the influence of those factors at home and at places of work which promote oncological diseases. Besides, the need of a rational regimen for oncological patients and the value of following prophylactic prescriptions after their treatment is completed is also emphasized.

The effectiveness of public education on cancer depends on correct organization and is assessed on the basis of results. Since it is intended, most of all and above all, to achieve the implementation of prophylactic measures and early detection of cancer, the active effort of medical workers must be supplemented by the participation of the population. In this connection, the oncological dispensaries in our country elaborate and suggest adequate organizational forms of anti-cancer medical propraganda to achieve certain objectives, and they cooperate and participate in this effort by involving their physicians.

In the effort to reach large masses of the population in the course of the education work a great role is played by groups of activists at enterprises and institutions, educational establishments, agricultural cooperatives and public organizations.

For achieving the objectives of the public education on cancer verbal, printed and visual methods are employed in Bulgaria. Most widespread is the verban method for it creates an immediate contact between the lecturer and the audience and leads to the elucidation and discussion of the questions that may be raised following the lecture. There are individual and group discussions, popular scientific lectures are delivered, question-and-answer meetings are organized, circles and seminars are arranged on specially selected oncological topics, talks are transmitted by the radio and television.

The visual method is used to illustrate lectures with a movie picture or by projecting slides, and in the form of popular scientific telecasts on oncology, as well as of posters, show cases, etc.

The oncological dispensaries can supply visual aids on the results of cancer control for local exhibitions on the achievements of public health.

Methodological instructions are published as an aid in guiding and organizing public education on cancer for the medical personnel of the general medical institutions who take part in lectures and talks arranged for the population.

The oncological emphasis in public health education gives satisfactory results, especially in organizing mass prophylactic examinations and monitoring oncological patients. At the same time, the propaganda with visual aids should be made more convincing. Health education should have a definite effect in terms of improving oncological assistance to the population of the country.

COORDINATION OF SCIENTIFIC RESEARCH ON THE PROBLEM
"SCIENTIFIC FOUNDATIONS OF ORGANIZATION OF CANCER
CONTROL"
I. Popov

The scientific council of the Institute of Oncology coordinates, approves and exercises control over the fulfilment of the plan of scientific research on the problem of malignant neoplasms. The plan is subject to approval by the Medical Academy and is approved by the Committee for Science, Technical Progress and Higher Education. In the section devoted to the epidemiology and prophylaxis of malignant neoplasms, provision is made regarding the elaboration of the problem of scientific foundations of organization of cancer control.

Scientific solution of the questions pertaining to the organization of cancer control is carried out mainly by the Scientific Research Institute of Oncology; some questions are solved jointly with the personnel of the Ministry of Health and the Scientific Research Institute of Social Hygiene and Organization of Health.

THE PROSPECTS OF A FURTHER IMPROVEMENT OF THE ORGANIZATION OF ONCOLOGICAL ASSISTANCE

I. Popov

The progress is the development of oncological assistance to the population cannot yet fully meet the requirements in specialized oncological assistance dictated by the prevalence of dispensary medical services.

A wide network of oncological dispensaries with small-size in-patient departments has played its positive role as a stage in the development of services of this kind and in establishing the monitoring method of observation of patients with malignant neoplasms. But today, when in the field of prophylaxis, early diagnosis and treatment of cancer more modern equipment and aids have come into use and new methods are being developed, the in-patient departments of the majority of oncological dispensaries no longer correspond to the modern level reached by the oncological science and practice.

The prognoses and conceptions developed on the basis of the dynamics of, and trends in, the incidence of malignant neoplasms demonstrate that the latter still constitute one of the main problems facing medicine and public health in our country. The conclusions reached have provided the basis for outlining the prospects of development of cancer control in Bulgaria. It is planned to introduce an integrated system of oncological assistance, one which would ensure uniformity of, and continuity between, the stages of detection, treatment and monitoring of patients with malignant neoplasms and precancerous diseases. For the implementation of this programme, it is necessary to have an advanced network of specialized oncological institutions with a staff of qualified oncologists. The general scheme of development of public health until the year 1990 contains provisions for turning several existing oncological dispensaries into large specialized diagnostic and treatment institutions. They will have departments for treating at certain cancer localizations and patients from various districts of the Republic will be concentrated in such dispensaries. Other dispensaries will also be further developed and will do valuable diagnostic and prophylactic work and treat those patients whose condition will not require the application of complex methods.

The planned development of oncological institutions will ensure regulation at different levels of diagnosis, treatment and prophylaxis of cancer in terms of quantity, quality and competence. A closer cooperation will take place with general medical institutions in providing assistance to oncological patients. The main oncological institutions will also function as the bases for training physicians and middle-level medical personnel of other oncological dispensaries and general medical institutions in their own areas.

It has been demonstrated in practice that assistance to patients with malignant tumours can be considered adequate only when a staff of competent specialists working in specialized institutions is supplemented by physicians with a knowledge of clinical oncology from other treatment institutions. Apart from that, modern material-technical base, and staff provision for oncological and some other main general medical institutions offering oncological assistance are also indispensable.

Table 1

Age-Sex Structure of the Population of Bulgaria for 1972

Age groups	Total	Urban population	Rural population	Men	Women
0 - 4	664.869	389.064	275.805	341.261	323.608
5 - 9	613.948	315.883	298.565	314.807	299.141
10 - 14	643.576	317.128	326.448	329.460	314.116
15 - 19	674.815	493.149	181.666	344.369	330.446
20 - 24	690.647	548.663	141.984	350.494	340.153
25 - 29	613.919	402.242	211.677	309.960	303.959
30 - 34	556.163	330.462	225.701	278.613	277.550
35 - 39	630.892	353.617	277.275	316.550	314.342
40 - 44	633.426	352.390	281.036	318.758	314.668
45 - 49	650.378	335.783	314.595	324.555	325.823
50 - 54	479.011	225.549	253.462	237.666	241.345
55 - 59	411.841	174.341	237.500	205.056	206.785
60 - 64	444.417	173.687	270.730	218.385	226.032
65 - 69	364.349	133.841	230.508	174.890	189.459
70 - 74	244.719	90.258	154.461	112.903	131.811
75 - 79	142.202	53.416	88.786	61.486	80.716
80 - 84	74.471	27.520	46.951	29.538	44.933
85 +	42.557	15.354	27.203	16.952	25.605
Total:	8.576.200	4.731.847	3.844.353	4.285.708	4.290.492

Table 2

The Number and the Incidence of Malignant Neoplasms in Bulgaria for the Period of 1970-1974

	Total			Urban population			Rural population		
	Absolute number	Per 100.000	Standardized	Absolute number	Per 100.000	Standardized	Absolute number	Per 100.000	Standardized
1970	17.435	205.36	–	8.296	186.76	–	9.139	231.82	–
1971	18.147	212.58	–	8.718	189.76	–	9.429	239.17	–
1972	18.422	214.80	–	9.018	190.58	–	9.404	244.61	–
1973	18.722	217.22	–	9.314	192.31	–	9.408	249.15	–
1974	19.128	220.40	–	9.667	196.59	–	9.461	258.63	–
1970-1974	91.854	214.21	196.04	45.013	190.26	186.79	46.841	243.78	154.66

Table 3

Incidence of Malignant neoplasms in Bulgaria
by Age and Sex for the Period of 1970 - 1974

Age groups	Men		Women	
	Per 100.000	Standard-dized rate	Per 100.000	Standardized rate
Total	231.37	181.31	195.90	145.97
0 - 29	15.27	8.45	14.66	8.11
30 - 39	52.25	6.91	78.70	10.41
40 - 49	152.96	18.34	192.13	23.03
50 - 59	406.30	36.36	359.32	32.15
60 +	1.061.26	111.01	689.76	72.14

Table 4

The Number and Incidence of Malignant Neoplasms in Bulgaria,
by Sex for the 1970-1974 Period

	Men			Women		
	Ab- solute number	Per 100.000	Stand- ard- ized	Ab- solute number	Per 100.000	Stand- ard- ized
1970	9.407	221.65	178.53	8.016	188.81	143.98
1971	9.798	229.635	182.34	8.297	194.33	146.33
1972	9.938	231.89	181.23	8.456	197.00	146.73
1973	10.113	234.91	181.72	8.528	197.68	145.29
1974	10.323	238.14	182.78	8.723	200.95	146.13
1970-1974	49.579	231.37	181.31	420.026	195.90	145.97

Table 5

Incidence of Malignant Neoplasms of Rare Localizations in
Bulgaria for the 1970 - 1974 Period

Localization	Abso-lute number	Per 100000 popu-lation	Stand rate
/200-209/Lymphoid and haemopoietic tissue	882	10.28.	
/153/ Large intestine	587	6.74	4.24
/185/ Prostate	542	6.22	4.31
/188/ Bladder	494	5.67	3.48
/182/ Corpus uteri	371	4.26	2.07
/183/ Ovary	431	4.25	2.91
/206/ Monocytic leukaemia	428	4.91	4.32
/157/ Pancreas	455	5.22	3.78
/172/ Melanoma	113	1.30	0.85
/186/ Testis	116	1.33	1.10
/189/ Kidney	189	2.17	1.15
/193/ Thyroid gland	203	2.33	1.58
/191-192/ Central nervous system	285	3.27	2.91
/201/ Hodgkin's disease	206	2.36	2.03
/150/ Oesophagus	97	1.10	0.79

Table 6.1

Distribution of New Patients with Malignant Neoplasms in Bulgaria, by Selected Localization for the 1970-1974 Period

Total Population

	All malignant neoplasms	Skin /172/	Lower lip /140/	Stomach /151/	Larynx /161/	Trachea bronchus and lung /162/	Rectum /154/	Breast /174/	Cervix uteri /180/
1	2	3	4	5	6	7	8	9	10
1970 Absolute number	17.435	3.000	519	2.726	372	2.307	569	1.252	524
Incidence per 100.000 population	205.36	35.33	6.11	32.10	4.38	27.17	6.70	14.74	6.17
1971 Absolute number	18.147	2.885	485	2.919	387	2.418	626	1.449	520
Incidence per 100.000 population	212.58	33.79	5.68	34.19	4.53	28.32	7.33	16.97	6.09
1972 Absolute number	18.422	3.006	507	2.726	443	2.591	625	1.350	560
Incidence per 100.000 population	214.80	35.05	5.91	31.78	5.16	30.21	7.28	15.74	6.52
1973 Absolute number	18.722	2.919	532	2.852	395	2.671	707	1.517	572
Incidence per 100.000 population	217.22	38.86	6.17	33.09	4.58	30.99	8.20	17.60	6.63
1974 Absolute number	19.128	3.038	572	2.711	402	2.566	777	1.579	605
Incidence per 100.000 population	220.40	35.00	6.59	31.23	4.63	29.56	8.95	18.19	6.97
1970 - 1974	91.854	14.848	2.615	13.934	1.999	12.558	3.304	7.147	2.781
Mean annual incidence per 100.000 population	214.21	34.63	6.10	32.49	4.66	29.27	7.70	16.67	6.49
Mean annual standardized rate	196.04	25.27	4.61	25.27	3.60	20.14	5.71	13.18	5.25

Table 6.2

Urban population

1		2	3	4	5	6	7	8	9	10
1970	Absolute number	8.296	1.147	177	1.117	174	1.099	266	768	348
	Incidence per 100.000 population	186.76	25.82	3.98	25.14	3.91	25.74	5.98	17.28	7.83
1971	Absolute number	8.718	1.166	155	1.171	190	1.153	310	871	330
	Incidence per 100.000 population	180.76	25.38	3.37	25.48	4.13	25.09	6.74	18.05	7.83
1972	Absolute number	9.018	1.246	179	1.128	219	1.219	306	876	379
	Incidence per 100.000 population	190.58	26.33	3.78	23.84	4.63	25.76	6.47	18.51	8.01
1973	Absolute number	9.314	1.209	169	1.229	190	1.287	373	956	379
	Incidence per 100.000 population	192.31	24.96	3.48	25.37	3.92	26.57	7.70	19.73	7.82
1974	Absolute number	9.667	1.268	208	1.162	217	1.288	410	1.004	381
	Incidence per 100.000 population	196.59	25.78	4.23	23.63	4.4	26.19	8.33	20.41	7.74
1970-	Absolute number	45.013	6.036	888	5.807	990	6.046	1.665	4.475	1.817
	Incidence per 100.000 population	190.26	25.51	3.75	24.54	4.18	25.55	7.04	18.91	7.68
		186.79	25.22	3.64	24.44	4.06	25.07	6.96	18.10	7.19

Table 6.3

Rural population

1		2	3	4	5	6	7	8	9	10
1970	Absolute number	9.139	1.853	342	1.609	198	1.208	303	484	176
	Incidence per 100.000 population	231.82	47.0	8.67	40.81	5.02	30.64	7.68	12.27	4.46
1971	Absolute number	9.429	1.719	330	1.748	197	1.265	316	578	190
	Incidence per 100.000 population	239.17	48.60	8.37	44.34	4.99	32.08	8.01	14.66	4.81
1972	Absolute number	9.404	1.760	328	1.598	224	1.372	319	474	181
	Incidence per 100.000 population	244.61	45.78	8.53	41.56	5.82	35.68	8.29	12.32	4.70
1973	Absolute number	9.408	1.710	363	1.623	205	1.384	334	561	193
	Incidence per 100.000 population	249.15	45.28	9.61	42.98	5.42	36.65	8.84	14.85	5.11
1974	Absolute number	9.461	1.770	364	1.549	185	1.278	367	575	224
	Incidence per 100.000 population	253.63	47.45	9.75	41.52	4.95	34.26	9.83	15.41	6.00
1970–1974	Absolute number	46.841	8.812	1.727	8.127	811	6.507	1.639	2.672	964
	Incidence per 100.000 population	243.78	45.86	8.99	42.30	4.22	33.87	8.53	13.91	5.01
		154.66	25.55	5.45	23.17	3.24	18.75	5.85	9.25	3.46

Table 7

Incidence of Malignant Neoplasms of Urban and of Rural
Population of Bulgaria by Age /Mean Rate for the 1970
-1974 Period/

Age groups	Per 100.000 total population	Per 100.000 urban population	Per 100.000 rural population
Total	214.21	190.26	243.78
0 - 29	14.98	14.31	16.23
30 - 39	65.44	71.54	57.14
40 - 49	172.50	188.76	153.72
50 - 59	382.67	426.67	348.21
60 +	863.57	1.039.72	757.25

Incidence of Malignant Neoplasms in Bulgaria and its
1970 -
Total

Administrative	Total	Skin /172/	Lower lip /140/	Stomach /151/
1	2	3	4	5
Blagoevgrad	187.07	41.28	6.83	34.90
Burgas	197.86	24.87	4.48	32.81
Yambol	207.03	35.25	6.78	39.84
Varna	216.30	35.58	6.32	32.34
Tolbukhin	187.54	20.45	7.78	33.61
G.Turnovo	290.04	43.71	7.40	49.55
Gabrovo	235.53	23.80	5.11	51.50
Vratea	274.72	61.43	11.59	33.25
Vidin	203.81	32.64	7.24	20.57
Mikhaylovgrad	208.23	40.77	6.50	23.29
Pleven	264.05	19.96	6.74	41.80
Lovech	245.48	45.36	6.07	33.66
Plovdiv	245.72	46.25	7.04	34.15
Pazardzhik	184.75	30.78	7.64	34.31
Smolyan	112.60	18.07	4.46	20.14
Ruse	220.94	32.70	3.84	39.49
Razgrad	158.84	27.33	5.54	26.32
Silistra	161.35	20.91	6.84	31.54
Sofia /City/	234.62	25.83	2.69	25.46
Sofia	191.91	30.32	7.33	28.06
Nyustendil	207.63	31.98	7.06	30.26
Pernik	202.10	22.88	5.63	25.98
Stara Zagora	234.12	45.98	6.70	36.26
Sliven	186.17	31.48	4.48	28.35
Khaskovo	241.00	49.61	8.10	36.44
Kurdzhali	121.19	14.48	4.11	23.27
Shumen	198.88	79.11	8.08	29.57
Turgovishte	192.83	34.29	6.35	33.83
Bulgaria	214.21	34.63	6.10	32.49

8.1

Administrative Districts, by Selected Localizations for the
1974 Period

Population

Lung /162/	Breast /174/	Cervix uteri /180/	Lymphatic and haemopoietic organs /200-209/
6	7	8	9
26.41	9.50	3.44	6.44
25.26	13.47	6.01	10.82
26.17	13.56	4.23	10.22
26.87	19.55	6.51	9.60
28.15	14.15	3.72	7.61
35.04	21.07	9.87	13.96
28.20	19.82	8.48	11.85
32.71	19.92	8.86	10.26
26.32	18.50	8.04	8.04
29.63	16.70	8.22	6.93
40.26	18.35	9.77	11.89
39.02	16.78	9.46	13.75
35.39	20.25	5.56	11.94
25.12	13.36	4.11	7.19
15.57	7.29	2.06	5.88
25.44	17.21	7.95	11.65
23.49	9.78	3.22	7.96
20.44	12.50	3.15	8.64
29.53	27.27	11.52	12.84
25.75	13.78	4.70	11.09
32.08	16.64	5.85	8.97
28.63	13.26	6.19	11.82
34.29	14.75	5.61	10.39
28.18	13.54	4.06	9.30
37.48	13.85	4.85	9.50
18.33	3.84	1.16	4.73
26.58	13.65	4.20	11.47
28.78	13.50	3.92	10.50
29.27	16.66	6.48	10.28

1	2	3	4	5
Blagoevgrad	188.75	34.75	4.52	27.89
Burgas	188.20	22.06	3.32	26.58
Yambol	151.10	19.90	4.35	25.50
Varna	193.31	27.50	4.46	24.29
Tolbukhin	187.88	19.48	7.35	29.23
G.Turnovo	221.91	27.23	3.61	37.80
Gabrovo	175.99	13.68	2.16	32.98
Vratsa	188.10	35.48	4.84	23.65
Vidin	141.50	15.89	3.07	10.25
Mikhailovgrad	144.80	20.39	2.44	12.84
Pleven	187.93	25.66	3.61	24.21
Lobech	156.10	24.25	2.63	18.98
Plovdiv	223.35	36.85	4.93	26.13
Pazardzhik	166.99	22.80	5.30	27.87
Smolyan	90.96	9.96	2.09	13.10
Ruse	201.69	26.10	1.92	31.66
Razgrad	125.83	19.82	3.60	14.71
Silistra	156.90	19.54	3.44	25.28
Sofia /City/	241.33	25.93	2.54	25.45
Sofia	157.13	20.95	5.74	20.78
Kyustendil	152.65	19.00	3.56	20.39
Pernik	162.42	15.03	3.60	19.65
Stara Zagora	165.89	25.78	4.34	23.39
Sliven	141.76	14.74	3.01	19.50
Khaskovo	80.15	36.22	5.87	25.69
Kurdzhali	111.83	18.26	3.93	18.54
Shumen	172.61	35.63	5.21	24.16
Turgovishte	160.64	24.03	3.16	26.24
Bulgaria	190.26	25.51	3.75	24.54

8.2

6	7	8	9
25.34	13.58	4.52	6.86
24.79	14.48	7.75	10.64
20.67	14.49	4.25	7.92
26.45	21.01	6.77	10.47
27.75	16.36	4.77	7.90
27.23	21.81	11.11	11.39
20.45	19.15	7.77	10.36
22.51	17.52	7.26	6.98
19.73	13.07	9.74	6.92
23.65	15.49	6.73	5.71
29.63	17.10	10.23	9.03
21.62	13.71	7.73	10.19
32.26	22.35	6.70	12.73
24.73	12.79	5.30	7.11
13.36	9.17	2.35	3.93
23.94	19.74	8.73	10.21
19.52	13.51	4.20	6.30
21.55	14.36	4.60	8.33
29.90	28.97	12.24	13.25
19.93	12.84	4.56	8.78
21.18	14.05	6.13	9.90
20.25	13.23	5.81	11.63
22.86	14.79	6.73	8.24
24.73	14.42	5.07	8.40
30.59	14.92	5.75	9.91
16.57	7.86	3.37	6.46
20.51	17.20	4.51	10.77
15.81	15.17	5.79	11.38
25.55	18.91	7.67	10.13

1	2	3	4	5
Blagoevgrad	192.19	46.34	8.61	40.34
Burgas	210.41	28.52	5.97	40.91
Yambol	261.71	50.27	9.26	53.86
Varna	265.46	52.85	10.30	49.57
Tolbukhin	187.26	21.24	8.13	37.21
G.Turnovo	342.09	56.30	10.30	63.31
Gabrovo	380.92	48.53	12.31	100.24
Vratsa	350.80	84.22	17.52	41.67
Vidin	254.48	46.26	10.62	28.97
Mikhaylovgrad	254.15	55.52	9.45	30.86
Pleven	332.86	59.99	9.58	57.70
Lovech	337.78	67.15	9.61	48.82
Plovdiv	283.61	62.16	10.61	47.74
Pzardzhik	204.99	39.87	10.31	41.65
Smolyan	127.98	23.84	6.14	25.15
Ruse	250.33	42.78	6.75	51.45
Razgrad	175.54	31.12	6.52	32.19
Silistra	164.39	21.85	7.48	35.83
Sofia /City/	172.20	24.88	4.01	25.48
Sofia	212.41	35.85	8.26	32.36
Kyustendil	212.41	45.46	10.69	40.52
Pernik	250.86	32.52	8.13	33.76
Stara Zagora	330.81	74.60	10.80	54.50
Sliven	234.88	50.64	6.17	38.48
Khaskovo	291.26	67.10	11.02	50.48
Kurdzhali	98.05	13.26	4.18	24.80
Shumen	221.69	42.13	10.57	34.28
Turgovishte	211.35	40.19	8.18	38.19
Bulgaria	2.436.87	45.84	8.99	42.28

8.3

6	7	8	9
26.85	6.34	2.60	6.11
25.87	12.16	3.75	11.05
31.56	1.26	4.34	12.47
34.04	16.42	5.97	7.76
28.47	12.35	2.86	7.38
41.00	20.50	8.92	15.93
47.13	21.45	10.20	15.47
41.67	22.02	9.01	13.14
31.67	4.58	6.66	8.96
33.96	17.57	9.30	7.82
49.86	19.38	9.36	14.48
56.99	19.96	13.06	17.42
40.68	16.69	3.64	10.61
25.57	14.02	2.74	7.28
17.13	5.96	1.86	7.26
27.71	13.33	6.75	13.85
25.51	7.89	2.73	8.80
19.63	11.61	2.16	8.85
26.03	11.44	4.81	9.03
29.17	14.34	4.78	12.44
43.40	19.33	5.55	8.02
38.93	13.30	6.65	12.07
50.48	14.69	4.01	13.43
32.12	12.52	2.90	10.34
46.49	12.46	3.67	8.94
18.90	2.54	0.45	4.18
31.86	10.57	3.92	12.08
28.37	11.27	2.91	10.00
33.85	13.90	5.01	10.45

Table 9

Incidence of Malignant Neoplasms in Bulgaria, by Selected Localizations and by Age for the 1970 - 1974 Period

Age groups	Total	Skin /172/	Lower lip /140/	Stomach /151/	Larynx /161/	Lung /162/	Rectum /154/	Breast /174/	Cervix uteri /180/
Total population									
Total	213.62	34.63	6.10	32.40	4.65	29.27	7.70	16.67	6.49
0-29	14.98	0.42	0.6	0.34	0.05	0.28	0.22	0.50	0.58
30-39	65.44	5.93	2.98	3.92	1.45	3.03	1.65	11.24	6.87
40-49	172.50	20.95	6.18	14.78	5.81	16.53	5.06	29.82	12.17
50-59	382.67	51.28	11.63	48.09	12.55	58.30	13.00	38.82	14.28
60+	863.57	163.93	23.00	160.02	14.87	129.06	34.49	41.68	12.25
Urban population									
Total	189.73	25.51	3.75	24.55	4.18	29.55	7.04	18.91	7.68
0-29	14.31	0.39	0.09	0.29	0.04	0.22	0.25	0.55	0.66
30-39	71.54	5.23	1.90	3.88	1.67	3.01	1.81	13.54	8.89
40-49	188.76	19.47	4.68	13.51	6.31	18.40	5.61	37.17	16.42
50-59	426.67	48.31	8.49	44.99	13.66	65.63	15.01	51.62	19.58
60+	1.039.72	168.80	19.27	172.21	17.57	157.47	43.72	66.22	18.38
Rural population									
Total	243.04	45.86	8.99	42.06	4.22	33.87	8.53	13.91	5.01
0-29	16.23	0.46	0.29	0.43	0.06	0.39	0.17	0.45	0.45
30-39	57.14	6.88	3.26	3.98	1.15	3.06	1.43	8.11	4.13
40-49	143.72	22.67	7.92	16.25	5.24	14.37	4.43	21.32	7.25
50-59	348.21	53.85	14.22	50.76	11.69	52.55	11.41	28.56	10.02
60+	757.25	161.05	25.26	152.06	13.24	111.99	28.92	26.37	8.55

Table 10.1

Incidence of Malignant Neoplasms in Bulgaria and Its Administrative Districts, by Age and Sex, for the 1970-1974 Period

Age groups Administrative districts	0-29	30-39	40-49	50-59	60+	Total	Standardized
1	2	3	4	5	6	7	8
Blagoevgrad	13.7	59.3	182.7	409.0	963.5	187.1	173.8
Burgas	16.6	65.3	176.2	398.9	911.6	197.9	170.0
Yambol	16.6	61.2	139.9	332.5	800.1	207.0	147.6
Varna	14.9	68.7	176.3	401.2	1038.5	216.3	183.0
Tolbukhin	14.1	63.0	144.3	385.6	875.2	187.5	159.4
G.Turnovo	15.7	72.6	185.2	400.8	894.3	290.0	169.9
Gabrovo	13.4	68.9	167.2	364.7	924.2	235.5	165.8
Vratsa	16.5	87.2	213.2	397.8	834.3	274.7	169.1
Vidin	15.9	63.7	142.1	191.5	512.8	2o3.8	1o4.9
Mikhaylovgrad	14.7	59.2	147.6	324.6	613.6	208.2	126.9
Pleven	12.8	70.6	180.2	367.6	904.7	264.0	165.5
Lovech	1o.4	58.4	153.7	332.4	780.5	245.5	143.2
Plovdiv	18.2	69.6	199.0	466.9	1009.6	245.7	190.6
Pazardzhik	18.1	67.3	151.4	360.5	840.0	184.7	153.5
Smolyan	12.5	42.9	119.9	297.8	625.0	112.6	119.1
Ruse	16.9	75.6	175.2	386.1	909.8	220.9	170.2
Razgrad	13.2	95.9	146.8	288.8	645.6	154.8	125.6
Silistra	15.6	57.5	138.2	339.6	669.9	161.3	133.3
Sofia/City/	18.2	76.6	209.1	438.3	1123.3	234.6	202.0
Sofia	13.4	63.5	155.5	357.4	659.9	191.9	135.4
Kyustendil	13.5	48.8	167.6	169.0	728.2	207.6	143.2
Pernik	14.7	58.7	163.1	365.3	777.4	202.1	149.5
Stara Zagora	14.4	62.0	175.7	403.5	929.7	234.1	170.6
Sliven	14.6	60.6	158.9	361.8	806.6	186.2	152.0
Khaskovo	16.5	74.1	163.7	397.9	984.4	241.0	177.1
Kurdzhali	9.2	42.7	127.6	368.6	674.4	1o1.2	129.6
Shumen	13.8	59.1	147.5	355.0	883.2	198.9	157.3
Turgovishte	14.5	56.3	157.5	284.4	705.2	192.8	133.6
Bulgaria	15.0	65.4	172.5	382.7	863.6	214.2	162.3

Administrative districts	M e n						
	0-29	30-39	40-49	50-59	60+	Total	Standardized
Blagoevgrad	13.04	60.09	169.77	441.84	1.258.07	215.28	206.64
Burgas	17.34	49.64	165.94	441.79	1.165.15	222.79	197.46
Yambol	17.02	44.09	158.29	396.43	989.66	235.10	173.21
Varna	15.48	56.01	158.77	408.40	1.187.07	221.20	195.72
Tolbukhin	15.59	57.26	142.01	426.31	1.046.48	207.38	185.42
G.Turnovo	13.72	59.36	157.45	411.01	1.028.69	304.75	178.69
Gabrovo	11.90	60.72	132.23	344.56	1.091.45	285.70	175.42
Vratsa	14.04	61.81	182.08	411.64	990.90	287.54	178.25
Vidin	14.52	47.79	123.04	286.22	612.63	217.44	118.79
Mikhaylovgrad	14.30	36.15	133.66	323.49	762.37	226.83	137.40
Pleven	13.82	61.65	152.97	391.31	1.110.42	290.62	185.30
Lovech	10.16	43.09	128.22	347.65	959.92	262.95	158.20
Plovdiv	18.94	62.71	192.22	529.21	1.282.02	274.26	223.06
Pzardzhik	14.19	51.89	147.31	383.21	1.067.24	205.70	178.29
Smolyan	13.86	33.87	113.99	325.32	878.13	126.94	146.77
Ruse	15.00	56.74	140.59	391.35	1.149.84	234.66	187.94
Razgrad	15.16	45.26	124.55	347.29	849.95	186.56	149.28
Silistra	18.45	34.29	128.34	364.81	825.84	176.09	149.15
Sofia/City	17.75	51.45	153.24	406.83	1.267.32	223.30	203.96
Sofia	14.12	52.59	147.85	377.73	816.43	211.04	151.67
Kyustendil	12.81	46.76	150.93	417.53	955.85	238.09	168.70
Pernik	11.48	44.24	138.22	415.34	954.66	216.47	165.79
Stara Gora	15.28	43.15	164.52	441.12	1.194.41	258.00	128.29
Sliven	16.52	60.02	159.14	417.08	1.042.71	214.53	199.62
Khaskovo	18.06	66.51	139.57	412.41	1.245.34	261.07	202.68
Kurdzhali	10.43	46.83	144.25	524.99	1.084.45	140.46	189.66
Shumen	14.68	44.17	136.80	365.04	1.069.98	215.92	174.94
Turgovishte	16.41	42.45	184.18	333.33	897.66	229.35	160.49
Bulgaria	15.27	52.25	152.96	406.30	1.061.26	231.37	181.05

10.2

Groups

				W o	m e n		
0-29	30-39	40-49	50-59	60+	Total	Standardized
14.46	58.58	195.74	375.86	695.20	157.30	135.06
15.75	81.79	187.24	355.35	676.15	171.88	134.30
16.12	78.44	141.53	272.04	625.28	178.27	116.55
14.32	82.16	195.13	393.80	903.68	208.53	158.28
12.55	68.92	146.64	343.52	715.79	165.59	128.43
17.64	85.41	211.90	390.80	774.22	273.91	148.02
15.15	77.81	201.83	385.72	779.71	232.42	147.10
19.12	111.53	243.75	384.62	696.47	261.12	151.33
17.45	77.65	159.35	296.45	422.54	190.83	103.17
15.20	80.58	161.22	325.68	479.65	190.02	110.46
11.84	79.35	207.58	343.99	722.58	236.79	145.46
10.73	73.95	178.88	317.51	623.79	226.17	121.39
17.37	76.41	205.79	407.77	782.70	215.08	150.92
9.84	74.61	155.50	338.29	637.81	161.91	121.30
11.07	51.06	127.26	266.50	413.88	95.73	88.93
19.02	95.39	211.21	380.71	698.35	205.97	145.04
11.18	65.42	167.90	232.88	466.21	132.20	97.53
12.74	80.45	148.35	314.74	530.92	146.13	109.14
18.63	103.63	264.68	470.44	999.96	245.38	187.34
12.57	74.53	163.30	337.77	517.06	171.86	129.71
14.30	50.76	182.86	325.57	531.51	177.25	111.62
18.45	73.08	189.10	317.43	615.36	187.10	126.01
13.39	81.96	187.27	366.89	704.17	209.18	136.55
12.60	61.12	158.60	307.80	595.78	153.91	114.92
14.84	81.54	188.18	383.61	767.88	220.20	144.60
7.86	39.31	112.14	209.47	373.13	66.36	75.13
12.89	73.25	158.17	344.83	718.07	181.48	130.90
12.58	68.64	131.94	238.43	530.27	156.88	100.63
14.66	78.70	192.13	359.32	689.76	195.90	135.43

Malignant Neoplasms in Bulgaria and its

Administ-rative districts	All malignant tumours Men per 100.000	Women per 100.000	M E N	Skin /172/ per 100.000	standard-ized rate
Blagoev-grad	215.28	157.30		38.2	35.67
Burgas	222.79	171.88		25.8	22.46
Yambol	235.10	178.27		37.8	26.76
Varna	221.20	208.53		35.4	30.96
Tolbukhin	207.38	165.59		22.5	19.61
G.Turnovo	304.75	273.91		42.6	24.30
Gabrovo	235.70	232.42		19.7	14.64
Vratsa	287.54	261.12		62.9	37.14
Vidin	217.44	190.83		32.7	17.46
Mikhaylov-grad	226.83	190.02		42.9	23.97
Pleven	290.62	236.79		45.2	27.87
Lovech	262.95	226.17		41.9	24.27
Plovdiv	274.26	215.08		46.1	41.65
Pazardzhik	205.70	161.91		30.0	25.60
Smolyan	126.94	95.73		20.9	23.89
Ruse	234.66	205.97		31.2	24.40
Razgrad	186.56	132.20		28.0	21.63
Silistra	176.09	146.13		20.7	17.21
Sofia/City	223.30	245.38		24.9	22.58
Sofia	211.04	171.86		27.6	18.92
Kyustendil	238.09	177.25		31.1	21.24
Pernik	216.47	187.10		21.4	15.56
Stara Zag.	258.00	209.18		41.7	32.43
Sliven	214.53	153.91		33.9	28.40
Khaskovo	261.07	220.20		43.6	33.18
Kurdzhali	140.46	66.36		17.7	24.85
Shumen	215.92	181.48		36.5	28.76
Turgoviste	229.35	156.88		39.7	26.58
Bulgaria	231.37	15.90		34.1	26.10

11

Administrative Districts, by Sex for the 1970-74 Period

Stomach /151/		Lung /162/		Breast /174/	
per 100.000	standard-ized rate	per 100.000	standard-ized rate	per 100.000	standard-ized rate
41.1	39.13	47.1	45.3	0.3	0.27
37.6	32.96	42.9	37.8	0.6	0.50
46.3	32.44	47.2	33.3	0.2	0.15
38.3	33.21	46.5	41.1	0.6	0.47
38.2	32.94	47.4	40.8	0.5	0.44
57.1	30.96	57.2	32.8	1.0	0.50
58.8	42.57	44.0	31.9	0.4	0.32
39.8	23.89	55.9	33.8	0.8	0.56
27.6	13.46	43.3	23.5	0.7	0.56
29.3	16.82	49.5	29.3	1.2	0.30
51.6	32.35	66.8	41.1	0.3	0.25
42.2	24.16	62.3	36.6	0.5	0.32
42.8	34.34	62.5	50.1	0.5	0.36
40.4	34.73	43.3	37.1	0.6	0.68
32.2	27.71	27.7	32.7	0.2	0.25
48.8	38.28	43.9	34.7	0.1	0.10
38.6	30.08	38.3	30.2	-	-
38.8	32.21	34.6	28.5	-	0.43
29.3	26.85	47.0	42.6	0.7	0.53
37.4	25.75	44.7	31.5	0.4	0.23
38.8	26.66	54.8	37.7	0.6	0.34
32.9	24.66	44.8	34.1	0.2	0.20
44.2	32.86	58.3	44.1	0.4	1.19
34.2	28.66	48.4	40.7	0.8	0.71
41.5	31.34	66.4	50.5	0.1	0.10
32.4	45.23	34.5	47.3	0.1	0.22
35.0	27.74	46.6	37.1	0.2	0.18
44.4	29.07	40.2	27.6	1.2	0.76
39.3	30.01	49.4	38.0	0.5	0.38

Table 11 /cont'd/

Administrative districts	WOMEN	Skin / 172/		Stomach /151/	
		per 100.000	standard-ized rate	per 100.000	standard-ized rate
Blagoevgrad		44.0	41.13	28.6	25.77
Burgas		23.5	19.08	27.9	22.62
Yambol		32.7	23.08	33.5	19.02
Varna		34.4	27.05	25.9	19.32
Tolbukhin		18.7	15.43	28.8	23.23
G.Turnovo		44.9	29.33	42.3	22.00
Gabrovo		28.1	17.29	45.7	27.53
Vratsa		60.2	27.00	28.2	19.39
Vidin		33.0	15.41	13.9	6.33
Mikhaylovgrad		38.5	21.45	17.0	9.07
Pleven		42.2	24.09	32.1	17.73
Lovech		48.8	24.14	24.9	12.78
Plovdiv		46.0	33.36	24.8	17.71
Pazardzhik		31.4	24.39	27.9	21.53
Smolyan		15.0	14.53	16.8	16.33
Ruse		34.1	23.95	29.9	21.05
Razgrad		26.4	19.82	14.7	10.85
Silistra		21.1	16.44	24.2	18.61
Sofia /City		26.7	21.60	21.4	17.37
Sofia		33.4	21.81	18.5	11.89
Kyustendil		32.9	20.74	21.6	13.42
Pernik		24.9	16.53	18.8	12.27
Stara Zag.		50.3	32.53	27.9	17.95
Sliven		28.9	22.17	22.6	17.09
Khaskovo		56.0	37.45	29.9	20.30
Kurdzhali		11.7	14.56	15.0	18.56
Shumen		41.8	31.16	24.0	17.49
Turgovishte		29.1	18.15	23.2	14.51
Bulgaria		35.0	24.50	25.5	17.61

Breast /174/		Lung /162/		Cervix uteri /180/	
per 100.000	standardized rate	per 100.000	standardized rate	per 100.000	standardized rate
18.6	17.48	4.6	4.3	6.9	6.50
26.9	23.09	5.8	4.6	12.3	10.75
26.6	19.19	4.9	3.2	8.6	6.35
39.3	32.91	9.8	7.9	13.2	11.23
28.2	24.33	8.0	6.6	7.2	6.28
40.3	27.14	12.1	6.8	18.1	12.48
40.1	29.52	10.3	6.7	15.1	12.21
38.5	25.29	8.3	4.9	17.4	12.96
35.2	22.27	9.9	4.7	15.9	10.63
32.5	21.07	9.4	5.5	16.7	11.95
36.1	24.77	12.6	7.1	19.1	14.51
33.4	22.11	13.7	6.8	19.0	12.81
39.3	30.40	8.2	5.9	10.9	8.66
26.2	22.04	6.7	5.3	8.3	7.03
15.2	15.43	1.6	1.7	4.4	4.44
34.8	27.06	6.0	4.3	16.0	12.67
19.1	15.93	9.2	7.0	5.9	5.03
24.6	20.43	6.0	4.7	6.3	5.58
54.1	45.18	10.9	8.8	23.0	19.10
27.4	20.29	5.7	3.5	9.4	7.33
32.3	23.30	8.7	5.5	11.1	9.07
26.9	20.42	1o.4	6.9	12.2	9.74
29.6	22.05	9.5	6.3	11.5	9.12
26.3	21.56	6.5	5.1	8.0	6.97
27.5	20.48	8.6	5.8	9.7	7.02
7.2	8.68	3.8	4.8	2.2	2.64
26.9	22.07	6.4	4.7	8.2	7.10
23.8	17.95	7.0	4.5	7.7	6.26
32.8	25.45	8.3	4.7	12.8	1o.34

Table 12

Prevalence of Patients with Malignant Neoplasms, According to the Data for the 1970 - 1974 Period, Provided by the Oncological Institutions of Bulgaria

| | Alive patients with malignant neoplasms registered in the oncological network at he end of each year | | | | | |
| | Total | | Urban population | | Rural population | |
	Absolute number	Per 100.000	Absolute number	Per 10.000	Absolute number	Per 100.000
1970	73.362	864.4	32.626	734.5	40.756	1.006.9
1971	79.075	926.3	35.249	767.2	43.826	1.111.7
1972	82.048	956.7	37.594	794.5	44.454	1.156.3
1973	85.708	994.2	40.292	830.6	45.416	1.204.7
1974	90.979	1.048.3	43.530	863.5	47.449	1.304.4

Table 13

Prevalence of Patients with Malignant Neoplasms, by Selected Localizations, According to the Data Provided by the Oncological Institutions of Bulgaria for the 1970-1974 Period

Alive patients with malignant neoplasms on registered in the oncological network at the end of each year

	/151/ Stomach		/162/ Lung		/174/ Breast		/180/ Cervix uteri	
	Ab-solute number	Per 100.000	Ab-solute number	Per 100.000	Ab-solute number	Per 100.000	Ab-solute number	Per 100.000
1970	5.098	60.0	7.313	43.7	7.868	92.7	3.415	80.4
1971	5.574	65.8	4.070	47.7	8.602	100.8	8.605	84.6
1972	5.524	63.2	4.184	48.8	8.982	104.7	3.847	89.7
1973	5.811	67.4	4.540	52.7	9.458	109.7	4.067	94.3
1974	5.794	66.8	4.679	53.9	10.142	116.9	4.402	101.3

Table 14

Distribution of Patients with Malignant Neoplasms of Selected Localizations the Time from Their Registration after the Diagnosis 1974

Sites	Number of alive patients with malignant neoplasms registered at the end of the year			
	Total	1-2 years	3-4 years	5 or more years
All malignant neoplasms		after	diagnosis	
Absolute number	71.933	30.973	11.936	29.024
Percent of the total number	100.0	43.91	16.6	40.3
out of the total number /151/ Stomach	3.095	1.941	410	744
	100.0	62.5	13.25	24.0
/174/ Breast	8.628	3.102	1.580	3.946
	100.0	36.0	18.3	45.7
/180/ Cervix uteri	3.783	1.207	545	2.031
	100.0	31.9	14.4	58.7

Table 15

Methods of Treatment of Patients with Malignant Neoplasms According to Data for 1974 Provided by the Oncological Institutions of Bulgaria

Localizations	Total	Patients with malignant neoplasms who have completed special treatment					
		of which					
		Surgical only		Radiotherapy only		Combined and chemotherapy	
		Absolute number	Percentage	Absolute number	Percentage	Absolute number	Percentage
All malignant neoplasms	18.281	4.217	23.1	5.859	29.3	8.705	47.6
of which /162/ lung	2.258	141	6.2	230	10.2	1.887	83.6
/174/ breast	3.071	506	16.5	578	18.8	1.987	64.7
/180/ uterus	1.494	434	29.0	85	5.7	975	65.3
/172/ skin	3.245	434	7.9	1.097	34.9	1.798	57.2
All other localizations	8.313	2.886	34.7	3.369	40.5	2.058	24.8

Table 16

Mortality from Malignant Neoplasms in Bulgaria for the 1970-
1974 Period /per 100.000 population/

Years	Total	Urban population	Rural population
1970	132.54	113.75	153.15
1971	136.49	116.67	159.58
1972	137.91	115.87	165.02
1973	138.55	116.60	166.68
1974	139.61	118.80	168.43
1970 - 1974	137.14	116.35	162.60

Table 17

Mortality from Malignant Neoplasms in Bulgaria, by Sex, for
the 1970-1974 Period

/per 100.000 population/

Years	Total	Men	Women
1970	132.54	155.63	109.46
1971	136.49	163.07	109.92
1972	137.91	163.36	112.46
1973	138.55	164.69	112.45
1974	139.61	164.62	114.64
1970-1974	137.14	162.35	111.86

Table 18

Mortality from Malignant Neoplasms in Bulgaria, by Selected Localizations for
the 1970 - 1974 Period
/per 100.000 population/

Years	All localizations /140 - 209/	Stomach /151/	Lung /162/	Breast /174/	Cervix uteri /180/
1970	132.54	33.44	24.97	6.35	1.93
1971	136.49	34.31	27.14	7.23	1.66
1972	137.91	34.13	27.28	7.38	1.98
1973	138.55	32.81	28.95	7.69	2.13
1974	139.61	32.90	27.90	7.06	2.00
1970 - 1974	137.14	33.53	27.27	7.31	1.94

Table 19

Mortality from Malignant Neoplasms in Bulgaria and its
Administrative Districts, by Selected Localizations for
the 1970-74 Period /per 100.000 Population/

Administrative districts	Total	Urban population	Rural population	
1	2	3	4	
Blagoevgrad	122.18	118.71	124.88	
Burgas	119.43	108.79	133.23	
Yambol	143.21	99.70	185.77	
Varna	128.63	112.53	163.04	
Tolbukhin	132.47	127.95	136.18	
G.Turnovo	161.84	122.16	192.18	
Gabrovo	139.07	103.12	226.86	
Vratsa	183.70	133.38	227.90	
Vidin	146.10	93.05	189.24	
Mikhaylovgrad	160.00	121.55	187.84	
Pleven	158.42	110.22	201.98	
Lovech	162.53	104.06	222.98	
Plovdiv	150.77	131.34	183.66	
Pazardzhik	127.94	113.42	144.49	
Smolyan	77.97	60.55	90.35	
Ruse	137.90	123.83	159.37	
Razgrad	115.37	93.10	126.64	
Silistra	115.90	118.39	114.19	
Sofia /City/	133.50	136.28	108.18	
Sofia	155.32	116.58	175.46	
Kyustendil	152.14	102.56	203.64	
Pernik	130.12	95.04	173.23	
Stara Zagora	142.93	98.36	206.10	
Sliven	128.98	107.82	153.19	
Khaskovo	146.90	116.98	185.97	
Kurdzhali	78.96	75.30	80.14	
Shumen	122.27	99.78	141.80	
Turgovishte	131.52	97.40	151.14	
Bulgaria	137.14	116.35	162.60	

Table 19 /cont'd/

	Stomach /151/			Lung /162/		
	Total	Urban popu- lation	Rural popu- lation	Total	Urban popu- lation	Rural popu- lation
	5	6	7	8	9	10
Blagoevgrad	39.36	34.17	43.40	25.58	26.13	25.15
Burgas	29.01	23.00	36.81	21.02	21.55	20.34
Yambol	43.28	28.98	59.15	25.50	19.70	31.18
Varna	28.92	20.17	47.62	24.87	30.71	27.32
Tolbukhin	34.36	26.47	40.82	26.66	26.84	26.51
G.Turnovo	41.18	25.98	52.86	27.45	21.81	31.76
Gabrovo	38.82	24.48	73.86	24.21	19.58	35.52
Vratsa	43.84	28.64	57.19	32.78	24.36	40.17
Vidin	25.86	13.32	36.05	28.85	19.22	36.68
Mihaylovgrad	35.03	25.28	42.08	31.43	23.86	36.91
Pleven	35.51	19.75	49.76	33.40	23.97	41.92
Lovech	34.73	18.80	51.18	36.34	20.56	52.63
Plovdiv	34.78	25.99	49.68	29.82	24.46	38.90
Pazardzhik	36.11	27.51	45.92	27.44	24.73	30.52
Smolyan	23.74	13.63	30.92	14.48	12.58	15.83
Ruse	38.19	30.53	49.89	25.57	24.85	26.68
Razgrad	32.97	18.92	40.08	21.68	18.92	23.08
Silistra	33.53	28.73	36.81	19.74	21.26	18.70
Sofia /City	22.80	22.23	28.09	24.73	24.78	24.28
Sofia	43.67	28.21	52.77	30.70	23.65	34.85
Kyustendil	38.64	18.21	59.86	35.10	21.97	48.75
Pernik	25.09	16.84	35.23	27.75	19.65	37.70
Stara Zagora	36.42	22.24	56.51	30.13	21.53	43.07
Sliven	29.79	19.02	42.11	26.91	26.16	28.13
Khaskovo	38.52	25.69	55.28	34.92	27.89	44.09
Kurdzhali	26.98	20.23	29.17	17.85	15.73	18.53
Shumen	32.48	23.81	40.01	25.77	21.72	29.29
Turgovishte	36.72	26.56	42.56	22.40	13.91	27.28
Bulgaria	33.53	23.64	45.70	27.27	23.54	31.85

| Rectum /154/ | | | Breast /174/ | | | Cervix uteri /180/ | | |
Total	Urban popu-lation	Rural popu-lation	Total	Urban popu-lation	Rural popu-lation	Total	Urban popu-lation	Rural popu-lation
11	12	13	14	15	16	17	18	19
4.01	3.35	4.53	3.76	4.23	3.40	1.02	1.46	0.67
4.61	3.74	5.74	1.92	6.90	6.52	0.72	0.93	0.44
5.44	3.28	7.55	5.15	5.98	4.35	1.52	1.15	1.88
4.66	3.76	6.56	8.42	8.58	8.06	1.95	1.95	1.94
4.55	4.41	4.97	4.15	8.08	3.77	0.99	0.91	1.05
8.24	6.25	9.77	14.8	8.75	8.71	2.64	2.36	2.86
7.66	5.47	13.01	7.35	6.76	8.79	1.94	1.72	2.46
6.86	4.56	8.88	9.06	8.12	8.89	3.33	3.27	3.37
9.31	6.40	11.67	8.85	5.12	11.88	4.13	4.61	3.75
8.39	4.48	11.22	7.10	7.74	6.65	3.59	3.05	3.98
6.69	3.73	9.36	8.69	8.31	9.04	2.85	3.37	2.39
7.67	4.39	11.o7	9.64	7.20	10.35	4.28	3.16	5.44
4.69	3.97	5.91	8.48	8.42	8.59	1.38	1.48	1.21.
3.72	3.37	4.12	7.00	7.11	6.87	0.96	1.08	0.82
2.72	1.57	2.98	2.61	3.40	2.05	0.43	0.78	0.18
4.80	4.54	5.19	8.29	8.62	7.80	2.74	2.95	2.42
4.23	2.10	5.31	4.53	3.90	4.86	1.81	1.80	1.82
3.38	3.16	3.54	6.42	5.74	6.89	1.63	1.43	1.77
6.16	6.34	4.41	10.58	11.70	3.81	3.00	3.28	0.40
5.13	2.70	6.57	7.20	8.61	6.37	1.75	1.68	1.79
4.64	3.16	6.17	6.86	0.59	7.82	2.01	1.78	2.26
7.73	5.81	10.10	7.18	5.49	9.36	0.77	0.80	0.73
5.50	3.63	8.28	6.13	1.04	7.41	1.61	1.59	1.63
4.48	3.32	5.80	7.87	8.24	7.44	2.11	2.69	1.45
5.54	5.13	6.07	6.02	6.40	5.43	1.45	1.59	1.27
1.92	1.96	1.90	2.37	3.09	1.36	0.27	0.84	0.09
4.60	3.30	5.73	5.17	5.39	4.98	0.64	0.69	0.60
4.27	3.16	4.91	8.42	6.32	6.55	1.15	0.94	1.27
5.42	4.44	6.61	7.31	7.77	6.63	1.94	2.13	1.71

Mortality from Malignant Neoplasms in Bulgaria and its

for the 1970-1974 Period

		Stomach /151/			Lung /162/	
	Total	Men	Women	Total	Men	Women
Blagoevgrad	39.36	45.34	33.44	25.58	43.67	7.63
Burgas	29.01	33.62	24.23	21.02	35.60	5.89
Yambol	43.28	50.67	37.86	25.50	43.95	7.23
Varna	28.92	33.40	24.29	24.87	39.95	9.29
Tolbukhin	34.36	37.33	31.35	26.66	44.73	14.01
G.Turnovo	41.18	49.47	33.17	27.45	45.55	9.95
Gabrovo	38.82	46.02	31.26	24.21	39.45	8.18
Vratsa	43.84	51.83	36.02	32.78	54.39	11.61
Vidin	25.86	34.40	17.74	28.85	47.35	11.22
Mikhaylovgrad	35.03	42.92	27.24	31.43	50.85	12.26
Pleven	35.51	43.71	27.00	33.40	56.28	10.89
Lovech	34.73	42.91	26.37	36.34	59.69	12.46
Plovdiv	34.78	43.13	26.71	29.82	57.51	8.94
Pazardzhik	36.11	43.21	28.94	27.44	46.79	7.88
Smolyan	23.74	26.67	20.48	14.48	25.43	2.30
Ruse	38.19	45.80	30.36	25.57	42.01	8.63
Razgrad	32.97	46.02	20.62	21.68	37.10	7.07
Silistra	33.53	41.60	25.55	19.74	33.61	6.04
Sofia /City	22.80	26.42	19.16	24.73	40.20	9.13
Sofia	43.67	56.26	35.00	30.70	50.76	10.45
Kyustendil	38.64	44.37	33.11	35.10	59.16	11.90
Pernik	25.09	29.22	20.79	27.75	44.38	10.39
Stara Zagora	36.42	45.43	27.17	30.13	51.79	8.53
Sliven	29.79	34.42	24.12	26.91	47.06	6.96
Khaskovo	38.52	43.88	33.20	34.92	60.82	9.13
Kurdzhali	26.98	37.22	17.82	17.85	33.15	4.16
Shumen	32.48	36.18	28.86	25.77	45.14	6.73
Turgovishte	36.72	46.53	27.24	22.40	36.19	9.08
Bulgaria	33.50	40.16	26.91	27.01	45.53	8.73

Administrative Districts, by Sex and Selected localizations
/per 100.000 Population/

Rectum /154/			Breast /174/			Cervix Uteri/180/
Total	Men	Women	Total	Men	Women	Women
4.01	4.48	3.56	3.76	0.13	7.38	1.02
4.61	4.53	4.71	1.92	0.09	13.64	0.72
5.44	6.14	4.76	5.15	0.00	10.27	1.52
4.66	4.49	4.84	8.42	0.09	17.03	1.95
4.55	4.77	4.17	4.15	0.00	11.51	0.99
8.24	9.80	6.75	14.8	0.12	17.06	2.64
7.66	7.97	7.34	7.35	0.20	14.89	1.94
6.86	6.73	6.99	9.06	0.13	17.81	3.33
9.31	9.19	9.43	8.85	0.23	17.06	4.13
8.39	10.00	6.81	7.10	0.00	14.13	3.59
6.69	7.84	5.56	8.69	0.00	17.24	2.85
7.67	9.71	5.60	9.64	0.18	17.52	4.28
4.69	5.44	3.97	8.58	0.00	16.70	1.38
3.72	4.60	2.84	7.00	0.26	13.83	0.96
2.72	1.65	3.22	2.61	0.00	5.52	0.43
4.80	5.27	5.01	8.29	0.00	16.85	2.74
4.23	4.56	2.75	4.53	0.41	8.45	1.81
3.38	4.23	2.56	6.42	0.00	12.78	1.63
6.16	6.56	5.76	10.58	0.23	21.04	3.00
5.13	5.36	4.91	7.20	0.00	14.08	1.75
4.64	5.34	3.96	6.86	0.41	13.09	2.01
7.73	8.88	6.55	7.18	0.00	14.69	0.77
5.50	6.15	4.95	6.13	0.10	12.32	1.61
4.48	5.40	4.25	7.87	0.17	15.63	2.11
5.54	5.14	5.95	6.02	0.14	11.07	1.45
1.92	2.33	1.56	2.37	0.00	4.16	0.27
4.60	5.87	3.37	5.17	0.16	10.1o	0.64
4.27	4.70	3.86	8.42	0.23	12.49	1.15
5.41	4.94	4.88	7.14	0.12	14.46	1.94

Table 20 cont'd

Administrative Districts	Total	Men	Women
Blagoevgrad	122.18	152.27	92.32
Burgas	119.43	142.04	95.95
Yambol	143.21	171.38	115.29
Varna	128.63	143.72	113.72
Tolbukhin	132.47	153.60	110.56
G.Turnovo	161.84	186.84	137.19
Gabrovo	139.07	157.99	119.15
Vratsa	183.70	215.79	152.26
Vidin	146.10	171.74	123.93
Mikhaylovgrad	160.00	191.32	129.07
Pleven	158.42	188.79	128.55
Lovech	162.52	193.37	130.97
Plovdiv	150.77	185.24	117.10
Pazardzhik	127.94	155.72	99.88
Smolyan	77.97	91.38	63.74
Ruse	137.90	157.25	117.96
Razgrad	115.37	149.24	83.29
Silistra	115.90	134.92	97.11
Sofia /City/	133.50	144.15	122.87
Sofia	155.32	181.48	125.52
Kyustendil	152.14	187.96	117.57
Pernik	130.12	150.88	108.46
Stara Zagora	142.93	177.20	107.75
Sliven	128.98	157.19	100.57
Khaskovo	146.90	179.14	114.80
Kurdzahli	78.96	113.99	47.62
Shumen	122.27	148.13	96.83
Turgovishte	131.52	157.68	106.25
Bulgaria	137.14	162.35	111.85

REFERENCES

1. A.S. Beshkov and E.V. Velev: /Geography of Bulgaria/. /In Bulgarian/ The Publishing House of the Bulgarian Academy of Sciences, Sofia, 1961.

2. J. Penkov and G. Khristov: /Economical geography of Bulgaria/. /In Bulgarian/ Publishing House "Science and Art", Sofia, 1975.

3. J. Stefanov et al.: Demography of Bulgaria. /In Bulgarian/ Publishing House "Science and Art", Sofia, 1974.

4. I. Popov et al.: /Collection of statistical data of cancer distribution in Bulgaria/. /In Bulgarian/ Inform. bulletin "Onkologia", 4/1972, 1-2/1973, Sofia

5. G. Mitrov et al.: /Prevention, early diagnosis and therapy of malignant tumours/. /In Bulgarian/ Publishing House "Medicine and Physical Culture", Sofia, 1974.

6. P. Khristov and I. Popov: /Organization and results in fight against cancer./ /In Bulgarian/ Publishing House "Medicine and Physical Culture", 1965.

7. The Ministry of Public Health: Collection of practical medical research materials/. /In Bulgarian/ Publishing House "Profizdat", Sofia, 1964.

8. The Ministry of Public Health: /Methodical guidelines of early diagnosis of malignant tumours/. /In Bulgarian/ Publishing House "Medicine and Physical Culture", of Sofia, 1973.

9. The Ministry of Health and the Ministry of Information. /Statistical collection "Zdraveopazvane"/. /In Bulgarian/ Sofia, 1974.

CANCER CONTROL IN CUBA

Z. Marinello and V. A. Kochnev

GEOGRAPHIC, ECONOMIC AND DEMOGRAPHIC CHARACTERISTICS OF THE COUNTRY; A HISTORICAL REVIEW ON THE DEVELOPMENT OF CANCER CONTROL

The Republic of Cuba is situated on the islands of Cuba /104,000 sq.km/, Pinos /2,200 sq.km/ and on more than 1,600 small islands in the Atlantic Ocean, the Gulf of Mexico and the Caribbean Sea. The territory of Cuba is 110,900 sq.km.

The length of the coastline is 5,746 km. There are numerous gulfs with beautiful bays: Cabanas, Mariel, Habana, Matanzas, Nuevitas in the north; Cienfuegos, Santiago de Cuba, Guantanamo in the south.

The relief of Cuba is mainly flat; mountains and hills occupy about one third of the territory.

In the west there are mountain-masses forming Cordillera--de-Guaniguanico. Numerous hills are situated along the main axis of the island /Habana-Matanzas, Bejucal-Madruga, Santa-Clara, Noroste de las Villas/. In the centre of Cuba there is the mountain-mass Guamaya with its highest peak Loma San Juan /1,156 m/.

The highest mountains are situated in the south-eastern part of the country. Along the southern coast there are the mountains of the Sierra Maestra with their highest peak Turquino /1,974 m/, the highest point in Cuba. To the east there are the mountains of the Sierra de Nipe /995 m/, Sierra del Cristal /1,231 m/, Cuchillas de Moa /1,139 m/ Cuchillas de Toa /1,011 m/, and Sierra del Purial /1,181 m/.

The climate is tropical, trade wind with a pronounced rainy season /between May and October/. The average temperature is 22.5°C in January, and 27.8°C in August, respectively. The lowest temperature is not below 5°C, the highest temperature reaches 40°C. The annual precipitation on the plains is 1,000--1,200 mm, while at the mountains 2,200 mm. The relative humidity in summer is 60-70 per cent during daytime and 80-90 per cent at nights; in winter the humidity is higher /85-90 per cent/.

The rivers in Cuba are mostly short and shallow. The Cauto, the largest river /370 km in length/ has its source in the Sierra Maestra. The fluctuations of the water level depend on the amount of precipitation /80 per cent of the precipitation falls within the autumn/. Many rivers have rapids; in the mountain areas there are disappearing and underground rivers.

Woods are preserved mainly in the mountain and boggy areas. In the course of exploitation of unused lands the woods have been mostly destroyed on the plains. However, some kinds of wood have been preserved including royal palm, therefore the plain landscape of Cuba resembles palm savanna.

According to the 1973 data the population of Cuba is 9,330,000; the Cuban comprise the main population group /95 per cent/, in the province of Oriente there is a group of aboriginal population of Indian origin mixed with the Cuban, but preserving some elements of their original culture. In the eastern areas there is a group of immigrants from Haiti. A small number of the Japanese and Chinese live on the island of Pinos and in the suburbs of Habana. The official language is Spanish.

The main mineral resources of Cuba are nickel, cobalt, iron ore, chromium, aluminium, copper, manganese, gold, cement, marble; the energetic resources include rather rich reserves of peat.

Cuba is an industrial and agricultural country, in which light industry predominates /textile industry, manufacture of agricultural products/; metallurgy has started developing only recently. Energetic resources are exploited; a number of thermal power stations with a total capacity above 1,000,000 kilowatts have been built.

The main agricultural products are sugar-cane, tobacco, coffee-beans, citruses, fruits, rice. Intensive cattle-breeding and poultry-raising are developed in the country.

The coastal waters are rich in fish; fishing is rather intensively developed.

Epidemiological data

Between 1970 and 1972 372,277 cases of cancer were registered in Cuba. Since 1968 an increase in the indices of cancer morbidity has been noted. It is obvious that factors as the improvement of diagnosis and the organization of health service influence the rates of cancer morbidity, however, there is an absolute rise caused by the actual increase of cancer cases.

In the structure of morbidity the first place is occupied by lung cancer /17.3 per cent/, skin cancer /9.3 per cent/ and breast cancer /7.5 per cent/. There are tendencies of increase in the indices of cancer morbidity of these three localizations. At present, in the frame of the National Cancer Register the study of the epidemiology of lung and breast cancers was started. Preliminary studies have shown that the industrial production hardly pollutes environment, in particular the air in Cuba.

Random-sample studies of lung cancer morbidity have allowed to establish that 95-98 per cent of patients with lung cancer have been smokers; smoking of cigars, cigarettes is widely spread, therefore epidemiological studies will be connected with the studies of the influence of smoking on the occurrence of lung cancer. Preliminary results of the investigation of epidemiological factors influencing breast cancer morbidity have shown that race as well as frequency or duration of lactation have not affected breast cancer morbidity. During the recent years epidemiological studies of Hodgkin's disease have been carried out and attempts have been made to determine the criteria of groups mostly threatened by lung and breast - cancer.

The history of cancer control in Cuba

Before the Revolution cancer control in Cuba was carried out by the Anticancer League which collected donations for the purchases of equipment and facilities, building of medical establishments, conducting of education campaign on cancer among the population.

It is quite obvious that the scope of activities of the Anticancer League was not sufficient for the organization of cancer control on a nation-wide basis.

Since 1923 the Cancer Institute /Curie Hospital/ and the Radium Institute in Habana were those two centres of cancer control which were relatively well equipped. However, the number of their beds and specialists could not fully satisfy the requirements in oncological aid. Personal donations were used for the treatment of malignant tumours and three oncological establishments were built outside Habana. Due to the absence of a uniform program of cancer control each above-mentioned oncological establishment functioned independently which decreased the possibility of conducting oncological aid to the population.

After the Revolution the revolutionary Government took charges of rendering support in conducting cancer control measures. In 1962, instead of the Anticancer Leagues, a national section of oncology affiliated to the Ministry of Health was set up with the responsibilities to provide oncological aid to the population and work out the prospective plans for cancer control.

The main tasks undertaken were as follows:
1. The decrease of the indices of morbidity and mortality from malignant tumours based on the improvement of methods of prophylaxis, diagnosis, and treatment of cancer.
2. Training of clinicians and research workers in the field of oncology.
3. To extend the education campaign on cancer.

In 1963, according to the decision of the Ministry of Health, oncology became a separate branch of medicine. At present, oncological aid to the population is provided by a network of specialized oncological establishments. The leading position in this field belongs to the National Institute of Oncology and Radiobiology. The specalized oncological establishments include oncological hospitals, provided with the necessary facilities and equipment for the treatment of cancer patients as well as "oncological units" /departments/ incorporated into general hospitals. At present a total number of 790 specialized oncological beds are available in the country. Moreover, some part of cancer patients are treated in general hospitals. The oncological hospitals are charged with consultative and organizational responsibilities.

In addition to therapeutic tasks oncological hospitals are entrusted with responsibilities to supervise for the organization of cancer control at the territory where the hospital is situated. The main structural departments of an oncological hospital or "oncological unit" are a radiotherapy department and a chemotherapy centre. In oncological hospitals surgery is done under special conditions, while in general hospitals which include "oncological units" surgery is carried out in the general surgical departments. Usually hospitals have small out-patient departments where specialists in oncology conduct their consultations. Moreover, oncologists consult patients in other medical establishments, carry out follow-up observation for patients treated for cancer, participate in the programs on cancer morbidity and mortality studies as well as in the studies on cancer epidemiology.

The National Institute of Oncology and Radiobiology founded in 1966 is the leading medical establishment in the field of oncology. In the organization of the National Institute three medical establishments including the Radium Institute, Curie Hospital and a hospital for the treatment of advanced cancer patients had been merged. The National Institute has 405 beds, 10 clinical departments, 37 laboratories and general service units. The National Cancer Register functions at the base of the Institute. In accordance with the program of its activities only patients with malignant tumours are treated at the Institute. The selection of patients for treatment is provided by a special service of "preliminary consultation" organized at the Institute.

During the recent years the possibilities of the Institute in the diagnosis of malignant tumours have been expanded, in particular radioisotopic diagnosis has developed. It is planned to expand and re-equip X-ray services.

Annually 2,000 major operations are performed for tumours of the breast, alimentary tract, respiratory tract, soft tissus. The same number of patients receive radiotherapy as well as chemotherapy.

At present, apart from the clinical department, 20 experimental and theoretical laboratories are engaged in the elaboration of mostly theoretical aspects of the problem of malignant tumours.

The National Institute is the main centre for the training of physicians and nurses in the field of oncology and radiotherapy.

In 1965 the National Society of Oncologists was organized. The scope of its activities is very extensive. The Society keeps close contacts with oncologists from remote areas, organizes the branches of the Society, publishes the journal of the Society "Cuban Archive of Oncology and Radiology". The monthly scientific meetings of the Society are devoted to actual problems of diagnosis and treatment of malignant tumours as well as to theoretical aspects of oncology and radiology. Joint meetings with of the societies of surgeons, gastroenterologists, urologists, etc. frequently take place. The Society actively participates in the organization of congresses. Thus, in 1978 the Congress of Cuban oncologists and the 1st Congress of oncologists from the countries of the Caribbean Coast were held. Oncologists of 9 countries took part in the Congress. The /Cuban/ National Society of Oncologists makes great efforts for the education of the population on cancer.

THE SYSTEM OF REGISTRATION OF PATIENTS WITH NEWLY DIAGNOSED MALIGNANT TUMOURS

In Cuba the registration of patients with newly-diagnosed cases of malignant tumours is compulsory. All medical institutions irrespective of their departmental subordination, as well as physicians who have diagnosed malignant tumour, must fill in a special document, the "Report on a Cancer Case".

The "Report on a Cancer Case" includes demographic information about the patient, his/her occupation, information about the medical institution where the diagnoses of cancer was established or confirmed, the localization of the tumour, its histology methods of confirmation of the diagnosis, stage of the process, treatment performed, No. of case history of the medical institution where the tumour was detected and the name of the physician /if the report is submitted directly by a physician/.

Before sending the "Report on a Cancer Case" to the regional statistical department, it is registered in a special register-book or card file of the medical establishment, this makes possible to specify and check /if necessary/ the information about a cancer patient detected in a given medical institution later. After appropriate registration and processing, the "Report on a Cancer Case" is submitted from the regional statistical departments to the department of oncological statistics of the Ministry of Health of Cuba, where it is coded and transferred to a punch card.

The department of oncological statistics sends the punch cards to the National Cancer Register, established in 1964.

In the National Cancer Register every information is transferred from the punch cards to punch tapes and is stored in a computer. In addition, the National Cancer Register has developed and completed an alphabetic card index, the ICD-code index /8th revision/ as well as archives of the Register and the archives of the "Report on a Cancer Case". The register separately stores the duplicates of the "Report on a Cancer Case".

Thus, the Register accumulates the materials about the annual number of patients with newly diagnosed malignant tumours and their distribution by localization. Apart from materials on cancer morbidity the department of statistics of the Ministry of Health sends the death certificates from malignant tumours, to the Register where they are properly processed.

The activities of the Register are mostly directed to the organization of the complete collection of the data on morbidity and mortality from malignant tumours, their statistical processing and of the study of epidemiological peculiarities of cancer distribution in Cuba.

The Register periodically publishes the materials on cancer morbidity and mortality by age, sex and standardized indices.

The National Cancer Register is closely connected with the department of national statistics, department of oncological statistics and the National Council on Oncology which are affiliated to the Ministry of Health of Cuba.

At present, the National Cancer Register obtains vast material on the statistics of malignant tumours. In accordance with the prospective plans the program of the activities of the National Cancer Register will be expanded, in particular it is planned to study the results of the follow-up of cancer patients and the efficiency of their treatment.

Some data on cancer morbidity and mortality in Cuba

The analysis of the averaged indices of cancer morbidity for 1970-1972 have shown a number of peculiarities concerning the different localizations and their structure. The comparison of the above indices with those for 1968-1972 has revealed the tendency for the decrease both in the total rates of morbidity and by the primary localizations: cancer of the stomach, skin, breast and cervix uteri. There was a slight rise in morbidity from lung cancer in both sexes. The total rate of cancer morbidity for the population in Cuba is relatively not high - 142.7 to 100,000 inhabitants /for 1970-1972/ as compared with the morbidity data in the European socialist countries. However, the calculation of standardized indices according to the European standards showed the increase of the rates by 15.4 % for males and 21.2 % for females. This is connected with the peculiarities of the structure of population in Cuba, where young persons form a large part of the population.

One of the peculiarities of the structure of cancer morbidity in Cuba is the high incidence of lung cancer /18 %/, the second place is occupied by skin cancer /9.8 %/, the third place by cancer of the breast /7.5 %/ while the cancer of the stomach occupies the fifth place only /4.7 %/ yielding the fourth place to tumours of lymphatic and haemopoietic tissues /6.5 %/.

107

There are also sex peculiarities in the structure of cancer morbidity in Cuba. The first place in cancer morbidity of males is occupied by lung cancer, 37.7 to 100,000 inhabitants; three times higher than the incidence of stomach cancer - 11.7 to 100,000 inhabitants.

In case of females the first place in the structure of cancer morbidity is occupied by the cancer of the breast, 21.7 to 100,000 inhabitants, which is characteristic now for many countries. The next places are occupied by the cancer of cervix uteri, 14.2 to 100,000 inhabitants and lung cancer, 13.2 to 100,000 inhabitants.

Of interest are the data characterizing cancer morbidity by main localizations according to counties. The comparison of these data with the total data for the whole country has revealed the counties with lower indices /Oriente, for example/, while for the counties of Habana and Maganzas the indices for all tumour localizations were found to the higher than those for the country as a whole. These results are connected not only with urbanization but also with the difficulties of registration of patients with malignant tumours in the remote and mountain districts of Cuba /e.g. Oriente/: this assumption is confirmed by the comparison of morbidity and mortality rates. In particular, there is no difference in these rates or they are almost similar for cancers the lung, stomach and oesophagus in the Oriente district.

The mortality rate of the population from malignant tumours is relatively low /99.2 for 1975/ and practically it did not changed during 5 years from 1970 to 1975. The analysis of mortality rates for 1972-1975 has revealed the main causes of mortality in the structure of malignant tumours - cancer of the respiratory tract, 26.3 % /88 % of them is lung cancer/ and malignant tumours of the gastrointestinal system, 25.7 % where the first place is occupied by stomach cancer /28.4 %/.

It should be emphasized that the main cause of death from malignant tumours in women is lung cancer /11.9 %/ followed by cancer of the breast /11.5 %/ and cancer of the stomach /4.8%/.

The evidence of the high level of registration of patients with malignant tumours is that morbidity rates taken as a whole exceed this respective coefficients of mortality. Only in some cases of certain age groups a slight predominance of the death rate is noted which speaks for the necessity to improve the organizational measures in cancer control in Cuba.

THE ORGANIZATION OF DETECTION AND EXAMINATION OF CANCER PATIENTS

The system of detection and examination of cancer patients involves the following steps:
1. First as a rule, the patient consults his local panel doctor at an out-patient department of the Health Service. In cases suspicious for cancer the local panel physician sends the patient for consultation to a surgeon and then he performs special examination using the diagnostic facilities available at the given out-patient department /laboratory tests, X-ray, endoscopic, cytological and other methods/.

If the diagnosis of a malignant tumour is confirmed, the patient is sent for treatment in a corresponding hospital. If the diagnostic facilities available at the out-patient department do not allow to make definite diagnosis, the patient is hospitalized and the examinations are carried out in a hospital. Then the patient may be moved to an oncological hospital or oncological unit of a general hospital or he may be treated at a hospital where he was examined.
2. In accordance to the adopted legislation a patient may take medical advice at any hospital where he will be examined and in case of indications he may be hospitalized for detailed examination and treatment.
3. For a number of years, mass prophylactic examinations of the population have been regularly conducted aiming at detecting tumours and precancerous lesions of the lung, buccal cavity and cervix uteri.

At present, the preparatory work for the implementation of the program for the early detection of breast cancer with the aid of mammography is under completion.

The system of mass prophylactic screenings for the early detection of malignant tumours may be presented in the following form: at present, mass prophylactic screenings cover all the working population of the country. It is planned to include pensioners and house-wives in the program of mass prophylactic screenings.

The organization of mass prophylactic screenings is provided by the committees of the Defence of Revolution. The aims of the committee is to provide maximal coverage of the population by prophylactic screenings. Each worker must obtain a "health certificate" which he receives after his fluorographic examination is done. In cases suspicious for cancer the worker is immediately sent to an oncological hospital, department of oncology in a general hospital or to a general hospital where he is subjected to detailed examination and if necessary to treatment.

Thus, fluorography of the chest is used as a method of mass prophylactic screening; persons selected for further examination are sent to a hospital without visiting an out-patient department.

In 1967 in Habana the program of preclinical detection of cancer of cervix uteri was started. Now this program covers the whole country.

Initially "the units of preclinical diagnosis" were set up where the members of the committee of the Defence of the Revolution sent all women older than 30 years for gynecological examination and for obtain Papanicolaou cytological smear. The success of the program allowed to extend it and entrust organizational functions to obstetric and gynecological consultation units, out-patient departments and hospitals.

In case of a negative Papanicolaou cytological smear, the next cytological smear is done 2 years later. In suspicious cases the cytological examination is repeated not later than 2 weeks and in an uncertain case the woman is sent to a gynecologist for consultation. The diagnosis should be confirmed within 3 months. In the presence of carcinoma in situ or invasive carcinoma the treatment should be started within a month.

Generally 500,000 women are examined annually. In the period of 1967-1973 1,686,930 cytological examinations had been performed. The results were as follows: 0.92 per cent with the suspicion for malignant tumour and 0.13 per cent with cancer of cervix uteri.

The program of early detection of breast cancer with mammography is on experimental trial. For 1976, 900 selected women were examined; in 100 of them breast cancer was revealed and in a number of cases the diagnosis of benign lesion was confirmed. Taking into consideration the high effectivity of the method it was decided to use it widely for the detection of breast cancer.

Among the programs of early detection of tumours it should be mentioned that the National Stomatological Service of Cuba takes an active part in the detection of buccal cancer.

THE ORGANIZATION OF HOSPITALIZATION AND TREATMENT OF PATIENTS WITH MALIGNANT TUMOURS

The system of planned hospitalization of cancer patients envisages that the patient consults first a local panel doctor who sends him to a general hospital, to a hospital with oncological unit or to an oncological hospital.

The sending of the patient to any medical establishment is to some extent determined by the site of tumour, the type of previous   treatment as well as local conditions and the presence of oncological establishments in the district.

A definite number of patients with malignant tumours are admitted to oncological hospitals from general hospitals where they have undergone examinations. The planned hospitalization covers about 60 per cent of the cancer patients subjected to hospital treatment.

A large group of patients /about 40 per cent/ appeal for medical aid directly to the hospital. Practically each inhabitant of the country may report to any medical establishment at the area of his residence and if necessary he will be hospitalized.

This tendency of direct application of patients to the

hospital for hospitalization is widely supported by the cancer education work among the population. The medical establishment which the patient visits is responsible for the selection of persons subjected to hospitalization. As a rule each hospital has an out-patient department. On the day of application to the hospital the patient is examined first by the "classifying physician" who decides about further examinations and laboratory tests required. In cases suspicious for tumour the patient is examined by an oncologist who fills in the case history and sends the patient for a detailed diagnostic examination which includes laboratory, X-ray, biopsy and other methods. After the completion of the diagnostic examination the patient is examined by the specialist who makes the final decision about the necessary hospitalization and determines the type of forthcoming treatment. If the question about hospitalization is decided positively, the patient should be admitted to the hospital within 12 days. This period is used for completion of the examination and preparation of the patient for surgery or radiotherapy. On admission of the patient to the hospital the plan of his treatment is worked out by the team of specialists.

If the patient is hospitalized in a general hospital and is subjected to radiotherapy, he is moved for the period of radiotherapy either to an oncological hospital or to a hospital with oncological unit. After radiotherapy the patient is moved back to the general hospital where his treatment is completed. Oncologists consult patients hospitalized in general hospitals, however the main elements of cancer treatment, surgery, chemotherapy and others are performed by the physicians of general hospitals.

The control for the treatment performed is provided by special commissions which analyse the causes of lethality, assess the surgical, radiologic, chemotherapeutic treatment modalities and scrutinize clinical documentation. These special control commissions are headed by the leading clinician or chief physician of the medical establishment.

Patients with advanced cancer are subjected to hospitalization; symptomatic treatment and care are provided in a hospital according to the adopted legislation.

FOLLOW-UP OBSERVATION OF CANCER PATIENTS

After the treatment performed for the malignant tumour the patient is subjected to periodic follow-up examinations which are most frequently carried out at the same medical institution where the patient was originally treated.

The follow-up observation is differentiated and it highly depends on the character of the tumourous process and the condition of the patient.

For most malignant tumours the follow-up observation is carried out for the whole life, however, for several localizations /skin tumours/ the checkups are conducted for 5 years, then the patient is excluded from the register.

During the first year after treatment the patients are examined every three months, then every six months for the period of 5 years; after the 5-year period the follow-up examinations are performed once a year.

A follow-up examination includes laboratory, radioisotopic, endoscopic and X-ray examinations and in some cases also immunological tests. The follow-up has all active character and contains the elements of prophylactic and therapeutic aid including radio-, chemo- and hormone-therapy, as well as surgery.

So far the recording of the results of follow-up observations has not been done at a national level. Nevertheless, it is planned to develop special registration forms and to concentrate the results of follow-up observations at the National Cancer Register. As the first step in this field the National Institute of Oncology and Radiobiology has developed the system of registration of the results of follow-up observation in the form of a registration card which includes information on the state of the patient, the assessment of the results of treatment, survival status and the methods of treatment applied for the period of the follow-up. All data are processed by a computer.

STUDIES ON THE EFFECTIVITY OF TREATMENT OF CANCER PATIENTS

The elaboration of the methods of measuring the effectivity of treatment of cancer patients is concentrated now at the National Institute of Oncology and Radiobiology.

The conventional method is the preparation of tables of survival according to tumour localizations /cancer of cervix uteri, endometrial cancer, breast cancer/. At present, several programs for an Olivetti P-101 computer and a CID-20IB mini-computer have been elaborated. These programs allow to evaluate the connection between two variables with the help of the χ^2_n- -test and determine the difference between the results of treatment in two groups of patients with Student's test. It is planned to use parametric for this purpose and non-parametric methods on the basis of multi-factor analysis.

Parallel with the theoretical studies devoted to the measurement of the effectivity of treatment of cancer patients, residents collect and evaluate the survival rates of patients treated at the National Institute of Oncology and Radiobiology.

Thus, 5-year survival rates for cancer of the cervix uteri according to stages are as follows:

$$\text{stage} \quad i - 80 \%$$
$$\text{stage} \quad ii - 57 \%$$
$$\text{stage} \quad iii - 40 \%$$
$$\text{stage} \quad iv - 17.4 \%$$

Cancer of the corpus uteri:

$$\text{stage} \quad i - 70 \%$$
$$\text{stage} \quad ii - 64 \%$$
$$\text{stage} \quad iii - 30 \%$$
$$\text{stage} \quad iv - 5 \%$$

Breast cancer:

stage   i - 5-year survival 72 %
            10-year survival 63 %
stage   ii - 5-year survival 53 %
            10-year survival 39 %
stage iii - 5-year survival 36 %
            10 year survival 21 %.

The results obtained correspond to international standards and this is an evidence of the high effectivity of treatment of cancer patients.

THE ORGANIZATION OF MEDICAL EXPERT COMMISSIONS FOR THE DECISION OF WORKING ABILITY AND FOR THE REHABILITATION OF CANCER PATIENTS

In accordance with the legislation each cancer patient receives a subsidy from the state during the whole period of his treatment; if the treatment is performed at an out-patient department, the patient receives 50 % of his salary; if the patient is treated at the hospital he receives 40 %. The length of the period while a patient is treated at an out-patient department - and, consequently, unable to work - cannot be more than 52 weeks.

On completion of the treatment according to the radical program, the patient can start his professional activities if his condition is satisfactory and he has no anatomical-functional defects. If, on completion of the radical therapy, the patient is unable to work and has some degree of disability, he is sent for an examination performed by a special medical commission which includes different specialists. This expert commission determines the degree of the patient's disability to work and gives recommendations for re-qualification, retiring on pension, etc.

If the patient is not completely cured despite the treatment performed or he stays in the hospital, he receives 40 % of his salary during the whole stay in the hospital.

If the commission recommends to retire on pension, the patient receives 50 % of his salary during his whole life.

There is a definite guaranteed minimum pension; if the salary of the patient does not reach this sum, the state pays additional allowance to reach the guaranteed disability pension.

Thus, the social help of the state for cancer patients is accomplished by the system of measures providing long state--paid treatment /52 weeks/ and disability pension for certain types of the disease and treatment performed.

In addition, there is a system of rehabilitation centres in Cuba where the patients are sent after special treatment. For cancer patients rehabilitation centres provide a complex of special physical exercises and, if necessary, prosthetic appliance.

TEACHING OF ONCOLOGY; TRAINING OF ONCOLOGISTS AND ALLIED MEDICAL PERSONNEL FOR ONCOLOGICAL INSTITUTIONS

The teaching of medical students is carried out at the medical universities at Habana, Santa Clara and Santiago de Cuba according to teaching programs worked out and approved by the department of Higher Education of the Ministry of Health and the Ministry of Higher Education.

Medical students are taught at the university for 6 years.

Teaching of oncology is included in the programs of clinical chairs. Special aspects of clinical oncology including diagnosis and treatment of malignant tumours are dealt with at lectures and practical sessions on surgery, medicine, obstetrics and gynecology, urology, etc. In the system of higher education in Cuba no provision is made for teaching oncology as a separate discipline and the chairs of oncology have not yet been established at the medical universities.

After 5 years of training medical students work for 1 year as interns at clinic at departments under the supervision of experienced specialists who are responsible for their practical training. There are two types of internship. The first one involves the training in one speciality according to the wish of the intern /surgery, pediatry or urology/ while the second type which is more preferred includes work in several - usually 3 to 4 - branches of medicine /surgery, therapy, gynecology, etc/.

On completion of the internship and receiving the diploma of a general practitioner a young doctor is usually sent for work to remote general hospitals.

Special training in oncology is given by a 3-year resident course. The training of residents in oncology is organized according to the decision of the Ministry of Health at the National Institute of Oncology and Radiobiology in Habana and in

116

oncological departments in Santiago de Cuba, Oriente and Camaguey.

The Ministry of Health has approved a uniform program for the training of residents in oncology. Each residents has a detailed individual program of training activities which includes lectures, practical work in an out-patient department, in different clinical wards in the department of statistics and epidemiology, in the laboratories of cytology and pathology, in the department of X-ray diagnosis and radiology, etc.

In the first days of training each resident gets a theme for his thesis, which he will elaborate during the 3 years of his training. On completion of the course of training the resident must submit his work to a special commission for evaluation. The thesis should include at least 100 type-written pages and should consist of an introduction, a review of literature, several chapters on the subject studied, conclusions and references.

At the National Institute of Oncology and Radiobiology the teaching department headed by the deputy director for training is responsible for the guidance and control of the training of residents.

One of the leading specialists of the Institute is appointed to supervise, consult and control a resident in his work on the thesis. The work of the resident is evaluated every month. According to the program on completion of the training period at the department the resident passes a test before a special commission approved by the director. The implementation of the respective parts of the training program and the thesis, the attendance at lectures, practical lessons, meetings of the Society of Oncologists and Radiologists, conferences, symposia, the participation in the work of social organizations are also assessed.

After the completion of the whole program of training the resident should pass an examination before a special commission approved by the Ministry of Health which consists of leading oncologists and other specialists.

For 15 days before the examination the resident works in

the department headed by the chairman of the special examination commission; who assesses his practical activity.

The marks received for the practical work, theoretical examination and the defence of the thesis are summarized according to a 100-point system. If the marks of a resident make up 100 points it is considered that he has successfully accomplished his training and he receives a diploma of a specialist in oncology; by the order of the Ministry of Health such a resident is given the rank of a 1st category physician and he has the right for an increase in his salary.

If the resident receives less than 70 points his specialization is considered as incomplete and he has the right to work as an assistant. A special examination commission decides whether such a resident can stand the examination again within a year. Nevertheless, such cases are very rare.

Highly-qualified specialists in oncology engaged in research or teaching activities with at least 5 years of practical work may be qualified by the National commission of the Ministry of Health, headed by the Minister. After a successful testimonial they receive the highest qualification rank, the second category specialist.

All residents who are trained in other towns of the Republic should undergo a special training at the National Institute of Oncology and Radiobiology for 6 months. It is planned to prolong this training period up to 1 year.

There are several programs for in-service training and out-service courses for improving the knowledge of oncologists and radiologists.

The large general hospitals, the regional oncological hospitals and the National Institute of Oncology and Radiobiology have medical schools where nurses are trained according to the programs worked out and approved by the Ministry of Health. On completion of the medical school nurses usually are assigned to work at the medical establishment where they were trained.

The secondary medical training is provided by a three--level system. There are medical schools with one-year courses which educate nurse-assistants. Such a school functioned before 1975 at the National Institute of Oncology and Radiobiology. Nurse-assistants work under the supervision of the nurses and attend 4-8 patients at the oncological clinics.

Medical schools with 2-year courses train qualified nurses. Qualified nurses attend 8-20 patients at the oncological clinics. In the medical universities there are 4-year medical schools training highly qualified nurses.

The National Institute of Oncology and Radiobiology has organized 2-year courses for training technicians in radio-physics. The students are taught many special subjects including electronics, radiation physics, statistics, histology, biochemistry, nuclear medicine, radiation protection, dosimetry, radiotherapy, etc.

The National Institute of Oncology and Radiobiology has introduced the service to students graduating from the University. At present 29 young graduates of the University work in the laboratories of the Institute.

During the last decade, 12 specialization courses have been arranged for the further training in oncology. On completion of these courses 305 graduates of the University, technicians and nurses have received diplomas of different specialities from biology of tumour cells and nuclear medicine to electrocardiology and care of oncological patients. The activities in this field promote the improvement of qualification of the staff of the Institute and the organization of a medical training centre in the country.

PUBLIC EDUCATION IN THE FIELD OF CANCER

It is well known that one of the most important factors influencing the efficacy of treatment of cancer patients is the detection of tumour at its early stages. This is connected to some extent with the sufficient information of the public on the first signs of this dangerous disease. Just for this reason public education in the field of cancer is of great importance. This work is done under the guidance of the Ministry of Health in Cuba which has a special department of public education, closely connected with the National Group of Oncology.

This group and the National Institute of Oncology and Radiobiology have information on cancer morbidity and mortality from different primary localizations of tumours which enable them to propose tendentions programs for the public education in the field of cancer.

The National Group of Oncology and the National Institute of Oncology and Radiobiology have analysed ten localizations of tumours leading to highest mortality, and worked out a national program on the early detection of tumours of the cervix uteri, buccal cavity, respiratory tract and breast. It was established that tumours at these localizations were detected in rather advanced stages. Therefore, there is a necessity to make the public realize the early signs of the disease.

First of all the groups of persons have been revealed among which education in the field of cancer should be conducted /groups mostly threatened by cancer/. These materials have been submitted to the department of public education of the Ministry of Health, where relevant instructions are worked out. These instructions are distributed among the medical institutions of the general health service. According to the instructions the leading authorities of the medical establishments should daily remind medical students, physicians and nurses to "medical alertness" to cancer detection. Stomatologists should examine the buccal cavity in the course of dental care, obstetricians and gynecologists prophylactically examine not only the cervix uteri but also the breast. In all patients visiting an out-patient department manual examination of the rectum and chest fluorography are performed. Physicians deliver lectures and speeches on the education of the public on cancer.

Social organizations such as Committee on the Defence of the Revolution, Federation of the Cuban women, trade unions of industrial and agricultural enterprises, the Society of the Red Cross, the National Society of Oncologists and Radiologists take an active part in this field.

An active role in public education in the field of cancer

120

and popularization of oncological knowledge is played by the means of mass media.

For several years a radioprogram "Health to the Cuban lands" have been broadcasted which is very popular. A large part of this program is devoted to the popularization of medical knowledge, in particular that of oncology.

The Central TV studio transmits a TV programme "Round table talks of scientists" for one hour daily in which problems of the health service are discussed. Oncologists take an active part in this programme which is thus used for public education in the field of cancer.

Great attention is paid to the problems of popularization of medical knowledge and cancer education of the public in the press.

The daily journal "Bohemia" is read the most and has a very wide circulation. It has a special health column in which various information is published, in particular on oncology.

The journal "Economic Views on Latin America" also opens its pages for the education of the public on cancer.

Lectures of leading oncologists are very popular and have high public attendance.

Special posters on oncological subjects and sheets of sanitary information have a wide circulation; since 1976 book series have been published entitled "Topics of Public Health". One of the editions of this series, "Woman and breast cancer" is very popular.

According to the decision of the Government on the labels of cigarette packs there is a warning that smoking is dangerous for health and leads to the development of lung cancer.

Popularization of this knowledge, the development of self--control habits lead to the fact that large number of practically healthy persons visit medical establishments for consultations and in some of them early stages of cancer are detected.

As an example of cancer education activities among the public the following publications should be mentioned.

THE METHOD OF SELF-EXAMINATION OF THE BREAST. Each year 400 women die from breast cancer in Cuba. In most cases these deaths are not inevitable, because the patients could be saved if they found the tumour and consult a physician at the beginning of its growth. It is a well-known fact that 95 % of breast cancer is detected by women themselves during the process of dressing, bathing, etc. Please help the physicians for your own sake. Learn to protect yourself. Perform self-examination of the breast.

Breast cancer can be cured in case of its early detection and timely treatment. One of the most effective methods of timely detection of breast cancer is self-examination of the breasts conducted by the woman herself. Therefore, each woman should learn to examine the breasts and should regularly perform self-examination for the whole life.

Self-examination is necessary to be carried out each month, the best time is the end of the periods; self-examination should be carried out in accordance to the instructions listed below:

During self-examination of the breasts the woman should look for definite abnormal signs. Having found one or several of these signs the woman should consult a physician. These signs are not always the evidence of cancer, they may reveal other benign lesions.

An adequate self-examination should be performed in 4 positions subsequently, keeping in mind the signs that may be revealed:
1. In front of the mirror in sitting or standing posture with arms lying along the trunk.
2. In front of the mirror with hands raised up.
3. In recumbent position with a pillow under the right shoulder raising the right hand behind the head, examine carefully the inner half of the breast near the nipple area with the left-hand figners.

Place the right hand along the trunk and examine the outer half of the breast and the axillary pit with the left-hand fingers.
In the same manner, examine the left breast.

Local changes that should be noted:
1. A nodule, a tumour or enduration in the breast.
2. Any deformation or change in the usual shape of the breast.
3. Asymmetric position of the breast or the nipples.
4. Retraction of the nipples.
5. Corrugation of the skin around the nipples.
6. Any discharge and bleeding from the nipples.
7. Any rash on the skin around the nipples.
8. Enlargement of the axillary nodes.
9. Any ulceration on the skin of the breast.

Certainly, these symptoms are not always the signs of cancer, however, you need consult a physician without delay and do not follow any other advice.

Visit the out-patient department of your district and the physician will decide what should be done.

WOMAN AND CANCER Your fate is in your hands.

In all likelyhood, you will not die from cancer as the majority of women will not either, nevertheless, some precautions should be taken and you may extend your chances for a long and stable cure from a malignant tumour.

Early diagnosis and timely treatment provide long and stable health. However, after the age of 35 the danger to develop cancer is increasing.

Cancer threatens most frequently the female genital organs, the breast and the gastro-intentinal tract.

<u>What should be done?</u> It is quite natural that sometimes you feel uneasy thinking about the possibility of having cancer. Each conscious woman should follow some pieces of advice:
1. Once a year visit your local out-patient department for prophylactic medical examination.
2. Visit the unit of preclinical detection of uterine cancer if you receive a summons from it.
3. Learn 7 signals of danger that may indicate cancer /any non-healing wound or ulceration, enduration in the breasts or in any other organ, nexplainable bleeding or suppuration, changes in a wart or mole, persistent cough or hoarseness, difficulties in swallowing, persistent "indigestion"/.

None of these signs are a definite symptom of cancer, but each sign, particularly postmenopausal bleeding, may point to cancer.

If one of the above-mentioned signs persists for more than 2 weeks, immediately visit your physician, do not wait for the appearance of pain. Persistent pain indicates a far advanced process. Learn to examine the breasts yourself. A doctor or a nurse will show you how to do it.

Self-examination of the breast takes only several minutes, it should be done once in a month.

Follow the advices of a doctor during pregnancy and after birth.

Do not take "home-made" drugs and do not perform "secret" treatment. You will waste your time and it will be late for you to visit the physician.

<u>Do not waste your time!</u> Cancer frequently develops without alarming symptoms and may rapidly spread in the organism. The hopes of recovery are greater, if the treatment is started earlier.

Intensive research studies are conducted for the revealing of the causes of cancer development and search is made for new, more effective methods of cancer treatment.

Periodic medical examinations, although they are very simple, allow to detect a large part of oncological diseases at their initiation by a physician.

The doctor will help you if you yourself wish it and offer the doctor the possibility of periodic examinations.

<u>Remember!</u> In a suspicious case visit an out-patient department, a consultation unit at a hospital or an oncological hospital.

Cuban people are struggling against cancer!

THE COORDINATION OF RESEARCH ACTIVITIES ON THE PROBLEM
"SCIENTIFIC BASIS OF CANCER CONTROL"

Since the foundation of the National Institute of Oncology and Radiobiology in 1966 a great deal of work has been done for developing the main trends of cancer research. Since 1966 the activities of the Institute have been fully oriented to the solution of the problem of malignant tumours.

In the first years research in the Institute was of applied character, included many different projects and it was not provided by the necessary budget any means and technical equipment, however, at present, the situation has been changed.

In the Institute is well provided with material resources, modern equipment and facilities, its staff has been reinforced by young specialists with special medical training or graduating from the University.

These attempts have resulted in the systematization of research programs, the development of the main problems to be implemented within 5 years.

20 basic laboratories have been organized in the Institute and their research activities are oriented for the solving of the following problems:

1. Etiology of Hodgkin's disease
2. Studies of carcinogenesis
3. Studies on diagnosis and treatment of malignant tumours
4. Radiobiology and radophysics applied to biomedicine and oncology.

Progress in research has been achieved in the following fields:

1. Development of nuclear medicine service and a national program of radiation protection.
2. Development of the system of information service and computer techniques as a basis for clinical research.
3. Organization of a laboratory of bioorganic chemistry for conducting studies in the field of experimental chemotherapy.

124

The international contacts of the Institute have largely expanded due to both the participation in the agreement on scientific and technical cooperation with the states of the CMEA and the active participation in the activities of international and Latin-American medical organizations.

Cuba is involved in the implementation of the program of the CMEA member-states on the following projects:

I. Scientific basis of the organization of cancer control
II. Experimental and clinical cancer chemotherapy
III. Epidemiology of lung cancer and its early diagnosis
IV. Early diagnosis of malignant tumours
V. Application of nuclear equipment for the diagnosis and treatment of cancer.

The Institute plans further development of oncological service to the population, training of specialists in the field of oncology, development of adequate models for diagnosis and treatment of cancer on a national basis.

The perspective long-term cooperation on the cancer control program involves the following problems:

1. Development of studies in the field of radiotherapy, in particular, the diagnosis of malignant tumours, pathology of tumours, computer techniques in oncology.
2. Development of biological, biochemical studies and studies on carcinogenesis.
3. Development of studies on scientific-technical information in the field of oncology.

Being the leading medical establishment in the field of oncology the Institute supervises the oncological network from scientific and methodological points of view, participates in its perspective planning, employs oncologists for research on statistics and epidemiology of malignant tumours.

The Institute works out programs for the training of oncologists specialized in surgery, radiotherapy, chemotherapy

of malignant tumours which provides for a high level of oncological aid to the population in the districts of the country.

PERSPECTIVES IN THE IMPROVEMENT OF THE ORGANIZATION
OF ONCOLOGICAL AID TO THE POPULATION

It is evident that a definite progress has been achieved
in Cuba in the organization of cancer control and prophylaxis
of malignant tumours. The establishment of specialized oncological institutions with a comprehensive program of their activities, which provides diagnosis and treatment of cancer patients
on a modern basis, has been completely justified. The organization of the National Institute of Oncology and Radiobiology as
well as the National Cancer Register have served as basis for
the development of cancer research in the field of clinical and
experimental oncology. The 5-year perspective plan covering a
wide scope of problems, incorporates a vast program of the
development and improvement of oncological aid to population.

1. The establishment of further cancer hospitals and oncological
units in the districts of the country allows to raise the level
of oncological aid to the population. It is planned to organize
oncological units in each district /a total number of 14 units/.

2. Training of highly qualified specialists in oncology and
radiobiology.

3. The elaboration of the program of early detection of tumours
of primary localizations by conducting of mass prophylactic
screenings for large groups of the population /it is planned
to start the implementation of such programs for the breast,
buccal cavity, lungs, larynx, stomach, rectum and prostata/.

4. The improvement of qualification and "oncological alertness"
of general physicians allows to raise the quality of early
diagnosis of malignant tumours.

5. Training in oncology of resident physicians specializing
in other fields of medicine. A 3-month course in oncology will

be included in their training program. A two-week course in oncology is introduced in the 6th year program of medical training of the interns.

6. Popularization of scientific knowledge in the field of oncology by the active participation of public organizations and means of mass communication in the education of the population on cancer.

7. The development of improved methods of treatment of malignant tumours.
a/ to carry out the discussion of all cases of unadequate treatment of cancer patients caused by poor training of the physicians in the field of oncology.
b/ to introduce a system of follow-up of cancer patients for the evaluation of the effectivity of treatment and survival rates.
c/ to increase the number of physicians specializing in oncology and radiology.

8. The elaboration of a more extended program of the activities of the National Cancer Register in the investigation of morbidity, mortality and epidemiology of malignant tumours.

9. The development of the program of prophylaxis of malignant tumours is based on:
a, the decrease in the number of precancerous lesions;
b, the control over the carcinogenic agents and their entering into the environment.
The latter include:
 i/ campaign against smoking
ii/ prevention of contacts with highly carcinogenic agents in the industry /tars, oils, soot, aromatic compounds, uranium ore, arsenic agents, ionizing radiation and others/.

The main studies of cancer research will be concentrated at the National Institute of Oncology and Radiobiology.
Applied studies directed to the solution of the problems mentioned above will be included in the program.

At the same time, basic studies on the problems of etio-pathogenesis of malignant tumours will be developed. In this connection a special role is played by the integration of research studies in the CMEA member-states as well as the elaboration of the uniform approaches to the solution of a number of problems, training of specialists in oncology in the CMEA member-states according to the uniform program.

The main task of the countries of the socialist camp is the search for the common ways and means, the exchange of views, the elaboration of common programs of fundamental research and their common implementation oriented to the solution of the problem of etiopathogenesis of malignant growth in the 20th century.

Table 21

Structure of the Population in Cuba by Age and Sex for 1970 and 1974

Age	1970			1974		
	Both sexes	Males	Females	Both sexes	Males	Females
1 - 4	950.821	486.509	464.312	1.121.684	648.052	472.632
5 - 9	1.168.886	597.646	571.240	1.222.820	639.265	583.555
10 - 14	812.576	416.588	395.988	1.094.102	445.583	648.519
15 - 19	767.808	390.162	377.646	763.113	417.343	345.770
20 - 24	721.949	365.458	356.491	763.113	390.889	372.224
25 - 29	652.606	332.441	320.165	698.754	355.602	343.152
30 - 34	561.917	287.132	274.785	625.201	307.111	318.090
35 - 39	464.568	234.383	230.185	514.872	250.679	264.193
40 - 44	428.080	215.870	212.210	450.513	230.897	219.616
45 - 49	374.218	191.232	182.986	395.348	204.537	190.811
50 - 54	346.754	179.344	167.410	358.571	191.850	166.721
55 - 59	314.523	161.984	152.539	330.989	173.243	157.746
60 - 64	263.724	141.828	121.896	275.824	151.723	124.101
65 - 69	228.733	127.450	101.283	261.285	131.709	129.576
70 - 74	91.733	51.610	40.123	104.788	52.822	51.966
75 - 79	83.822	43.486	40.336	95.753	48.267	47.486
80 - 84	54.487	28.891	28.596	65.667	33.102	32.565
85 and older	45.288	21.575	23.713	51.737	26.080	25.567

Table 22

Distribution of the Population in Cuba According to the Administrative
Districts 1971 and 1974

Administrative districts	1971			1974		
	Total population	Males	Females	Total population	Males	Females
Cuba	8.691.660	4.455.779	4.235.881	9.194.134	4.698.754	4.495.380
Pinar del Rio	555.898	291.586	264.312	500.771	308.379	282.392
Habana	2.354.939	1.163.671	1.191.268	2.454.902	1.218.951	1.235.951
Matanzas	508.181	262.980	245.201	535.410	275.958	259.452
Las Villas	1.380.063	7.133.326	666.737	1.448.256	743.954	704.302
Camaguey	826.767	4.348.840	391.927	879.373	458.833	420.540
Oriente	3.065.812	1.589.376	1.476.422	3.285.422	1.692.679	1.592.743

Table 22

Absolute Number of New Cases and Incidence of Malignant
Neoplasms in Cuba for 1970-1972

	Absolute number	Incidence per 100.000 population	
All malignant tumours	37.277	142.7	100.0
Buccal cavity /141-149/	1.758	6.7	4.7
Esophagus /150/	884	3.4	2.4
Stomach /151/	2.277	8.7	6.1
Rectum /154/	897	3.4	2.4
Larynx /161/	1.006	3.9	2.7
Trachea, bronchi, lungs /162/	6.713	25.7	18.0
Skin /172, 173/	3.661	14.0	9.8
Breast /174/	2.800	10.7	7.5
Cervix uteri /180/	1.807	6.9	4.9
Other sites	12.988	49.8	34.9
Lymphatic and haemopoietic tissues /200-207/	2.436	9.3	6.5

Cancer Morbidity by Age and Sex in Cuba

Tumor localization and ICD Code	Males							
	Under 30	30-	40-	50-	60-	70 and over	Total	Standard rates *
All malignant tumours 140-209	11.2	31.7	105.4	306.5	622.3	2.245.6	158.6	182.9
All tumours except tumours of lymphatic and haemo-poietic tissues 140-199	5.0	24.0	93.3	284.7	604.5	2.164.5	147.1	170.7
Lymphatic and haemopoietic tissues 200-207	6.2	7.8	12.1	21.8	17.8	81.1	11.4	12.2
Lips 140	0.1	0.5	2.0	5.9	6.4	28.7	2.1	2.4
Esophagus 150	0.0	0.5	3.7	9.2	22.3	69.8	4.9	5.7
Stomach 151	0.2	2.1	7.2	18.1	54.2	177.2	11.7	13.6
Rectum 154	0.1	0.9	2.2	6.6	14.5	55.1	3.6	4.2
Trachea,bronchi lungs 162	0.2	2.4	20.0	75.8	163.2	578.4	37.7	44.2
Breast 174		0.1	0.2	0.9	0.2	5.0	0.3	0.3
Cervix uteri 180	-	-	-	-	-	-	-	-

* European standard rates

for 1970-1972 /Incidence per 100.000 Population/

Females

Under 30	30-	40-	50-	60-	70 and over	Total	Stand-ard rates[x]
10.9	36.5	171.0	335.0	372.4	1.545.0	126.2	153.0
6.9	56.3	163.2	322.2	361.3	1.486.3	119.0	144.9
4.0	2.7	7.7	12.7	11.0	58.7	7.2	8.1
-	0.1	0.1	0.9	2.2	4.2	0.4	0.4
0.0	0.1	1.2	3.6	7.5	32.7	1.9	2.2
0.1	0.7	3.3	9.6	24.6	93.6	5.6	6.7
0.1	0.6	2.5	7.9	13.0	47.5	3.3	4.4
0.1	0.8	9.2	29.5	56.1	212.9	13.2	16.4
0.7	9.2	53.3	75.4	42.3	193.6	21.7	26.9
0.6	8.9	32.2	47.5	22.1	126.5	14.2	17.4

Cancer Morbidity According to the Administrative

/Absolute Number of New Cases   and

Cuba and administrative Districts	Lips /140/		Esophagus /150/		Stomach /151/		Trachea, bronchi, lung /162/	
	A	B	A	B	A	B	A	B
Cuba	327	1.3	884	3.4	2.277	8.7	6,713	25,7
Including: Pinar del Rio	17	1.0	42	2.5	125	7.5	320	19.2
Havana	142	2.0	230	3.5	762	10.8	2.533	35.9
Matanzas	33	2.2	52	3.4	138	9.1	482	31.6
Las Villas	34	0.8	190	4.6	376	9.1	1.351	32.6
Camaguey	45	1.8	121	4.9	280	11.3	767	30.9
Oriente	54	0.6	221	2.4	578	6.3	1.211	13.2

A = Absolute number
B = Per 100.000

25

Districts of Cuba /by Selected Sites/
Incidence per lOO.OOO Population/

Skin /172, 173/		Breast /174/		Cervix uteri /180/		Lymphatic and hemopoietic tissues /200-207/	
A	B	A	B	A	B	A	B
3.661	14.O	2.800	10.7	1.807	6.9	2.436	9.3
112	6.7	115	6.9	102	6.1	119	7.1
1.367	19.4	1.293	18.3	668	9.5	816	11.6
404	26.5	198	13.O	91	6.O	134	8.8
363	8.8	479	11.6	258	6.2	475	11.5
608	24.5	170	6.9	137	5.5	250	10.1
761	8.3	522	5.7	542	5.9	635	6.9

Table 26

Number of Deaths and Mortality /per 100.000 population/ from
Malignant Neoplasms in Cuba for 1970-1975

	1970	1971	1972	1973	1974	1975
Number of deaths from malignant neoplasms	8.446	8.604	8.929	8.962	9.006	9.265
Mortality per 100.000 population	99.7	100.0	102.1	100.5	97.9	99.2

Table 27

Mortality /per 100.000 Population/ from Malignant Tumours by Selected Localizations Age and Sex in Cuba for 1973 - 1975

	ICD code /8th revision/	Absolute number	per 100.000 population
All sites	140-209	27.393	99.3
Buccal cavity and larynx	141-149	1.030	3.7
Gastro-intestinal organs	150-159	7.092	25.7
Esophagus	150	759	2.8
Stomach	151	2.015	7.3
Intestines	152-153	1.704	6.2
Rectum	154	674	2.4
Respiratory organs	160-163	7.253	26.3
Trachea, bronchi lungs	162	6.357	23.0
Connective tissue and bones	170-171	383	1.4
Skin	172-173	257	0.9
Breast	174	1.578	5.7
Female genital organs	180-184	2.112	7.7
Cervix uteri	180	557	2.0
Endometrium etc.	182	1.129	4.1
Tumours of lymphatic and haemopoietic tissues	200-207	2.401	8.7

Table 27 /cont'd/

	Males					
	Under 30 years	30-39	40-49	50-59	60 and over	Total
All sites	8.5	18.5	59.6	1.196.8	935.0	116.0
Buccal cavity and larynx						
Gastro-intestinal organs						
Esophagus		0.2	2.1	8.8	33.2	4.1
Stomach	0.1	1.1	3.9	15.0	85.0	9.8
Intestines						
Rectum						
Respiratory organs						
Trachea, bronchi lungs	0.1	2.4	16.2	60.6	287.1	33.7
Connective tissue and bones						
Skin						
Breast	-	0.1	0.2	0.4	1.3	0.2
Female genital organs						
Cervix uteri						
Endometrium etc.						
Tumours of lymphatic and haemopoietic tissues	5.3	60.0	9.6	19.5	46.9	10.8

Females					
Under 30 yrs	30-39	40-49	50-59	60 and over	Total
6.7	27.8	85.6	201.4	559.5	81.3
-	0.3	1.1	2.7	11.4	1.4
0.1	1.4	2.4	8.6	40.1	4.8
0.2	1.3	6.7	24.9	101.1	11.9
0.2	5.4	22.4	42.7	60.6	11.5
3.1	3.2	6.4	13.4	28.6	6.6

Number of Deaths and Mortality /per 100.000 Population/ from

Districts

Administrative Districts	Lips /140/		Buccal cavity and larynx /141/		Esophagus /150/		Stomach /151/		Rectum /154/	
	A	B	A	B	A	B	A	B	A	B
Cuba	27.935	99.3	1.030	3.7	759	2.8	2.015	7.3	674	2.4
Pinar del Rio	1.400	79.0	48	2.7	38	2.1	103	5.8	26	1.5
Havana	9.888	134.3	433	6.0	243	3.3	613	8.3	311	4.2
Matanzas	1.688	105.1	49	3.1	39	2.4	115	7.2	46	2.9
Las Villas	4.749	109.3	175	4.0	142	3.3	318	7.3	103	2.4
Oriente	6.694	67.9	220	2.2	202	2.1	619	6.3	118	1.2
Camagüey	2.838	107.6	92	3.5	93	3.5	245	9.3	68	2.6

Malignant Tumours in Cuba According to the Administrative for 1973-1975

Trachea, bronchi lungs /162/		Skin /172-173/		Breast /174/		Cervix uteri /180/		Tumour of lymphatic and hemopoietic tissues /200-207/	
A	B	A	B	A	B	A	B	A	B
6.357	23.0	257	0.9	1.978	5.7	557	3.0	2.401	8.7
325	18.3	15	0.9	67	3.8	19	1.1	132	7.5
2.278	30.9	37	1.2	706	9.6	230	3.1	769	10.4
436	27.1	17	1.1	98	6.1	24	1.5	132	8.2
1.281	29.5	40	0.9	258	5.9	54	1.2	384	8.8
1.290	13.1	72	0.7	323	3.3	173	1.8	731	7.4
732	27.8	23	0.9	84	3.2	55	2.1	246	9.3

141

Table 29

Highest Age-Incidence and Highest Age-Mortality
by Sex and Selected Tumour Localizations

Tumour localization and sex	ICD Code /8th revision/	Age of patients	Age of dead patients
<u>Males</u>			
Buccal cavity and larynx	140-149	66	67
Esophagus	150	73	69
Stomach	151	67	72
Rectum	154	66	72
Trachea, bronchi, lungs	162	67	69
Skin	172,173	67	82
Lymphatic and haemo-poietic tissues	200-209	66	71
<u>Females</u>			
Buccal cavity and larynx	140-149	67	69
Esophagus	150	60	70
Stomach	151	66	73
Rectum	154	62	69
Trachea, bronchi, lungs	162	66	67
Skin	172,173	57	87
Breast	174	52	
Cervix uteri	180	52	53
Lymphatic and haemo-poietic tissues	200-209	65	62

REFERENCES

1. Маринелло Видауретто. "Организация боръбы против рака в
   республике Куба". В кн.: Труды VIII Международного противо-
   ракового конгресса, Москва, 22-28 июля 1962 г., Гос.изд.
   мед.лит., М.-Л., 1963, стр. 94-97
   Marinello Vidauretto. "Cancer Control Organization in Cuba"
   In: The works of the VIIIth International Cancer Control
   Congress, Moscow 22-28 July, 1962. Meditsinskaya literatura,
   M.-L., 1963, pp. 94-97.

2. Registro Nacional del Cancer. Republica de Cuba, Ministerio
   de Salud Publica, grupo de estadistica del Instituto Nacional de Oncologia y Radiobiologia. La Habana, 1969.
   National Cancer Register. Cuba. Ministry of Health. Statistical Group of the National Institute of Oncology and Radiobiology. Havanna, 1969.

3. G. Halley. Cuba. In: Cancer Incidence in Five Continents.
   Editors: J. Waterhouse, C. Muir, P. Correa. IARC scientific
   publications No 15, Vol. III, Lyon, 1976, pp. 168-171.

4. Informe Anual. Republica de Cuba. Editado e impreso por el
   Centro Nacional de Information de Ciencias Medicas. Minis-
   terio de Salud Publica, La Habana, 1976.
   Annual Report. Cuba. Edited and published by the National
   Information Centre of Medical Sciences. Ministry of Health,
   Havanna, 1976.

5. Cuba: La Salud en la Revolucion. Editor: Olga R. Ruis,
   Editorial Orbe, Instituto Cubano del Libro, La Habana,
   1975, 178 p..
   Cuba: Public Health and Revolution. Editor: Olga R. Ruis,
   Editorial Office Orbe, Cuban Institute of Book, Havanna,
   1975, 178 pp..

6. Sistema de Informacion estadistica del Programa para el
   Diagnostico Preclinico del Cancer Uterino. Direccion National de Estadistica del Ministerio de Salud Publica.
   Revista Cubana Adm, Salud 2, 1, 1976, pp. 91-101.
   Statistical information system for the program of preclinical diagnosis of uterus cancer. National Statistics Department. Rev. Cub. Adm. Salud 2, 1 1976, pp. 91-101.

7. Alert Silva: Algunos aspectos de los tumores malignos de los ninos en Cuba. Revista Cubana Pediatrica, Vol. 45, Nos. 4,5,6, 1973, pp. 401-420.
Alert Silva: Some Aspects of Malignant Tumours in Cuban Children, <u>National Centre of Information of Medical Sciences,</u> Cuba, 1973, Vol. 45, Nos. 4,5,6, 1973, pp. 401-420.

CANCER CONTROL IN CZECHOSLOVAKIA

GEOGRAPHIC, ECONOMIC AND DEMOGRAPHIC ASPECTS AND THE DEVELOPMENT
OF CANCER CONTROL IN CZECHOSLOVAKIA
J.Durkovsky, V. Dvořak, V. Plesko and J. Stach

Czechoslovakia is a federal state which consists of two national republics - the Czech Socialist Republic /ČSR/ and the Slovak Socialist Republic /SSR/. Czechoslovakia covers the total area of 127,877 sq km /of which the ČSR is 78,863 sq km and the SSR 49,014 sq km/. On January 1, 1975 the total population of the Republic was 14,738,311 /of which 10,023,768 inhabitants live in the ČSR and 4,714,543 inhabitants in the SSR/. Density of the population is 115 persons per sq km. Administratively the Czech Socialist Republic is divided into 8 counties /regions/: Northern, Western, Southern, Middle and Eastern Bohemian County, Northern and Southern Moravian County and the City of Prague, the capital of Czechoslovakia and the ČSR. The Slovak Socialist Republic is divided into 4 counties: The Western, Middle and Eastern Slovak County and the City of Bratislava, the capital of SSR. Each county as well as the capitals are subdivided into 8-14 districts.

The following meteorological data for Prague and Bratislava for the 1954-1974 period give an idea of the country's climate conditions: the mean annual temperature varied in Prague from +7.8°C /1956/ to +10°C /1974/, in Bratislava from +9.3°C /1956/ to +11.4°C /1961/. The mean annual precipitation in Czechoslovakia was 826 mm in 1974 /778 mm in the ČSR and 906 mm in the SSR/.

The mineral wealth of the country is characterized by mining of brown coal, lignite, manganese, lead and copper ores, mercury, antimony, tin, wolfram, graphite, magnesite, kaolin, ceramic clay, pitchblende and also by thermal springs.

Industrial production in 1974 could be illustrated with cast iron - 8,905,000 tons, steel - 13,640,000 tons, rolled metal - 9,563,000 tons, products of heavy, medium and light machine industry, lorries, cars, tractors, locomotives, railway wagons, electric motors, oil engines and products of light industry /sewing-machines, vacuum cleaners, refrigerators, washing machines, photocameras, radio sets, television sets, bicycles, knitted goods, footwear, glass, etc./.

The characteristic data of transport for 1974 are: railways - 13,241 km, highways - 73,538 km, length of navigable rivers - 458 km, internal air routes - 5,706 km, external air routes - 103,917 km.

The main agricultural products are: wheat, barley, rye, oats, maize, potato, sugar beet, fodder, leguminous plants, vine, vegetable oil, flax, hemp, tobacco, hop, fruits, various vegetables and products of animal husbandry as meat, milk and eggs.

Demographic data

The age structure of the population in 1974 was the following:

Age groups	
0 - 14	23.2 per cent
15 - 39	37.1 per cent
40 - 59	22.2 per cent
60 and over	17.5 per cent

The median age /the age which divides the average age of all members of the population into two numerically equal groups/ was 31.5 years. The mean age was 35.1 years. The sex ratio was 1,053 women to 1,000 men. The main demographic parameters: the birth rate is 19.8 per 1,000; death rate 11.7 per 1,000; the natural increase of the population 8.1 per 1,000; marriage rate 9.6 per 1,000 population; divorce rate per 100 marriages 21.6; the infant mortality rate /the death of children under one/ 20.4; the new-born mortality /the number of death per 1,000 live-born children dying before reaching the age of 28 days/ was 15.4 in 1974.

The social structure of the population:

workers	60.4 per cent
employees	27.9 per cent
member of agricultural cooperations	8.5 per cent
small cooperating producers	1.7 per cent
small farmers	1.0 per cent
free professions	0.5 per cent

In the national economy 7,357,000 persons were employed /5,714,000 in the productive and 1,643,000 in the nonproductive section/, mainly in the industry - 2,828,000, then in the agriculture - 1,058,000, building industry - 875,000 persons, etc. There were 812,000 secondary and high school students and apprentices.

DEVELOPMENT OF CANCER CONTROL

It should be noted that cancer control in Czechoslovakia has a long tradition. As far back as 1905, a group of well-known physicians in Prague created a "Society for Establishment and Management of Sanatoria for Patients with Malignant Tumours, Especially Cancer". The main task of the society was to organize treatment and charitable assistance for cancer patients and only to a smaller extent to elaborate large-scale cancer control measures.

A rise in the incidence of cancer and mortality from malignant neoplasms in the 20s and 40s forced the organizers and leaders of the society to introduce changes and to pay attention also on the study of the etiopathogenesis of tumours and development of methods for better treatment. A well-known Czech pathologist, Professor Hlava and the pioneer of the modern radiology and roentgenology, Professor Jedlička elaborated new objectives for the Society which at that time was called "Czechoslovak Society for Research and Control of Malignant Neoplasms in Prague". The so-called "Bioptic Station" was organized under the guidance of the Society. For a long period the station became a wide base for the study of modern oncological histology and it still fulfils an important function as a consultative, research and arbitration centre.

An experimental department for tumour research was set up in the Ist Pathological-Anatomical Institute in Prague. And, finally, the Society organized the so-called cancer dispensary, which had been functioning successfully until the creation of the Institute of Oncology.

The Moravian physicians followed the Prague example and founded a similar society in Brno. Despite all the obstacles, the necessary financial resources were collected and used for the building of the Institute of Oncology in Brno 1935, with very modern equipment for that period of time. The Prague Society created also an institute of this kind, which was opened in 1936. A similar society, though not so active, was established in Bratislava. It was not until 1951 that the Ministry of Health in Bratislava created the Cancer Research Institute. For a long period this institute remained the leading research centre in oncology in the whole Czechoslovakia. Its research departments were later, in 1969, incorporated in the Slovak Academy of Sciences /SAS/ as the Institute of Experimental Oncology. From the clinical part, which was located in a new building, the Oncological Institute of Slovakia was created. In 1954, the Prague and Brno Institutes became specalized treatment centres with research units, and as Institutes of Oncology are still existing. Thus, Czechoslovakia has three main bases for a comprehensive study of problems of malignant neoplasms.

In 1952 the government declared the large-scale control of diseases with mass occurrence and especially the prevention of these diseases by means of mass screening as preferential task. This decree signified, in fact, the beginning of work aimed at a new concept of the control of malignant tumours. The situation in the field of cancer control in Czechoslovakia was analysed and the knowledge was completed by experiences accumulated abroad; among others also from the oncological assistance rendered to the population in the USSR.

It was decided that, in addition to the oncological institutes, in each county hospital oncological service will be rendered in the form of oncological departments and out-patient clinics. This program was fulfilled in the majority of county hospitals by January 1, 1954, and in those rare cases where it could not be realized, cancer consultation rooms were established.

It was obvious that the oncological institutes and oncological departments of county hospitals will present integral parts of the general organization of curative and preventive health services in Czechoslovakia.

In the past years the conditions for complex oncological treatment were not equal in the counties of Czechoslovakia, and the possibilities of surgical treatment of patients with malignancies were better as compared to that of radiotherapeutic methods. Therefore it was necessary to increase the possibilities of modern radiotherapy and chemotherapy.

The out-patient clinics of oncological departments concentrated their efforts to the control and prophylactic activities. The county oncological departments and cancer consultation rooms were later reinforced by the network of district cancer consultation rooms covering usually the area of one or more districts. The activity of the cancer consultation rooms covered up not only the registration and analysis of notified patients but also their continuous follow-up. District cancer consultation rooms were guided by the county oncological departments in county hospitals or by county cancer consultation rooms. Cancer consultation rooms organized also the first screenings and activities in the field of public education about cancer in close co-operation with the general health services.

This way the out- and in-patients oncological departments were established in the country and in 1953 the compulsory notification of malignant neoplasms was generally introduced.

The development of scientific research and accumulation of experiences in the field of cancer control required the further reorganization of oncological assistance to the population. These actual needs were accomplished by the Ministry of Health in 1966 and further improved in 1975.

The whole oncological policy and simultaneously the management and care for the cancer patients were divided into two separate branches: radiotherapy and clinical oncology.

The practical application of this reorganization in the field of radiotherapy was equal in the whole Czechoslovakia, namely the performance of radiotherapy was concentrated in radiological departments on an in- and out-patient basis.

These departments took over the structure, organization and charge of the previous departments of oncology in the field of treatment of patients.

Departments of radiotherapy were established and still exist in every county hospital /hospital of the IIIrd type/ and in many district hospitals /IInd type hospital/. Their standard equipment includes a sufficient amount of radium, machines for depth and superficial radiotherapy, cobalt and cesium units. Some large departments and institutes have betatrons and are able to use radioisotopes in the treatment of malignant neoplasms, while the diagnosis with isotopes is performed in the department of nuclear medicine.

The main scope of clinical oncology was to ensure the prompt and precise diagnosis of cancer in its early stage, specialized and high-quality treatment of all patients with malignant neoplasms together with long-term follow-up, care for patients with terminal stages of disease, analysis of the organization of cancer control and of epidemiologic and other aspects of malignancies /cancer incidence and mortality, effectiveness of diagnosis and treatment, etc./

The basic principles of the new policy in the field of ʼclinical oncology were completely respected in the whole Chechoslovakia, while their practical application showed some differences in the two national republics.

In the Czech Socialist Republic, in all county and greater district hospitals the so-called Centres of Clinical Oncology were set up and made responsible for the coordination of diagnosis and treatment of individual localizations and types of malignant neoplasms. The basis of Centres of Clinical Oncology are the radiotherapy departments in county and district hospitals, they exist as separate units only in hospitals where the mentioned departments are not available. Under the methodological guidance of the chief physician of the Centre, teams of specialists elaborate for each patient /irrespective of the specialized department of the hospital to which he is admitted/ a comprehensive plan of his examination and treatment and, finally, determine which institution should follow up the patient after the accomplishment of the treatment. The Centres of Clinical Oncology at the district and county level are functioning on an out-patient basis using the beds and hospitalization possibilities of the given hospital, especially the beds of departments of radiology, surgery, etc.

Within this structure, special attention is paid to the chemotherapy of malignant tumours. A new statute has been adopted regarding the senior consultant for chemotherapy of malignant tumours who works at the district or county level and who is also obliged to take an active part in working out the plan of importation or production of cytostatics and especially of their distribution with a view to make their use more rational.

The statute of the senior consultant was introduced also for the oncological problems of surgery, pediatrics, gynecology and medicine. Senior consultants exert their activity in all Centres of Clinical Oncology in County hospitals and in selected district hospitals.

On the other hand in the Slovak Socialist Republic in accordance with the new policy in the field of clinical oncology the so-called Policlinical departments of Clinical Oncology /out-patients clinics of clinical oncology/ were established in all districts and counties. Their activity consists of providing methodological guidance for physicians and paramedical personnel, of ensuring cooperation among specialists in cancer diagnosis and treatment, of the follow-up of patients with malignant and premalignant diseases, of the registration and analysis of the incidence as well as of an active participation in screening programs and public education about campaigning.

The senior consultants for chemotherapy, oncological surgery, gynecology, medicine and pediatrics are established in every county hospital and also in selected district hospitals.

Finally, in every county of the Slovak Socialist Republic the County Institutes of Clinical Oncology were established which may provide a comprehensive diagnosis and therapy of cancer patients and take part in the organization and in providing the methodological guidance for the district out-patient departments of clinical oncology within each particular county. The Institute of Clinical Oncology in Bratislava is the leading, specialized methodological centre for malignant neoplasms in the Slovak Socialist Republic.

At every level, the mentioned institutions of clinical oncology in SSR, as opposed to the system in ČSR, are not established in the departments of radiology, but operate as independent units.

In 1976 also the new detailed cancer notification forms were prepared and introduced together with a new system of compulsory registration of cancer patients in the whole Czechoslovakia.

Despite the fact that new tasks have been established in the field of clinical oncology, oncological assistance cannot be intensified and its quality improved unless the training of physicians in clinical oncology is increased.

The system of education and training of specialists students of medicine and of paramedical personnel in oncology will be described in details later on. Another important part of cancer control program is public education about cancer. In this field the work is based on the existing organizational structure and is carried out in a close cooperation with the Centres of Clinical Oncology in ČSR and similar institutions in SSR. Problems of public education about cancer in this country will be discussed later.

The new organizational structure of oncological assistance is considered as a transitional step to its more perfect form. Thus, control of malignant neoplasms will become an integral part of the general prophylactic and treatment activities. The above-mentioned system of Centres of Clinical Oncology, pro-

vision of highly qualified clinical staff physicians and teams
of experienced specialists - all these are directed towards
enhancing the alertness to cancer problems among physicians of
various specialities, which, as it may well be considered, can
contribute in the future to an earlier diagnosis and adequate
comprehensive treatment of cancer patients, resulting in the
increase of the number of cured patients according to the level
of knowledge.

Particularly the further extension of cancer screening
with a special attention to the high-risk groups of population
is prepared.

Great attention is paid also to the projects of modernization of diagnostic and therapeutic equipment and to the development of new anticancer agents.

Thus, the development of clinical oncology had great influence on the improvement of cancer prevention, diagnosis and
treatment as compared to the past when radiotherapy was the
only discipline responsible for cancer care.

The actual situation in oncology could be summarized with
the following data: on December 31, 1976, in Czechoslovakia
there were 3 oncological institutes with 481 beds for cancer
patients, with 92 doctors, 33 oncological in-patient departments in hospitals of the IInd and IIIrd type with the total
of 1,326 beds and 85 doctors and 125 out-patient departments
with 92 doctors. There were 16 doctors in districts with consultation rooms only in the hospitals of the IInd type.

The number of beds for oncological patients per 10,000
population is 0.9. On December 31, 1974 in the Czechoslovak
Socialist Republic there were 197 physicians engaged in oncology, among them 81 were women.

The number of different institutions of the oncological
network in Czechoslovakia together with the distribution of
beds and physicians is shown in Table 30.

The distribution of physicians working in oncology in the
years from 1965 to 1974 is illustrated in Table 31.

153

Table 30

Oncological Network in Czechoslovakia

Year	Out-patient establishment			In-patient establishment			Oncological institutes		
	Number of departments	physicians in out-patient departments	physicians in consultation centres	Number of departments	beds	physicians	Number of institutes	beds	physicians
1965	103	64,51	15,64	30	1126	68,01	3	455	73,77
1968	103	68,20	14,15	31	1154	63,04	3	455	70,16
1969	110	71,34	16,39	31	1153	70,38	3	485	80,77
1970	115	73,77	15,44	31	1153	72,81	3	455	83,10
1971	116	81,90	15,19	31	1203	75,55	3	469	84,55
1972	116	81,16	15,29	31	1205	79,42	3	469	86,50
1973	127	88,24	14,36	31	1295	76,30	3	481	89,53
1974	128	86,71	14,11	33	1330	81,15	3	481	92,90
1975	125	92,03	15,87	33	1326	84,64	3	481	95,88

Table 31

Distribution and Number of Physicians Working in Oncology

Years	Institutions of the Ministry of Health	Institutions of other Ministries	Total number	Proportion of women
1965	157	11	168	41
1968	147	18	165	51
1969	135	29	164	55
1970	141	30	171	64
1971	161	18	179	70
1972	167	21	188	76
1973	171	18	189	83
1974	178	19	197	81

Specialized oncological assistance is made available at the rate of 0.06 physicians per 10,000 population.

Basic data illustrating incidence and mortality of the population of Czechoslovakia from malignant neoplasms

The age- and sex structure and other demographic parameters as well as basic data illustrating the time- and geographic distribution of the incidence of malignant neoplasms in men and women together with their proportional structure during the last years in Czechoslovakia are shown in the annexed tables.

The following remarks should be added to the present tables:

The distinction between the urban and rural population is not made in Czechoslovakia due to which the main parameters of the incidence of oncological diseases for the country can be studied as a whole only. The analysis of the incidence of malignant neoplasms in Czechoslovakia shows that the number of newly diagnosed patients with malignant neoplasms is annually increasing. This can be attributed to a longer life expectancy while, on the other hand, there is an absolute increase in the incidence of cancer of the lung, skin, large intestine and rectum in some age groups of males and cancer of the breast, large intestine and rectum in females. Cancer of the stomach is diminishing in both sexes while females exhibit a lower incidence of cancer of the uterine cervix. Mortality from malignant neoplasms has increased only inconsiderably in the recent years which can be attributed to the improvement in diagnosis and treatment of malignant neoplasms.

The proportion of patients under the observation of the oncological network is increasing, however, in the course of a differentiated approach to the analysis of the available data, we shall see that the results of treatment of tumours in visceral localizations cannot be considered satisfactory yet, while the results of treatment of cancer of the skin, the breast and the uterine cervix have undoubtedly improved.

SYSTEM OF REGISTRATION OF PATIENTS WITH PRIMARILY DIAGNOSED MALIGNANT NEOPLASMS
V. Dolejsi and R. Rubes

In 1952 the compulsory notification and registration of newly diagnosed cases of malignant neoplasms was introduced in Czechoslovakia. From this time the whole system of notification and registration was constantly developed, and in the meantime various aspects of basic data on oncological patients were stressed and more or less thoroughly described in the notification forms, while the main principles of notification remained the same for a long period /see later/.

The first compulsory notification form for patients with malignant neoplasms used in whole Czechoslovakia till 1976-1977 included 11 items /see Supplement 2/.

As it can be seen, the first part of items of this notification form was reserved for the basic identification data of the patient /first and family name, date of birth, patient's permanent residence with address, occupation - for retired persons previous occupation - and the detailed description of the place of work /factory, transport, agriculture, etc./. The next item was reserved for the topography of the malignant tumour, containing information on the primary localization with the indication of its spread. In the case of cancer of the breast, uterine cervix and body as well as of the malignant neoplasms of ovary, the clinical extent of the diseases was recorded, while in the case of stomach cancer it was necessary to specify the part of stomach involved /cardia, pylorus, other or unknown part/. The TNM classification data were not generally required, but slowly introduced and progressively reported from some counties and for the majority of localizations, while in the gynecological localizations the system of FIGO classification persisted for some period.

One item was designated also for the detailed description of the histological structure of the tumour.

In item 8, it was necessary to specify exactly what kind of treatment has been applied and in item 9 the suggested subsequent therapy was described. Item 10 gave information on what occasion the disease was detected /at a mass prophylactic examination, or when the patient came to see the doctor in connection with symptoms that worried him or in the course of examination in connection with another disease/. The last item was intended for reporting some additional data /complementary information, death of patient, etc./.

The oncological report has to be filled in in three copies by the treatment institution which has detected the malignant neoplasm and transmitted to the oncological institution at the level of district within a week after the detection or within two weeks in case of histological verification. In the district institution the report is verified, supplemented /especially if the district institution had undertaken the therapy/, then the respective parts of the report are transmitted to the oncological institution of the county hospital with an out-patient clinic. There the report is verified again, supplemented in connection with the treatment offered by the latter and coded for machine processing. The coding of tumour topography is done in accordance with the latest revision of the International Classification of Diseases, Injuries and Causes of Death; in case of histology tumour differentation is described. Coding is also used to designate the final method resorted to in completing the patient's examination and also for subsequent items. The notification form is then sent for a statistical analysis at the county, republic and state lavel. The main registered data arranged by region, sex, age, detailed diagnosis and group of diagnoses are regularly published in "Malignant Neoplasms" issued annually by the Institute of Medical Statistics of the Ministry of Health. The results of the analysis of the incidence of malignant neoplasms by counties and federal republics are used as basis for the organization of oncological assistance to the population and of long-term planning.

Mortality from malignant neoplasms is studied only on the basis of death certificates which are filled in by the physician.

In connection with the introduction of the new organization and structure of oncological assistance, the system of notification and registration of oncological patients has been thouroughly revised recently. As a result of this analysis a new system of notification form was developed and introduced in the first half of 1976 in the ČSR and during 1977 also in the SSR. The new system of notification conforms to a maximum extent to the requirements of cancer registry. In this new form of the compulsory notification of malignant neoplasms a "suspicion of a malignant neoplasm" was reintroduced in order to give the patient an opportunity to be hospitalized for the determination of the diagnosis.

The main document of this recently introduced system is the "Notification of malignant neoplasm". Topography of tumours is classified in details /4-digits ICD-O 1976/, the TNM system is compulsory, provision has been made for the possibility of histological and cytological classification and coding in addition to a merely descriptive approach. The report also provides for the possibility of making entries about the subsequent treatment of the patient and for the better description and evaluation of methods of treatment /surgery, irradiation, chemotherapy, immunotherapy and hormonal treatment/. Provision has been made to indicate in the report the treatment institution which is obliged to follow up the patient /see Supplement 3/.

Notification Form

1. Full name of patient:

2. Date of birth:

3. Permanent address: No ... Street
                              District
                              Region /City or County/

4. Occupation: _____
                    /for retired persons, previous one/

5. Place of work:

6. Diagnosis /localization and clinical stage of disease/:

   _____

7. Results of histological examination:

8. Treatment performed:

9. Treatment recommended: /additional treatment, follow-up,
   and so on/ _____

10. Disease detected - In the course of prophylactic exami-
    nation. - The patient visited the doctor because of his
    symptoms:

    The disease was detected by chance /in connection with
    examination for another disease/

11. Special remarks:

Date   Stamp of the institution
                                 and signature of the
                                      physician

Notification of
malignant tumour

Stamp of medical
establishment

Surname, name:	maiden name:	Year of birth, registration number:

Domicile
permanent address:

Domicile
temporary address:

Main occupation:	1. working
Present occupation:	2. pensioner by age, working 3. pensioner by age, not working
Date of first visit to a physician:	4. pensioner by disability, working
Time necessary for establishing the diagnosis /in months/:	5. pensioner by disability, not working 6. other

Diagnosis:

TNM classification:		T	N	M

Clinical stage of disease:	1 stage I 2 stage II	3 stage III 4 stage IV	5 stage O 6 systemic disease	7 metastases from unknown site of primary tumour 8 stage was not determined 9 stage unknown

Most valid basis of diagnosis	1 histology 2 surgery	4 cytology 8 roentgen explora-tion	16 endo - scopy 32 labora-tory analyses	64 autopsy O clinically clear

Histology:	Degree 1 degree I 2 degree II 3 degree III	Histological classification:

Cytology:	Cytological classification:

Method of treatment:	Disease is considered: 1 detected early 2 detected in time but in advanced stage 3 detected late 4 detected at autopsy

==

Surgery:	Radiotherapy	
Date:	Date of the beginning:	
Type of operation: 1 extirpation of tumour 2 simple removal of the organ affected by tumour 3 radical operation with removal of regional lymph vessels and nodes 4 major radical operation 5 radical removal of nodes /block dissection/ without removal of primariy tumour 6 palliative 7 exploratory laparotomy 8 other operation 9 type of operation is unknown 0 operation was not made	1 roentgeno-therapy 2 teletherapy $^{60}Co/^{137}Cs$ 3 therapy with electron radiation 8 therapy with high-energy radiation 16 therapy with closed radiation $^{60}Co/^{137}Cs$ 32 therapy with open irradiators 0 patient was not treated	Type of radiotherapy: 1 radical on primary tumour 2 radical on on regional nodes 3 radical on primary tumour and regional nodes 4 regional therapy 5 palliative therapy 6 type is unknown 1 preoperative therapy 2 postoperative therapy 3 therapy before and after operation 4 independent therapy
Operation performed in:	Radiotherapy performed in:	

Chemotherapy:	Immunotherapy:	Hormonotherapy:
Date of the beginning and place:	Date of the beginning and place:	Date of the beginning and place:
Type: 1 using one preparation 2 using several preparations simultaneously	Type: 1 specific 2 unspecific 3 combined 4 not employed 5 no information	1 yes 2 no 3 no information

/cont'd/

3 using several preparations successively 4 not employed 5 no information Preparation:	Preparation:	Preparation:
Functional elimination of endocrine organ: 1 ovary 2 suprarenal glands 3 hypophysis 4 thyroid gland 5 testis Method of elimination: 1 operation 2 radiation 3 medicaments	Causes of the absence of treatment: 1 state of the disease not requiring treatment 2 local dissemination of tumour 3 generalization of the process 4 contraindications not related to tumour process 5 refusal of treatment by patient 6 death 9 other reasons Date of death:	Establishment and department where dispensary treatment will be carried out: Date of notification Stamp and signature of physician

ENTRY OF OUT-PATIENT DEPARTMENT OF CLINICAL ONCOLOGY /Hospital of IInd type /district//	Registration No. of report

Suspicion was reported: 1 yes 2 no 9 unknown	Date of report:
Dispensary observation for precancerous disease performed: 1 yes 2 no 9 unknown	
Project of treatment was respected: 1 yes 2 no 9 unknown	Mailed to the department of cliniccal oncology
Number of tumours in the same patient:	of the county /in hospital of the IIIrd type/: Date:
Disease was registered as: 1 early diagnosed 2 exactly detected but advanced 3 lately detected	

Establishment where patient
was treated:

Stamp and signature of
physician of out-patient
department of clinical
oncology

Entry of out-patient department
of clinical oncology hospitals
with out-patient clinics of
IIIrd type in town, county

Registration No. of report

Establishment
where the follow-up
will be performed:

Date of report:
Mailed to the Institute of Health Statistics Date:

Stamp and signature of
physician of out-patient
department of clinical
oncology

The system of transmitting the report remains, in principle, the same. The only difference consists in the fact that the report is concluded only after the completion of the first treatment. A progressive feature of the new form is the introduction of the so-called form of control notification to be used for regular information on the condition of the patient on the basis of follow-up investigations. The report enables one to make judgements about the effectiveness of treatment, to determine optimal methods of treatment, to receive information about the economic effect of treatment after the return of patients to work as well as information on the death of patients and its causes.

Information on each patient will be processed with the aid of modern technique of computerization. Such information will be supplemented and can be used for statistical processing and analysis at any time. Naturally, this voluminous documentation can be successfully used in arriving at optimal variants of prophylactic and treatment measures.

ORGANIZATION OF DETECTION AND EXAMINATION OF PATIENTS WITH MALIGNANT AND PREMALIGNANT DISEASES

V. Kubec

A. <u>The system of examination of patients suspected of having malignant tumour</u>

To allow the reader better comprehension of the system of detection and examination of persons suspected of oncological diseases it seems necessary to explain the basic principles of the organization and structure of the health service and medical assistance in Czechoslovakia. The basic institution of the medical assistance forming the periphery of the whole health network is the medical station offering the general curative and preventive medical assistance on an out-patient basis /ambulatory/ for the population of a limited territory /one village or more smaller settlements or one part of town/ or for employees of some enterprises /factory, etc./. A general practitioner with physicians specialized in pediatry, gynecology plus obstetrics and stomatology, together with paramedical personnel form the staff of the lowest medical institution.

To this level of medical assistance corresponds the hospital of the Ist type which serves the territory with the population of up to 50,000 and provides medical assistance in four basic fields of medicine: internal medicine, surgery, obstetrics plus gynecology and pediatry.

Because of rather good transport facilities and relatively small distances the number of hospitals of the Ist type remained limited and the majority of patients who need hospitalization or more specialized examinations or diagnostic procedures are directed to hospitals of the IInd type or district hospital, situated usually in the administrative centre of the district. The hospital of the IInd type serves a territory with the population of about 150-200,000. This hospital has 12 departments in addition to the four basic ones, available in the hospital of the previous type.

The hospital of the IIIrd type or county hospital is in many cases the education base of the medical faculty and serves a territory with a population of 1-1.5 millions. It has in-patient departments and out-patient units not available in the hospital of the IInd type /urology, oncology, resuscitation, occupational diseases, etc./. These hospitals provide the basis for scientific research and postgraduate education for physicians and are supplied with all facilities necessary for diagnosis and treatment of malignant neoplasms.

It must be also explained that all medical institutions, i.e. hospitals, out-patient units, sanatories, stations of public health, etc. at the concrete level form together an administrative organization called Institute of National Health, e.g. "District Institute of National Health" at the level of district, "County Institute of National Health" in the administrative Centre of county and "City Institute of National Health" in big cities.

The oncological patient is usually seen for the first time by the general practitioner or by an other physician at the medical station of his residence or place of work. When symptoms indicative for malignant neoplasms are present the examining physician fills in the respective document and transmits the patient to a medical establishment of higher type where the diagnosis is confirmed or excluded. The latter institution is obliged to notify the medical station of the results of examination. The medical station is obliged to follow up the patient and make steps for his hospitalization, further investigations and treatment, if necessary.

Most of the patients suspected of having malignant neoplasms are subjected to examination on an in-patient basis in hospitals of the IInd or IIIrd type.

Methods of Examination

In the diagnosis of cancer and in the evaluation of the treatment results a complexity of factors is taken into consideration, namely:

a/ clinical course of the disease;

b/ objective changes observed in the course of physical examination;

c/ evidence obtained by biopsy, roentgenoscopy, radioisotope and ultrasound diagnosis, thermography, endoscopy, haematological, biochemical, immunological and other methods of investigation, including exploratory surgery.

The possibilities of using some or other methods of investigation depend on the type of hospital to which the patient is referred to.

In hospitals of the Ist type only the basic methods /laboratory and roentgenologic/ are available.

Hospitals of IInd type possess facilities for more extent investigations, while the entire range of diagnostic methods is available in hospitals of the IIIrd type only.

Apart from the conventional methods of investigation, contrast media, including angio- and lymphography, are used in the following sites:

- digestive tract
- trachea, bronchus and the lung
- breast

- bones and soft tissues
- urinary tract
- lymphatic nodes
- central nervous system.

In the recent years a significant progress has been made in the diagnosis by using fiberoscopy in the following sites:
- digestive tract
- upper and lower part of the respiratory tract
- lower part of urinary the tract.

The histological verification of malignant neoplasms is considered as basic principle. The entire network of medical institutions is well equipped for histological investigations, with an adequate staff of specialists. Necessary steps are being made to establish cytologic investigations on a larger scale in both the diagnostics and the evaluation of the treatment results.

Haematologic and biochemical laboratory tests made in all county and district hospital /IIIrd and IInd type/ constitute the basic form of examination of each patient and are completed by necessary specialized biochemical investigations.

Radioactive isotopes are used on a very wide scale and are routinely applied in the diagnosis of tumours of the following sites:
- thyroid gland
- brain
- bone
- liver
- lung
- kidney
- lymphatic nodes.

Such examinations are available in selected district hospitals /IInd type/ and in all hospitals of the IIIrd type.

Special Investigations

The ultrasound diagnosis of tumours based on Doppler's principle has found a wide application in neurology, ophthalmology, surgery, gynecology and pediatrics, often in combination with isotope scintigraphy. It should be noted, however, that the ultrasound equipment is available only in some hospitals of the IIIrd type.

During the last years, possibilities in diagnostics have been increased by means of thermovision, especially in diagnosis of the breast tumours and of the neoplastic processes of lymph nodes.

Among the special investigations, the measurement of tissue-impendance seems to be promising. "DIACA", produced in Czechoslovakia are apparatus has found a wide application in the diagnosis of tumours accessible by means of endoscopy, mainly tumours of the rectum and cervix uteri.

Immunologic methods have been also developed; they have found application in diagnosis of certain types of tumours.

The length of time necessary for the final diagnosis of malignant tumours has not been established or limited in Czechoslovakia.

Specialized oncological institutes are practically not used for initial diagnosis of malignant neoplasms; these functions are entrusted to the general medical network. In the oncological institutes the special diagnostic procedures are developed and used for the better localization of tumours and for the better determination of their extent, thus allowing for the application of special treatment techniques or control during treatment.

B. Screening

The methods of mass screening for early detection of malignant neoplasms and precancerous diseases have been determined by the methodological instructions of the Ministry of Health.

At present, screening is conducted in three forms:

1/ screening made in special departments of out-patient clinics belonging to the network of general health services;

2/ screening made in patients admitted in hospitals of all categories;

3/ mass screening of the population.

Ad 1/. In the specialized departments of out-patient clinics examinations are performed by physicians in all patients who

168

attend the clinic, no matter what their complaint is. The aim
of these examinations is to detect early stages of malignant
neoplasms and precancerous conditions. The extent of such
examinations depends on the diagnostic capacity of an out-patient clinic.

Ad 2/. The age groups of patients subjected to prophylactic
examinations during every hospitalization are:

- males aged 40 and over;
- females aged 30 and over.

Unless prophylactic examination has been performed on a
patient in the age group indicated above, he cannot be discharged from the hospital. The examination consists of the
following steps:

- roentgenoscopy of the lung;
- basic biochemical and haematological analyses;
- physical examination of the abdominal cavity;
- palpation of accessible lymphatic nodes;
- inspection of the skin;
- inspection of the mouth;
- in males, examination of the rectum by palpation,
- in females, gynecological and breast examination.

Ad 3/. Beside detection of malignant diseases and precancerous
lesions, mass screening of the population also includes detection of cardiovascular disorders and diabetes. The mass screenings are carried out on a large scale in all medical stations
and specialized departments of hospitals and out-patient institutions. In this respect the close cooperation with public
organizations involving voluntary activists in the organization
of the examinations is of a great benefit. The Director of the
local Institute of National Health, who relies on the methodological guidance of the Centre of Clinical Oncology, is responsible for the preparation and conduct of the examinations.

The age groups encounter:

- males aged 40 to 64;
- females aged 30 to 64.

The examinations are directed toward the detection of
tumours of the lung, digestive tract, lymph nodes accessible

to palpation, skin, mouth and prostate in males, and that of the breast, skin, digestive tract, genital tract, first of all uterine cervix, and lymph nodes accessible to palpation in females.

All examined persons are submitted to roentgenography.

The experience shows that the number of persons in the selected age groups represents about 40,000 per 100,000 population.

Screening is carried out once in two years, which means that during one year out of every 100,000 persons approximately 20,000 are subjected to the examination.

I. The first step of prophylactic examinations is laboratory investigation which includes:

a/ examination of blood consisting of the determination of blood group and of sedimentation rate;

b/ analysis of urine with the aid of Labstix /determination of pH, proteins, glucose, ketons and blood in the urine/; stool examination for occult bleeding with the aid of hemocult test;

c/ investigation of the gastric secretion with Gastrotest tablets.

II. In case of achlorhydria, the second step is the determination of LDH activity in blood serum to detect pernicious anaemia and the examination of gastric secretion after the administration of histamine.

Each citizen subjected to prophylactic examination fills in an extensive questionnaire containing personal and anaemnestic data. The questions are serving the purpose of detection of the disease in eventual high risk persons. For each examinee, a special documentation is kept where physicians, the members of the diagnostic team make their entries. Then the collected evidence is summarized, and measures for the second stage examination are recommended by the leading physician of the Centre of Clinical Oncology.

Once a month each local Institute of National Health prepares reports on the progress of mass screening; the reports are processed and analyzed by the Ministry of Health of the ČSR and SSR.

The prophylactic oncological examinations constitute a main element of the oncological programme of the Ministry of Health in this country.

ORGANIZATION OF HOSPITALIZATION AND MEDICAL ASSISTANCE FOR PATIENTS WITH MALIGNANT NEOPLASMS
V. Kubec

One of the main efforts of clinical oncology is to secure a high-quality treatment without delay for the patients with malignant neoplasms.

The existing system of medical institutions, including also three specialized oncologic institutes with the total of 481 cancer beds, are the basis for the organization of hospitalization.

The capacity of clinical and radiological bases of the oncological institutions in the country determines the specific features of organization of hospitalization.

Organization of clinical oncology

The multidisciplinary nature of clinical oncology calls for coordination, precise and reliable organization of all the elements of its activities.

With this in view the next measures were established:
1. The Ministry of Health has set up a consultative committee of experts which elaborates proposals regarding various aspects of clinical oncology.
2. The consultative councils are operating at the level of each County Institute of National Health which supervise the quality and results of treatment in patients with malignant neoplasms and elaborate proposals for the improvement of this work.
3. All hospitals of the IInd and IIIrd type /district and county hospitals/ have centres of clinical oncology; methodologic guidance is exercised by the Centre of Clinical Oncology of the county hospitals established in the residence of the local Institute of National Health. The centres are closely connected with the radiotherapeutic department or with other departments where oncological patients are treated /if radiotherapeutic departments are not established/.

171

The principles of hospitalization of patients

Patients with malignant neoplasm are admitted to departments of the local general hospitals. In Czechoslovakia special beds for oncological patients are available only in the oncological institutes in Brno, Bratislava and Prague. The nature and localization of the disease is decisive for the admission of the patient to a specialized department of the hospital.

The highest proportion of oncological patients is treated at radiology departments where they constitute almost 100 per cent of patients. A high percentage of oncological patients is admitted to surgical, gynecologic, internal medical, pneumologic, otorhinolaryngologic, pediatric and other departments. The duration of hospitalization varies considerably, depending on the nature and localization of the disease and the methods of treatment used. As a rule, the patient remains at the radiology department for 28 days, at the surgical department for 15 days.

The main principle of hospitalization of oncological patients consists in their admission to those medical institutions the equipment and facilities of which allow the diagnosis and treatment of malignant tumours at an adequate and complex level. All questions arising in the process of elaborating and selecting the methods of treatment as well as in the course of treatment are decided upon in consultation with a team of specialists. A plan of treatment is elaborated and put forward by a group of specialists of the centre of clinical oncology and the method of treatment is approved by the head physician of the department to which the patient had been admitted. The head physician of the specialized department is responsible for the patient's treatment. If the head physician does not agree with the proposed treatment, his reasons must be thoroughly documented.

The specialized department to which the patient is admitted is responsible for the completion of the treatment and, in accordance with the rules, to ensure the institution where the follow-up will be performed.

172

The completion of treatment is undertaken by the departments of the respective hospitals. In cases which require a long period of hospitalization, after the specialized treatment the patient is referred to the hospitals for aftercare. If, for some reasons, the patient cannot be admitted to another treatment institution, the responsibility for completion of his treatment and repeated hospitalization is entrusted to the institution where the primary treatment had been performed.

In the course of treatment and follow-up, the detailed examination of the patient is performed periodically by a team of specialists. The team of physicians working in specialized departments is guided by the physician responsible for clincal oncology. Such teams were established mainly in county hospitals /IIIrd type/ with the best conditions for the complex therapy of oncological patients. In the complex therapy of in- and out-patients a great role is played by physicians specialized in chemotherapy of malignant diseases.

The secondary prevention of malignant neoplasms represents an integral part of the newly established oncological program in this country. It is based on the active detection of early stages of malignant neoplasms and precancerous conditions as a measure allowing for a change in the structure of patients regarding the stage of the disease. Among the responsibilities of clinical oncologists and specialists in individual fields of prevention and therapy, regular analyses of advanced stages of the disease and of cases detected too late are included. These analyses are used as a basis for the elaboration of measures aimed at improving the quality of diagnosis in those fields of medicine which are related to oncology.

The level of rendered assistance is evaluated on the basis of the results of treatment. In a majority of counties and districts, the evaluation of results is made continuously but the methods for the assessment of therapeutic efficiency has lacked uniformity so far. The elaboration of uniform system based on a new and more extent system of registration of patients with malignant neoplasms started in 1976.

In the future it is planned to educate specialists in clinical oncology on a large scale for teamwork in specialized institutions with the aim to improve the therapeutic efficiency. It is proposed that such a large-scale institute specializing in multidisciplinary approach should serve the majority of oncological patients in a region with a population of 2-2,5 million.

THE SYSTEM OF TREATMENT OF MALIGNANT NEOPLASMS ON AN OUT-PATIENT BASIS

V. Kubec

In the modern, complex treatment of patients with malignant neoplasms it is sometimes difficult to distinguish exactly between the treatment performed on an in-patient basis /hospitalized patients/ and that on an out-patient basis /not hospitalized patients/. During recent years the proportion of patients treated on an in-patient basis has been steadily increasing and only the relatively small part of patients is treated completely without hospitalization, mainly the cases where surgical procedures are not involved in the complex of treatment methods.

On the other hand the number of therapeutical interventions performed on an out-patient basis is also increasing as the result of introduction of modern therapeutical principles mainly of a complementary nature.

In case of malignant neoplasms the treatment on an in--patient basis and that on an out-patient basis are as a rule combined.

1. The methods of treatment applied in case of hospitalization are mainly the following:

radical surgery

complex methods of radiotherapy

complicated procedures of chemotherapy.

2. The methods of treatment applied on an out-patient basis are as follows:

minor surgical interventions

radiotherapy

maintenance chemotherapy

hormonetherapy

other procedures

rehabilitation.

Ad 1. Nearly all, more or less radical, surgical interventions require hospitalization. Surgical interventions and complicated radiotherapy are performed at higher-level hospitals, i.e. selected district hospitals /hospital of the IInd type/ and all county hospitals /hospital of the IIIrd type/. Hospitalization is also made for application of interstitial and intracavitary radiotherapy and for application of radical external radiation and isotopes.

Complex chemotherapy, especially when several preparations are administered simultaneously, also needs hospitalization. In Czechoslovakia, hospitalization has been practised in case of repeated courses of chemotherapy.

Ad 2. Among surgical interventions, the removal of skin carcinoma and recurrent neoplasms in the easily accessible localizations is performed on an out-patient basis. Also a greater part of radiotherapy, especially superficial X-ray therapy is performed on an out-patient basis. In the last years, the majority of treatment institutions have adopted nonconventional fractionation, i.e. application of large fractions in longer intervals. This is of great importance for out-patients living far from hospitals.

Long-term courses of chemotherapy are solved by:

a/ referring the patient to a hospital of the Ist or IInd type for maintenance chemotherapy;

b/ provision of daytime beds for out-patients in the specialized departments of county hospitals /IIIrd type/ for chemotherapy. This method is coming quickly into a wide use and is very effective, because if applied rationally, it enables six out-patients to be treated during one day.

Thus, in case of the shortage of beds in radiotherapy units radiation treatment can be widely used on an out-patient basis. Radiotherapy is performed in patients living at a distance of about 75 km from hospital if the transport conditions are good.

Hormonetherapy is, as a rule, available in all medical institutions.

Rehabilitation occupies an important place in the out-patient treatment of patients with malignant neoplasms. Patients after radical surgery or radical radiotherapy are subjected to it. It is effected, as a rule, in rehabilitation departments of the district hospitals.

STUDY OF THE EFFECTIVITY OF TREATMENT IN ONCOLOGICAL
PATIENTS

P. Cepcek, V. Cerny and A. Godál

Specific problems of the study of treatment efficiency of
chemotherapeutic agents.

Since the special methods of treatment of tumour diseases /chemotherapy, hormonal treatment, immunotherapy/ are mostly empirical, assessing of their efficiency is connected with specific problems. An expedient assessment of new therapeutic substances, applied individually or in combination in treatment schedules should be based on the following criteria:

1. toxicity and effectivity in preclinical experiments;
2. tolerance and toxicity in clinical conditions;
3. effectivity in clinical conditions;
4. clinical applicability.

Toxicity and efficiency in preclinical conditions are determined by the degree of acute and chronic toxicity in different kinds of laboratory animals and the degree of response to treatment in cases of fast- and slow-growing tumours.

The determination of tolerance and toxicity in clinical conditions is made in the first phase of clinical investigation in patients with advanced tumours.

The efficiency in clinical conditions is studied on a selected range of tumours in the second phase of clinical investigation.

Clinical applicability is studied in the third phase of the clinical investigation.

All of the three phases represent an object of the compulsory work which is required by the protocols worked out separately for each phase in accordance with conventional rules. With each phase the complexity of the investigation of the investigation increases.

The criteria on which the work is based in the first phase are those of the statistical assessment of tolerance shown by the patients under treatment, toxicity and its effect on individual tissue systems. The evaluation of the parameters is made, where it is possible, numerically /haematological toxicity/ or quantitatively /no, insignificant, medium, important changes/. The first phase is intended to determine the maximum value of the tolerable doses of the given substances, individually or in combination, or the limits of treatment schedules.

In the second phase the objective of the work consists in selecting the so-called "signal tumours" for the study of the effectivity of treatment and the choice of criteria for an objective assessment of the treatment.

The criteria are given by:

a/ the degree of regression of the signs of tumour disease /the degree of response/;

b/ duration of regression /duration of response/.

The degree of response is determined by the quantity of remissions.

Remission is considered complete if there is a regression of all symptoms of the disease detected in the course of the comprehensive examination. Insignificant manifestations of toxicity caused by the treatment are usually tolerated.

Partial remission is a condition when the improvement cannot be qualified as complete remission, and regression of the representative tumour masses exceeds 50 per cent.

Improvement signifies a condition when the tumour masses show signs of diminishment but not to the extent to reach the criterion of partial remission on the one hand, or the criterion of "stationary disease", on the other.

Stationary disease is the reduction of the size of the tumour masses less than 25 per cent.

Progression of the disease implies the increase in the symptoms of tumour disease as revealed in the course of post--treatment examination.

The contents of the criteria are well determined in case of solid tumours. For systemic diseases /leukemia, myeloma/, methods of assessment are more complicated.

The duration of response is evaluated on the basis of duration of various degrees of remission and the duration of survival of patients.

The duration of remissions is evaluated within the following limits. The beginning of remission /as of the moment of appearance of signs meeting the criteria of remission/ and the end of remission /the appearance of regression of the disease or renewal of the tumour growth after its diminishment or the appearance of new localizations of tumour/.

Besides, a mean duration of remissions, and maximum and minimum durations of remissions are evaluated in patients to whom the given substance has been administered.

The survival of patients as a result of the given method of treatment is a less characteristic criterion /usually because of the need to use of other, subsequent treatment/. It is measured from the beginning of the evaluated treatment to its completion or to the death of the patient, i.e. as an average survival rate, or on the basis of the maximum and minimum survivals /in months/ or as an average of 1, 2 and 5-year survivals rates.

The object of study in the third phase are the possibilities for clinical application of the given method of treatment; a new substance is used as a rule already in combination with other substances, or the study of a new treatment schedule is made with the method of the so-called "pilot study" or with the method of controlled clinical study.

Methodologically, the "pilot study" is a simple procedure. It is aimed at obtaining general information about the efficiency and tolerance of the therapeutic method under study. It is applied without a control group of patients.

The method of controlled clinical study implies a comparison between one or several chemotherapeutic methods and the control group of patients treated with an optimal, already known method. The procedure involved here is rather complicated but it gives an opportunity to obtain objective data necessary for a subsequent application of the results of this work into practice.

The object of study is evaluating the effectivity of clinical therapy with drugs is either a new substance /chemically difined or having a biological nature /individually or a rational combination of such substances, or schedules of their application, and recently also the effectivity of the whole treatment complex. The purpose of such an evaluation is the optimisation of the given treatment as such and, especially, its curative effect.

The second and more real possibility involves the elaboration of the optimal combination of the given method of treatment with other methods /complex modality treatment/. The experience shows the effectivity of such a system of comparison in case of cooperation of several institutes within one county or on an international basis.

Study of the effectivity of surgical therapy in patients with malignant tumours

Surgical methods have great possibilities of application in the therapy of malignant tumours. All surgical interventions in oncology depend on the clinical and pathomorphological findings, on the biological nature and pattern of metastatic spread of individual types of malignant neoplasms, but mainly on their localization. The method of surgical intervention must be decided individually for each patient.

Rational performance of operations with saving the organs without extensive sacrifice of tissue necessitates a good knowledge of the pathophysiology of malignant tumours. It is, however, generally known that radical surgical intervention with the removal of the whole organ or of the greater part of tumour with regional lymphatic nodes results in better control of the tumour.

In many cases surgical intervention is limited by the extent of the disease and is of palliative character. Such interventions enable diminishing of the tumour extent and are beneficial in combination with other methods /radiotherapy, hormonal, immuno- and chemotherapy/.

For the evaluation of the results of treatment and their comparison on a larger basis, uniform criteria must be generally accepted and respected for the classification of the extent of malignant tumour. The TNM-system of classification of malignant neoplasms /UICC/, despite certain shortcomings, characterizes the degree of tumour development and extension rather adequately. To assure perfect classification all available methods of examination have to be used by specialists for individual localizations.

Beside the performance of adequate and most suitable surgical intervention completed with other methods of therapy the follow-up of patient is of great importance in oncology, especially during the first two years after the intervention, when the mortality is culminating not only in advanced cases, but also in patients in the Ist and IInd clinical stage of the disease. The survival time is, however, not the only criterion for the evaluation of different surgical and other method of treatment. In this respect the postoperative course of the disease, individual symptoms and complications arising in consequence of extended surgical intervention, the damaging of tissues as a result of radiotherapy, or of haemopoiesis by chemotherapeutic agents, or various unfavourable conditions arising after hormone therapy and finally the side-effects of immunotherapy are of importance and must be taken into account in the evaluation of therapeutic results.

The regular follow-up of patients in the postoperative period is very necessary mainly in some slowly growing or lately diagnosed tumours where good results could be obtained also by repeated surgical removals of tumours. The surgery of early-found relapses could hinder the extension of tumour to neighbouring anatomical structures or organs. Especially in such cases the combination of surgery with other methods of treatment could improve and prolong the time of survival. Like in the classification, also during the follow-up of patients all accessible methods of examination, mainly radiographic, endoscopic and radioisotopic, must be used.

In our opinion it is extremely important for every method of treatment, be it surgical or other, that treatment should be given only in in-patient institutions which are capable of ensuring complex care, i.e. treatment, regular examinations and assessment of the condition of patients with a view to their further treatment.

Controlled clinical experiment can be successfully used in the surgical treatment of the common localizations of malignant neoplasms /the stomach, lung, breast, female genital organs/. In these experiments national and international cooperation should be welcomed. The study of the effectivity of surgical, combined and comprehensive treatment of patients with malignant neoplasms can be most successful and may give most accurate results only under the conditions of such an integrated cooperation.

ORGANIZATION OF MEDICAL DETERMINATION OF DISABILITY
AND THE REHABILITATION OF ONCOLOGICAL PATIENTS
L. Makovická

In Czechoslovakia the determination of disability attributed to sickness is an inseparable part of the duties of every general practitioner and specialist. They continuously receive the necessary aid and special assistance from medical experts engaged in the problems of disability. The competent physician is at the same time the chairman of a special advisory committee. The members of this committee are recruited from general practioners and specialists as temporary advisors if necessary. This committee meets once a week at every medical station /serving a certain territory or enterprise/ evaluates the health status of the patients with temporary disability and decides upon the further prolongation of this period. Similar committees are also constituted in every hospital for patients treated on an out-patient basis or for final decision in difficult or disputable cases which could not be resolved at the lower level of the medical service.

It is a duty of every physician or of the documentation centre of the respective hospital to keep detailed medical documentation for each patient, with all data related to the patient's health condition, its dynamics and disability.

The estimation of the disability of a particular patient with oncological disease cannot be made on a formal basis. When judging an oncological case the physician must consider the nature, development or stabilization of the patient's disease and his condition. All circumstances need to be taken into account. The patient's eventual return to work must be decided on the basis of a close cooperation of all specialists of the expert team, including the psychologist, social worker and the competent physician, with regard to the patient's own interest as well as the interest of his relatives and of the whole society.

When the disease was diagnosed and effectively treated in an early stage there is a possibility for the patient to return cured to his work. But if extensive anatomo-functional disturbances developed in consequence of a radical surgical intervention or radiotherapy, this should be duly taken into account and the transfer of the patient to a more convenient kind of work should be recommended. The physical state of oncological patients after their return to work is usually balanced. Patients with haematologic malignancies should return to their work, be it for a short time, during remissions, provided they are in a condition to perform is. Premature disability gives rise to depressions of the patient; besides certain apprehensions of social nature may arise due to decreased standard of living.

Health and labour rehabilitation of oncological patients is very important for their return to normal life. Especially the condition of patients with extensive functional disturbances after surgical treatment needs to be rehabilitated already on the first days after the surgical intervention. In rehabilitation emphasis should be made on assisting the patient in adjusting himself quickly to the new conditions and achieving personal independence for the longest period possible.

Analysis of disability by selected nosological groups of diseases is made regularly in Czechoslovakia by treatment institutions of all categories.

More profound analyses of disability caused by oncological diseases including such parameters as functional disturbances, methods of treatment and perspectives of survival and the quality of life are in progress.

ORGANIZATION OF MEDICAL ASSISTANCE FOR PATIENTS WITH ADVANCED TUMOURS

V. Kolár and Z. Mechl

The specialized organization of control of tumour diseases constitutes an integral part of the statewide prevention and treatment services of health institutions. Although the assistance to patients with advanced stages of tumours is connected with many complexities and differences in various countries, there are several generally accepted principles in this field of problems.

Patients with advanced tumours can be divided into two categories:

a/ patients in whom even the generalization of the process still holds a promise of complete remission or, at least, a considerable improvement of their life conditions,

b/ patients in incurable stage of disease.
Ad a/ It is obvious that the first group of patients needs a special medical care on a large scale of modern methods of treatment, i.e. surgical intervention, radio- and chemotherapy, often in combination, or, if necessary, also immunotherapy. The therapeutic procedures used in this situation are mainly radical and very complicated not only for the patient but also for the medical staff. The patient should be admitted into a specialized institution which possesses all the necessary equipment and facilities. If the treatment is successful, in some cases the therapy can be later continued on an out-patient basis, but the patient should be constantly followed up by the institution which had started the treatment.

183

Ad b/ It has been established that patients with widely disseminated tumours may exhibit a considerable variety of symptoms. From the point of view of further treatment patients can be divided into two groups:

1/ patients presenting no special complaints, despite a wide dissemination of the tumour;

2/ patients in whom the dissemination resulted in severe subjective and objective troubles.

The patients in the first group may receive help at home during a considerable period of time; often, they are not confined to bed and can perform some domestic works. It would be sufficient for them to be seen from time to time by a physician or a nurse, to receive symptomatic therapy and psychotherapy. The physician or the nurse could organize the special control examination of such patients in the nearest medical institution or arrange their admission to a hospital, if some other special examination and the elaboration of a new system of treatment are necessary.

A majority of patients in the second group can be treated at home for some time though their hospitalization may be necessary from time to time. Because they need only symptomatic therapy, it would be necessary to reserve a certain number of beds for them in the nearest general hospital.

In the resolutions passed in Geneva in March 1965, the WHO Committee of Experts for the Treatment of Malignant Tumours has indicated the necessary conditions for planning the treatment of patients with advanced malignant tumours in an area with a population of 1 million. The Committee has made calculations not only of the necessary number of beds but also of the equipment, the number of physicians and the requirements for the lasting hospitalization and follow-up of such patients.

It is obvious from this report of experts that the problem of the organization of the long-term management of these patients together with periodical examinations and treatment could not be considered adequately solved. These patients have minimum requirements on highly specialized medical procedures but need continuous care and help furnished by general practitioners and especially by nurses.

184

In a majority of patients with advanced tumours even a partial remission, which might make their life more tolerable and lengthen their survival, cannot be achieved. On the contrary, the treatment possibilities are limited too often to symptomatic treatment only. The tumour itself, its considerable dissemination and the previous anti-tumour therapy weaken the resistance of the organism, which is reflected in a greater susceptibility to infection. The progressing disease leads to cachexia combined with anaemia, absence of appetite and diminished nutrition, which, in its turn, results in metabolic disturbances, disturbances of ion exchange and inhibition of protein metabolism. It is difficult but necessary to treat these complications because they immeasurably increase the physical and psychic suffering of the patient.

By removing or considerably alleviating pain, it is possible to effectively influence the psychic condition of the patient, to remove fear and anguish and to achieve, thereby, a favourable effect upon his physical condition. Sooner or later, a chronically ill patient will have doubts as to the possibility of his recovery, though it should be recalled that a majority of patients firmly believe in it. It is a common knowledge that the efficiency of treatment can be enhanced by a good psychic condition of the patient and the latter's confidence in the physician. Even if the ineluctable approach of the terminal stage cannot be stopped, it is our duty to do all we can to relieve the patient in this last minutes of pain, anguish and fear.

For patients in the advanced stage of tumour development, opiates will still remain indispensable. The danger of development of habit is not so great as is ususally pointed out and for a patient whose days are numbered this can well be neglected. Refusal of opiates administration when other drugs have no effect any longer, can only mean lack of understanding of the physical and psychic condition of the patient and an indolent attitude to his suffering.

TEACHING OF ONCOLOGY, TRAINING OF ONCOLOGISTS AND
PREPARATION OF PARAMEDICAL PERSONNEL IN ONCOLOGY
V. Thurzo

Basic education of medical students

A uniform system of training of medical students in oncology has not been established in Czechoslovakia yet. At the
Medical Faculty of the Komensky University in Bratislava and
at the Faculty of General Medicine of the Charles University
in Prague oncology is taught as a separate discipline. Nevertheless, because of the different circumstances and conditions
in both faculties the contents of teaching of oncology in not
identical.

Medical Faculty of the Komensky University in Bratislava

The teaching of oncology as a separate discipline started
in 1962. The separate Chair of Oncology and Radiology was constituted at the Research Institute of Oncology. The structure
of the chair in the mentioned period of time was as follows:

Oncology	Radiology	
Experimental	Radiotherapy	Nuclear medicine
Clinical	Radiodiagnosis	

Until 1968 all lectures and practical training were performed in the frame of pathology, internal medicine and gynecology.

From 1968 the Chair of Oncology organized separate lectures and practical training on the following topics:

1/ experimental oncology   - 2 academic hours
2/ clinical oncology   - 5 academic hours
3/ radiotherapy   - 5 academic hours

Lectures are read during 6 weeks /one lecture each week/
in the fourth year /summer semester/.

The lectures and practical training are based on the
interdisciplinary nature of both experimental and clinical
oncology. Oncology is closely associated with a great number
of different branches of medicine. Experimental oncology includes the knowledge of natural sciences /physics, molecular

biology, etc./. The lectures on experimental oncology give
recent information concerning the malignant transformation of
cells, etiology and development of tumours from the viewpoint
of viral, chemical and physical carcinogenesis, the biology of
tumour growth as well as immunology and epidemiology of cancer.

Lectures on clinical oncology are based on the interdisciplinary approach to diagnosis and therapy and they concern
the main principles of the methods of diagnosis and therapy.
Special problems relating to clinical cases are managed at lectures on other branches of medicine /surgery, gynecology, radiology and other/.

At all lectures, the importance of oncology as a social
problem is stressed; this is done, in the first place, with a
view to attract special attention to the development of oncological alertness both among physicians and the population.
Special examination from oncology is required.

The staff of the Chair of Oncology and Radiology at the
Medical Faculty of the Komensky University in Bratislava is
formed by the head of chair who is professor of experimental
oncology and 4 senior lecturers.

Faculty of General Medicine of the Charles University in Prague

At the Faculty of General Medicine there is an Oncological
Department, which was constituted in 1973 on the basis of a
former Oncological Division of the Radiology Department, and
is a part of the Chair of Radiology. Thus, at this faculty
there is no separate Chair of Oncology but there is a specialized Oncological Department. The staff of the department includes three persons responsible for teaching: 1 assistant
professor and 2 senior lecturers. There are 5 more physicians
who also take part in teaching.

The training starts in the fourth year of the studies;
during one semester ten lectures and 4 academic hours of practical training are given. Lectures are read on clinical oncology and radiotherapy.

At the Faculty of General Medicine of the Charles University in Prague a number of oncological laboratories of various

institutes and hospitals /Departments of Oncology, Gynecology, Institute of Medical Chemistry, Institute of Biology/ also participate in education.

At other medical faculties in Czechoslovakia teaching of oncology is carried out within the framework of basic theoretical and clinical branches of medicine during the entire period of study.

Postgraduate education of physicians in oncology

Earlier the postgraduate training of physicians in clinical oncology was carried out in the form of a two-week course organized once a year. Approximately 20 physicians were trained annually.

The courses were organized by the chief specialist for oncology at the Ministry of Health, while the lectures and practical training were performed in the Institute of Oncology in Bratislava.

Lately the courses were organized by the Chair of Radiology of the Postgraduate Institute for Physicians and Pharmacists with the successive participation of all district oncologists. The program consisted of the so-called "oncological minimum" containing basic aspects of clinical oncology.

At the present time, new concepts of clinical oncology have been approved in the ČSR and the SSR.

In the SSR the concept of postgraduate preparation in clinical oncology comprises the following main specializations: surgery, gynecology, radiology, internal medicine and pediatrics.

At the Postgraduate Institute for Physicians and Pharmacists the Chair of Clinical Oncology was constituted. Its task is the education of specialists in clinical oncology, who will act as senior consultants of clinical oncology at the departments of surgery, gynecology, internal medicine and pediatrics of the hospitals of the IInd and IIIrd type and as heads of out-patient departments of clinical oncology 14-28 day courses were organized during recent years.

Training of paramedical personnel

For nurses working in district oncological out-patient centres and oncological departments 14-day courses are organized by the Postgraduate Institute for Paramedical Personnel, while lectures and practical training are conducted at the Institutes of Oncology. Secondary schools for paramedical personnel do not offer any preparation for work in oncological establishments. In such schools special education is given only to technical assistants in department of radiology.

PUBLIC EDUCATION ABOUT CANCER
J. Fremmer and M. Taufrova

The problems of prevention of malignant tumours are closely connected with the health education of the population. The role of such an education is determined by the fact that a part of the population remains ignorant of factors related with these diseases as well as of early symptoms of cancer and the possibility of its cure, if detected in time.

Especially important is the prevention of cancer through the adequate education of the widest range of the population to the oncological alertness and to the collaboration with the medical staff in organizing preventive measures. The importance of attending prophylactic examinations should be emphasized in the educational work. If the educational work is directed to certain population groups selected according to some principles /place of work, age, sex, possible localization of precancerous diseases or malignant tumours/ its efficacy can, thereby, be enhanced.

Organization and structure

In increasing the efficiency of educational work a great role is played by the scientific methodological assistance rendered by the health education departments of county and district medical institutions which represent specialized organizational and methodological centres for public health education in the given area. Their main objective consists in working out plans of educational work for various groups of the population in a close cooperation with the centres of clinical oncology and other institutions engaged in the campaign against cancer. A properly prepared plan has to be based on the assessment of the level of the sanitary knowledge of the population and has to respect the sanitary, political, cultural and social situation in the given country or district. Departments of health education participate in providing for the implementation of the programmes and measures in the field of public education about cancer; in particular, they pay much attention to the study of the efficacy of various forms and methods in this work. Besides, the departments of health education offer professional consultations, aids and the necessary materials for educational work to medical workers engaged in health education and also other organizations taking part in integrated cancer control measures /organizations of commerce, general education, culture, agriculture and public catering, industry, water economy and others/. They conduct publishing activities, according to the needs of the given country or district in this field, are engaged in the distribution of educational materials and check their utilization and effects obtained. All the measures indicated above are carried out within the framework of the postgraduate activities aimed at raising the qualifications of physicians and para-medical personnel in the methods of educational work in the field of cancer control.

The public health education departments systematically cooperate with the mass media and the institutions and organizations having relation to the health protection /local national committees, trade union organs, the Czechoslovakian Red Cross, etc./.

The Institutes of Health Education in Prague and Bratislava are the highest specialized methodological centres for public health education. They are engaged in determining the extent of primary knowledge of the population on cancer in introducing and assessing the efficiency of new forms and methods of public education about cancer and in publishing standard texts for the special courses of medical workers on the methods of health education in oncology which emphasize the questions of prevention of oncological diseases and contain advices for the patients. They take part in increasing the qualifications of medical workers and maintain a close contact with the central organs of mass organizations, with the mass media and foreign organizations and institutions dealing with similar problems.

Public education on cancer in medical institutions

Health education in oncology is intended to reach a wide range of the population, and therefore receives great attention in every medical institutions.

Educational work on cancer is carried out especially by physicians in medical stations, in maternity consultation centres, and in specialized departments of hospitals and out-patient clinics, rehabilitation departments, in rest homes for children and adults, both in night and day sanatoria and other institutions.

Health education outside medical institutions

The organization of education on cancer depends also on the selection of the population /school-children, students or groups of adult population/.

It is obvious that, in terms of achieving a correct orientation of the attitude of the wide range of the population to cancer, the education of youth on cancer plays an important part as a measure intended to free the youth from prejudices and mistakes causing fear of cancer, using all suitable forms and places.

Education on cancer among other groups of the population can be carried out at enterprises, factories, offices, schools, PTA-meetings, factory clubs, recreation and reading rooms, factory trade union meetings, sport-clubs, rest homes and tourist camps, cultural institutions, etc.

Methods

Among the methods of educational work on cancer practised in the medical institutions the method of conversation seems to be the most promising between the physician or the nurse and the patient. In this case the educational work can be rendered very concrete because of the psychic condition of the patient who, as a rule, suffers of depression and awaiting calming. The discourse is also very important in communicating with the relatives of the patient who had been discharged from the hospital.

Among the group methods of the patients' education on cancer the most effective ones are the talks and reports completed by films, slides, tables, graphs and literature /e.g. dealing with the problems of correct nutrition, way of living, personal hygiene, hygiene of the environment both at home and at work, the hazards of smoking and alcohol consumption/ or judiciously selected leaflets, wall newspapers and posters. One of the purposes of the talks conducted in medical institutions consists in creating such an atmosphere which might induce the feeling in the patients that their health would benefit from hospital treatment. Medical workers should convince the patient that whatever is prescribed for him by the treating physicians is in his own interest and for his own good.

Among the many forms, the method of discourse word performed outside of the health institutions and oriented towards the healthy population is the most effective, especially those which rest upon the personal influence of the physicians and paramedical personnel. Very important form is the discussion organized in the form of questions and answers. This form can be applied in small groups of people which allow a close contact /employees of a factory, or other establishment, etc./. But in this case too, it is always necessary to find a correct way for explaining the problems and excluding scepticism and cancerophobia among the audience.

A less effective form of health education in oncology is the lecture, especially in a heterogenous group of listeners /age, sex, occupation/. The use of films and slides to accompany a verbal description is very important. These methods together with illustrated books and leaflets which briefly inform the reader, /e.g. on the first symptoms of the disease

or the methods of self-examination of the breast/ greatly facilitate the explanation of various problems and questions.

The experience suggests that the most efficient is the
selection of one question instead of many and leaving sufficient time for discussion. A film supplementing the material
offered by the lecture is shown before the discussion.

Presentation of films without an introduction or adequate
comments is not advised in the public education on cancer. An
exception in this respect are the films exhorting the audience
to attend the prophylactic examinations. Their considerable
mobilizing value is beyond any doubt.

The results of the research conducted by the Institutes
of Health Education in Prague and Bratislava in 1968-1975
demonstrated that in the general part of public education on
cancer emphasis should be oriented toward the increasing of the
basic knowledge of the population about cancer and its prevention, on the information concerning internal and external etio-
pathogenetic factors related to cancer and the legislative
measures leading to the elimination of carcinogenic factors
from out environment. The educational work should motivate the
population to seek medical aid in case of the appearance of
alarming symptoms.

Special emphasis is placed on familiarizing the population
with the exogenous factors which increase the risk of malignant tumours.

Especially important is the health education at certain
factories where the risk of occupational cancer is high and
where the absolute exclusion of harmful agents in the place
of work is not possible. In such situations the health education is obliged to find the right way between the present
state and the possibilities. It is very important in these
situations to orient the health education to the maximum use
of the methods of individual protection.

The verbal presentation is used successfully in fighting
against cancerophobia, incorrect views regarding the infectious
nature of cancer, its heredity and utilization of various
domestic means for its treatment. Information of the population

on the activities of the socialist health system in cancer control is also of great importance.

The remaining methods and forms of health education /printed material and visual methods/ including the mass media /press, radio, television/ also play their educational role. Campaign against cancer through the press is used on a wide scale; therefore, much attention is paid to achieving a high methodological level of the articles and the development of a close cooperation between the departments and institutes of health education and journalists. Apart from the newspapers, magazines and monthlies which have a country-wide circulation, the newspapers published on the district, town, and factory level are also involved in the health education of the population on cancer. Short articles by local, well-known physicians in the given district and use of the local experiences and materials can have an effective influence upon all groups of the population.

Radio broadcasts are used to inform the population about reliable, scientifically based and confirmed news in the fields of cancer diagnosis and treatment, the state of development of oncological assistance as well as for preparation of mass prophylactic measures. Special editorial boards of the Czechoslovakian Radio closely cooperate with the Ministry of Health and the Institutes of Health Education in preparing the detailed plans of radio programmes in the field of health and health protection. Brief reports through local factory broadcasting centres, especially in the period of preparing mass prophylactic examinations or health-improvement measures, are very efficient.

On the basis of an agreement between the Ministry of Health and the Czechoslovakian Television, public education through television has been increasing in the recent years. The oncological theme finds its place in special programmes and also in TV serials having attractive names /e.g. "School for Parents" or "School of Youth"/. These films are intended, after they are shown on TV, to be used in lectures and other kinds of health education. The advantage of telecasts consists in the fact that they offer a wide opportunity for various visual methods. The contact of the lecturer with his spectators by phone is very popular.

Fro a more effective utilization of the printed material and the visual methods in the fight against cancer it is arranged that the contents of the public educational booklets supplement the lecture and physicians or the nurse could distribute them immediately after the lecture. The same is valid on broad-sheets which are intended to inform the population on some selected questions /e.g. the broad-sheet, which contains information for women with regard to the importance and technique of self-examintion of the breast/. The broad-sheets can be used in special rooms of health education. Attendance of prophylactic examinations by the population can be also promoted by posters situated in places most frequented by the public. For this purpose, wall newspapers or exhibitions, which illustrate recent diagnostic and treatment methods and results achieved in the country or district in the control of malignant tumours, can also be successfully used.

Likewise, the courses for activists of the Czechoslovakian Red Cross can greatly contribute to the anti-cancer campaign.

It is the duty of all medical workers to carry out activities in cancer prevention. In cancer prevention the work of health organizations and services has a large ethical value and is also significant for the national economy. In this intensive fight for the health and prolonged longer life of people and for a further enhancement of trust of the entire population in the socialist health system, the educational work will always have an important place.

COORDINATION OF SCIENTIFIC RESEARCH ON THE PROBLEM
"SCIENTIFIC BASIS OF ORGANIZATION OF CANCER CONTROL

J.Somodi

Research in medicine, biology and other related fields has a relatively long tradition in our country. In the past studies and investigations connected with the problem of cancer were performed only occasionally and were dispersed in institutes and laboratories of various organizations /universities, industry, establishments and institutes of the Ministry of Health, Academy of Science, etc./. It was only in the recent years that the uniform organization and central coordination of medical research have been established by the creating the Council for Medical Research with a wide scope of activity and full competence.

Development of research in oncology in Czechoslovakia

Until the year 1950 the research in oncology was conducted only sporadically, mainly at the Oncological Institute in Brno and at some medical faculties. At those times excellent scientists worked in oncology in our country but without adequate research possibilities and conditions.

The year 1951 may be considered as the beginning of organization of oncological research in Czechoslovakia. In this year the Research Institute of Oncology was established in Bratislava by the decree of the Ministry of Health and the Headquarters of Medical Research of Czechoslovakia. This Institute consisted of experimental and clinical divisions and of the department for the organization and methodology. The experimental laboratories formed a considerable part in this newly created institute.

At the same time small experimental departments were constituted at the Institute of Oncology in Prague and Brno.

Various activities of scientific institutions which were created in those years became an integral part of cancer research. Among them the Research Institute of Pharmacology and Biochemistry in Prague started working on screening and synthesis of cytostatics, the Institute of Organic Chemistry and Biochemistry of the Czechoslovak Academy of Sciences in Prague initiated an intensive study on problems pertaining to the biochemistry of tumours with emphasis upon the possibilities of chemotherapy. Virology and immunology of tumours was the main research task of the Institute of Experimental Biology and Genetics in Prague.

In a number of university laboratories that declared their commitment to problems involved in cancer new research programmes were initiated already in the preceeding years.

The main efforts were directed towards the questions of biology, immunology, morphology and biochemistry of tumours, and other disciplines contributing to permanent and early diagnosis of tumours.

The initial difficulties caused by the insufficient number of well-experienced specialists in biochemistry, experimental biology and other related fields of science were relatively quickly surmounted by the aid of the leading institutions and suitable conditions have been established on a large scale for the organized and coordinated oncological research.

The actual structure of oncological research in Czechoslovakia

The research in oncology as well as in other fields of medicine and related areas in accomplished under three different organizational sections:
1. State plan of basic research
2. State plan of technical development
3. Research program in medicine and pharmacology

1. The state plan of basic research includes mainly fundamental, more or less theoretical, research projects; it is organized by the highest scientific institution in this country, the Czechoslovakian Academy of Sciences, and performed mainly in the particular institutes of this organization. Oncological research performed in the framework of this plan is included in the principal problem "Research in the Pathological Conditions of the Cell in Relation to the Malignant Growth". Chairman of the scientific council of the mentioned project is Academician V. Thurzo.

Five particular topics are investigated within the framework of this problem:

The study of the mechanism of the malignant transformation of the cell by oncogenic viruses containing RNA. The whole work on this topic is coordinated by the Institute of Experimental Oncology of the Slovak Academy of Sciences in Bratislava.

The study of the molecular nature of the cell transformation in animals. Particular investigations in this field are coordinated by the Scientific Research Institute of Experimental Biology and Genetics of the Czechoslovakian Academy of Sciences in Prague.

The function of the oncogenic viral genome in the cell and its regulation. This partial project is also coordinated by the above-mentioned institute in Prague.

Immunology of tumours. Coordinated also by the same institute in Prague.

Biology of the tumour cell and tumour growth. Individual parts of the research programme are coordinated by the Institute of Pathology of the Purkyně's University in Brno.

2. In the frame of the State plan for the development of the science and technics a special state program was established by the government for the 5-year-period 1976-1980 as "complex research of diseases caused by malignant growth". This plan is conducted and sponsored by the Ministry of Development of Science and Technics and enables to investigate a very wide spectrum of important problems in oncology, such as the etiology of tumours, and their prevention, and concentrates resources and efforts not only in the institutes and laboratories oriented to medical research but also in the research institutions of physics, chemistry, biochemistry, biology and ecology. The programme consists of eight particular sections /each section having numerous individual parts/:

Viral and chemical oncogenesis. The main executive organ is the Institute of Experimental Oncology of the Slovak Academy of Sciences in Bratislava.

Immunology of tumours. The main executive organ is the Institute of Molecular Genetics of the Czechoslovakian Academy of Sciences in Prague.

Diagnosis of tumours. The main executive organ is the Institute of Biophysics of the Faculty of General Medicine at the Charles University in Prague.

Experimental and clinical chemotherapy of tumours. The main executive organ is the Institute of Experimental Oncology of the Slovak Academy of Sciences in Bratislava.

Surgical and combined treatment of tumours. The main executive organ is the 2nd Department of Surgery of the Faculty of General Medicine at Charles University in Prague.

Radiotherapy_of_tumours. The main executive organ is the Institute of Clinical Oncology in Bratislava.

Epidemiology_of_malignant_neoplasms. The main executive organ is the Institute of Experimental Oncology of the Slovak Academy of Sciences in Bratislava.

Scientific_foundations_of_organization_of_cancer_control. The main executive organ is the radiotherapy department of the county hospital in České Budějovice.

3. Research programme for medicine and pharmacology is organized by the Ministry of Health of ČSR and SSR, separately in the two national republics but the common centres for some special problems in clinical oncology were established in various medical institutes, laboratories, hospitals and other establishments with a state-wide advisory competence. This research is oriented mainly to the actual problems of cancer diagnostics, treatment and control with very close relations to the practical application and use of the results. The research within this framework is coordinated and lead by the "Head board for problems in oncology" of the respective Ministries of Health.

Publication and circulation of results

The results of the studies and investigations obtained in oncology are regularly published in domestic or foreign scientific periodicals.

"Neoplasma", the only official international oncological journal in the socialist countries has its editorial board at the Institute of Experimental Oncology of the Slovak Academy of Sciences in Bratislava. "Neoplasma" publishes papers on experimental and clinical oncology, oncological statistics and reports in English from domestic and foreign institutes and reports on the results of the joint scientific programme relating to "Malignant Neoplasms" of the CMEA member-states.

In every third year the Institute of Experimental Oncology of the Slovak Academy of Sciences compiles a bibliography of papers originate in Czechoslovakia which contributes to the worldwide circulation of information about the activities of scientific workers of Czechoslovakia in experimental and clinical oncology.

Table 32

The Age - Sex Structure of the Population in Czechoslovakia in 1970 and 1974

Age groups	1 9 7 0			1 9 7 4		
	Men	Women	Total	Men	Women	Total
Total	6.983.458	7.350.158	14.333.616	7.155.000	7.531.000	14.686.000
0-4	549.819	524.340	1.074.159	626.000	599.000	1.225.000
5-9	559.097	534.784	1.093.881	551.000	528.000	1.079.000
10-14	587.618	564.975	1.152.593	554.000	526.000	1.080.000
15-19	655.259	630.039	1.285.298	614.000	587.000	1.201.000
20-24	628.404	610.657	1.239.061	657.000	629.000	1.286.000
25-29	512.989	504.483	1.017.472	601.000	585.000	1.186.000
30-34	418.880	417.199	836.079	484.000	479.000	963.000
35-39	443.484	446.923	890.407	402.000	408.000	810.000
40-44	465.214	480.756	945.970	444.000	454.000	898.000
45-49	473.259	508.552	981.811	449.000	478.000	927.000
50-54	269.290	291.993	561.283	444.000	487.000	931.000
55-59	400.708	443.166	843.874	245.000	278.000	523.000
60-64	377.270	433.207	810.477	377.000	439.000	816.000
65-69	289.917	369.042	658.959	310.000	389.000	699.000
70-74	185.376	281.483	466.869	214.000	311.000	525.000
75-79	98.697	173.006	271.703	114.000	204.000	318.000
80-84	46.940	90.301	137.241	48.000	101.000	149.000
85+	21.237	45.242	66.479	21.000	49.000	70.000

Table 33

Incidence of Malignant Neoplasms in Czechoslovakia /All Localizations Combined/ for the 1970-1974 Period

	Total population					Men					Women				
	1970	1971	1972	1973	1974	1970	1971	1972	1973	1974	1970	1971	1972	1973	1974
Absolute number	39.590	39.553	42.371	42.747	44.249	21.115	20.678	22.095	22.584	23.693	18.475	18.875	20.276	20.163	20.556
Per 100.000 population	276.20	274.87	292.93	293.59	301.30	302.36	294.97	313.60	318.43	331.14	251.36	255.77	273.30	269.99	272.95
Standardized rate	276.2	277.9	287.9	285.3	292.7	302.36	291.96	311.91	315.75	326.71	251.36	254.13	270.43	266.23	267.83

Table 34.1

Distribution of Patients with Malignant Neoplasms in Czechoslovakia by sites, for 1970 and 1974 Period

/ Men /

Localization	ICD /8th rev./ Code Number	1 9 7 0		1 9 7 4	
		Absolute number	per 100.000 population	Absolute number	per 100.000 population
All malignant neoplasms	140-209	21.115	299.21	23.693	331.2
Lip	140	449	6.36	417	1.8
Tongue	141	72	1.02	94	1.3
Salivary gland	142	63	0.89	64	0.9
Other parts of oral cavity	143-145	115	1.63	104	1.5
Pharynx	146-149	123	1.74	166	2.3
Oral and pharyngeal cavity	140-149	882	11.64	845	11.8
Esophagus	150	185	2.62	201	2.8
Stomach	151.0	238	3.37	251	3.5
Pylorus	151.1	458	6.49	347.	4.8
Other unspecified parts of stomach	151.8	699	9.90	959	13.4
Site unspecified	151.9	1.539	21.81	1.260	17.6
Small intestine	152	39	0.55	49	0.7
Large intestine, excluding rectum	153	844	11.96	998	13.9
Rectum	154	1.092	15.47	1.352	18.9

Site	Code				
Liver	155	345	4.89	377	5.3
Gallbladder and bile ducts	156	238	3.37	258	3.6
Pancreas	157	582	8.39	680	9.5
Peritoneum and unspecified digestive organs	158-159	202	2.86	209	3.0
Digestive organs and peritoneum	150-159	6.471	91.68	6.940	97.0
Nose, middle ear	160	54	0.77	46	0.7
Larynx	161	552	7.82	611	8.5
Trachea, bronchus, lung	162	5.218	73.94	6.081	85.0
Other and unspecified respiratory organs	163	136	1.93	131	1.8
Respiratory organs	160-163	5.960	84.46	6.869	96.0
Bone	170	123	1.74	117	1.6
Connective and other soft tissue	171	129	1.83	144	2.0
Melanoma of Skin	172	202	2.86	288	4.0
Other skin	173	1.386	19.64	3.168	44.3
Breast	174	45	0.64	37	0.6
Bone, connective tissue, skin, breast	170-174	1.885	26.71	3.754	52.5
Prostate	185	1.118	15.84	1.307	18.3
Testis	186	162	2.30	173	2.4
Other and unspecified male genital organs	187	93	1.32	66	0.9

34.2
/ Men /

Localization	ICD /8th rev/ Code Number	1 9 7 0		1 9 7 4	
		Absolute number	per 100.000 population	Absolute number	per 100.000 population
Urinary bladder	188	875	12.40	949	13.3
Other and unspecified Uro-poietic organs	189	512	7.26	540	7.5
Urinary and male genital organs	185–189	2.760	39.12	3.035	42.4
Eyes	190	52	0.74	61	0.9
Brain	191	282	4.00	309	4.3
Other parts of nervous system	192	36	0.51	46	0.6
Thyroid gland	193	65	0.92	60	0.9
Other endocrine glands	194	22	0.31	35	0.5
Ill defined sites	195–199	1.582	22.48	410	5.7
Other and unspecified sites	190–199	2.043	28.96	921	12.9
Lymphosarcoma and reticulum cell sarcoma	200	303	4.29	325	4.6
Hodgkin's disease	201	280	3.97	264	3.7
Other lymphoid tissue	202	36	0.51	66	0.9
Multiple myeloma	203	92	1.30	131	1.8

Lymphatic leukaemia, lymphadenosis	204	228	3.23	278	3.9
Myeloid leukaemia, myelosis myeloleukaemia	205	160	2.27	182	2.6
Monocytic leukaemia, monocytic leucosis	206	2	0.03	7	0.1
Other and unspecified leukaemia	207	40	0.57	49	0.7
Polycythemia ver, myelofibrosis	208-209	33	0.47	27	0.3
Lymphoid and haematopoietic tissue	200-209	1.174	16.64	1.929	18.6

Table 34.3

/ Women /

Localization	ICD /8th rev/ Code Number	1 9 7 0		1 9 7 4	
		Absolute number	per 100.000 population	Absolute number	per 100.000 population
All malignant neoplasms	140-209	18.475	249.32	20.556	272.9
Lip	140	71	0.96	63	0.9
Tongue	141	10	0.13	18	C.2
Salivary glands	142	63	0.85	63	0.8
Other parts of oral cavity	143-145	41	0.56	34	0.4
Pharynx	146-149	47	0.63	52	0.7
Oral and pharyngeal cavity	140-149	232	3.13	230	3.0
Esophagus	150	46	0.62	68	0.9
Stomach	151.0	74	1.00	120	1.6
Pylorus	151.1	329	4.44	257	3.4
Other unspecified parts of stomach	151.8	403	5.44	562	7.4
Site unspecified	151.9	1.150	15.52	886	11.8
Small intestine	152	36	0.49	43	0.6
Large intestine, excluding rectum	153	827	11.16	985	13.1
Rectum	154	843	11.38	999	13.3

Liver	155	265	3.58	267	3.5
Gallbladder and bile ducts	156	579	7.81	683	9.1
Pancreas	157	372	5.02	529	7.0
Peritoneum and retroperitoneal tissue and Unspecified digestive organs	158–159	313	4.22	304	4.0
Digestive organs and peritoneum	150–159	5.237	70.68	5.703	75.7
Nose, nasal cavities, middle ear and accessory sinuses	160	43	0.58	44	0.6
Larynx	161	32	0.43	33	0.4
Trachea, bronchus and lung	162	536	7.23	561	7.5
Other and unspecified respiratory organs	163	71	0.96	79	1.0
Respiratory organs	160–163	682	9.20	717	9.5
Bone	170	95	1.28	90	1.2
Connective and other soft tissue	171	98	1.32	104	1.4
Melanoma os skin	172	213	2.87	296	3.9
Other skin	173	1.366	18.43	3.256	43.2
Breast	174/1	404	5.45	529	7.0
	172/2	504	6.80	704	9.5
	174/3	482	6.50	552	7.3
	174/4	220	2.97	206	2.7
	174/9	1.164	15.71	1.249	16.6

Table 34.4

/ Women /

Localization	ICD /8th rev/ Code Number	1970		1974	
		Absolute number	per 100.000 population	Absolute number	per 100.000 population
Bone, connective tissue, skin and breast	170-174	4.546	61.33	6.986	92.8
Cervix uteri	180/0	123	1.66	128	1.7
	180/1	430	5.80	414	5.5
	180/2	405	5.47	445	5.9
	180/3	384	4.78	310	4.1
	180/4	74	1.0	76	1.0
	180/9	309	4.17	218	2.9
Chorionepithelioma	181	18	0.24	8	0.1
Other uterus	182/0	826	11.15	934	12.4
	182/1	157	2.12	251	3.3
Multiple myeloma	203	83	1.12	137	1.8
Lymphatic leukaemia, lympha- denosis, lymphoid leucosis	204	125	1.69	194	2.6
Myeloid leukaemia, myelosis myeloleukaemia	205	154	2.08	163	2.2

Monocytic leukaemia monocytic leucosis	206	4	0.05	3	0.0
Other unspecified leukaemia leucoses	207	36	0.49	45	0.6
Polycythaemia vera and Pyelofibrosis	208-209	19	0.26	23	0.3
Lymphoid and haematopoietic tissue	200-209	841	11.37	1.076	14.3

Incidence of Malignant Neoplasms in Czechoslovakia and its

for 1970

Counties (administrative regions)	140-209 Sites Combined		140-149 Oral cavity and pharyngeal cavity		150-159 Digestive organs and peritoneum	
	m	w	m	w	m	w
1 9 7 0						
Czechoslovakia whole	299.2	249.3	11.65	3.13	91.70	70.67
CSSR /whole/	329.3	273.1	9.22	3.15	99.79	78.04
Prague /capital/	222.7	232.6	8.70	3.92	48.71	41.40
Middle Bohemian	313.8	253.8	7.94	3.55	91.70	72.34
Southern "	440.8	330.6	10.29	2.67	134.99	111.99
Western "	416.9	347.4	14.18	1.30	130.47	95.94
	337.6	260.2	7.93	3.60	98.55	72.52
Northern "	281.6	220.7	10.17	2.63	77.40	52.68
Eastern "	321.9	265.7	9.79	2.56	97.73	75.31
Southern Moravian	440.9	406.4	5.61	1.68	165.66	134.52
	365.2	297.9	12.84	3.63	120.38	92.37
Northern "	412.9	283.9	7.27	2.07	129.42	88.41
	319.1	278.0	6.41	3.33	100.80	86.91
SSR /whole/	234.8	196.7	16.85	3.08	74.41	54.36
Bratislava /Capital/	259.8	253.9	12.03	3.20	75.03	57.88
Western Slovakia	234.7	193.7	15.63	1.84	75.23	55.44
Middle "	242.6	204.03	18.77	3.53	76.08	55.27
Eastern "	220.6	178.1	17.34	4.13	71.32	51.11

Administrative Regions /Countries/ by Localization and Sex
and 1974

160-163 Respiratory organs		174-189 The breast, urinary and genital organs		170-173 Neoplasms of bone and soft tissues, melano-ma, the skin 190-199 Unspecified sites		200-209 Lymphoid and haematopoietic tissues	
m	w	m	w	m	w	m	w

1 9 7 0

84.46	9.20	39.75	101.41	55.02	53.55	16.64	11.35
99.06	9.52	43.25	111.92	60.04	57.94	17.99	12.52
70.56	8.52	27.84	122.16	56.83	52.30	10.05	4.26
106.38	7.27	46.28	118.53	50.25	44.08	11.23	8.07
142.16	10.40	55.49	114.07	78.87	68.92	19.02	22.58
143.23	10.37	39.71	168.54	75.16	60.93	14.18	10.37
123.47	9.96	37.95	111.54	47.29	49.54	22.37	13.01
105.19	6.85	29.07	110.63	43.60	37.75	16.17	10.18
91.04	6.41	46.21	112.96	58.57	18.55	11.70	11.70
108.36	17.94	56.05	156.94	83.45	80.15	21.80	15.13
92.67	12.82	52.12	100.95	65.72	75.56	21.48	12.57
111.79	11.05	48.72	93.25	80.71	63.55	29.08	25.56
81.97	10.13	44.19	97.55	64.75	62.94	20.96	17.18
53.25	8.50	32.27	78.14	44.32	43.82	13.74	8.76
58.04	7.23	42.47	128.25	57.33	46.04	14.86	11.18
54.69	7.01	31.13	78.67	46.25	43.02	11.72	7.74
55.16	8.18	33.10	79.67	43.13	48.08	16.33	9.59
48.14	11.11	30.47	63.64	40.20	39.52	13.13	8.57

Table 35 /cont'd/

Counties (administrative regions)	140-209 Sites Combined		140-149 Oral cavity and pharyngeal cavity		150-159 Digestive organs and peritoneum	
	m	w	m	w	m	w

1 9 7 4

Czechoslovakia whole	331.2	272.9	11.8	3.0	97.0	75.7
CSSR /whole/	372.3	307.9	10.0	2.9	107.7	86.2
Prague	357.8	351.2	7.2	3,7	101.8	77.5
Middle Bohemian	341.8	287.2	9.3	3.3	90.7	79.5
Southern "	451.9	352.5	14.2	2.1	133.4	115.9
Western Bohemian	377.1	283.1	10.1	2.0	99.3	76.9
Northern "	317.4	254.9	10.9	3.1	89.8	67.0
Eastern "	330.4	283.0	11.1	1.3	88.9	76.7
Southern Moravia	417.9	338.0	9.7	3.8	127.1	99.0
Northern "	381.4	304.6	9.5	2.5	119.0	93.8
SSR /whole/	245	197.1	15.7	3.5	74.5	53.1
Bratislava	280.0	11.4	11.4	2.3	93.1	83.6
Western Slovakia	266.3	213.2	17.6	4.4	78.2	54.3
Middle "	255.9	188.7	13.4	2.8	78.2	53.3
Eastern "	197.8	154.9	17.0	3.5	61.3	43.4

160-163 Respiratory organs		174-189 The breast, urinary and genital organs		170-173 Neoplasms of bone and soft tissues, melanoma, the skin 190-199 Unspecified sites		200-209 Lymphoid and haematopoietic tissues	
m	w	m	w	m	w	m	w

1 9 7 4

m	w	m	w	m	w	m	w
96.0	9.5	43.0	108.2	64.8	62.2	18.6	14.3
113.1	10.7	48.5	123.3	72.6	68.7	20.4	16.1
108.6	15.9	48.0	170.1	75.2	72.7	17.0	12.3
114.4	8.0	53.2	129.8	60.1	52.7	14.1	13.9
135.0	13.5	58.1	118.6	83.4	75.3	27.8	27.1
147.0	11.1	41.6	125.3	59.3	53.8	19.8	14.0
112.8	8.4	34.5	116.1	55.8	48.8	13.6	11.5
92.6	8.7	42.3	111.5	76.0	72.4	19.5	12.4
116.7	10.9	57.5	117.1	82.3	86.0	24.6	21.2
101.0	11.2	48.7	108.3	78.9	71.8	24.3	17.0
60.2	6.9	31.4	75.5	48.5	47.9	14.7	10.2
67.2	12.9	29.1	125.7	60.8	79.5	18.4	14.0
64.5	6.8	33.0	86.9	56.8	50.2	16.2	10.6
68.6	6.6	32.5	714	46.5	45.7	16.7	8.9
43.9	5.6	28.6	52.8	37.2	39.3	9.8	10.3

Table 36

Incidence of Malignant Neoplasms in Czechoslovakia all Localization Combined by Age and Sex for 1970 and 1974

Age groups	1970 Men		1970 Women		1974 Men		1974 Women	
	Absolute number	per 100.000 population	Absolute number	per 100.000 population	Absolute number	per 100.000 population	Absolute number	per 100.000 population
Total	21.115	302.36	18.475	251.36	23.693	331.14	20.556	272.9
0-4	69	12.55	60	11.44	77	12.30	53	8.8
5-9	55	9.84	38	7.11	57	10.34	51	9.66
10-14	57	9.70	53	9.38	50	9.03	53	10.08
15-19	97	14.80	79	12.54	91	14.82	84	14.31
20-24	147	23.39	129	21.12	139	21.16	105	16.69
25-29	140	27.29	172	34.09	155	25.79	201	34.36
30-34	203	48.46	288	69.03	246	50.8	133	69.5
35-39	365	82.30	507	113.44	314	78.1	484	118.6
40-44	660	141.87	968	201.35	692	155.9	899	198.0
45-49	1.209	255.46	1.551	304.98	1.222	272.2	1.482	310.0
50-54	1.120	415.91	1.144	391.79	2.128	479.0	2.023	415.4
55-59	2.580	643.86	2.139	482.66	1.766	741	1.435	516
60-64	3.692	978.61	2.592	598.33	3.869	1.026	2.812	641
65-69	4.223	1.456	2.831	767.12	4.571	1.475	3.171	815
70-74	3.389	1.828.18	2.675	950.25	4.377	2.045	3.210	1.032
75-79	1.914	1.939.27	1.827	1.056.03	2.493	2.190	2.348	1.151
80+	1.195	1.752.79	1.422	1.049.11	1.445	2.090	1.811	1.207

Table 37

Mortality from Malignant Neoplasms in Czehoslovakia for the
1970 - 1973 Period

Y e a r s		Number of deaths from malignant neoplasms		
		M e n	W o m e n	Total population
1970	Absolute number	17.919	13.510	31.429
	Per 100.000 populations	256.59	183.81	219.27
1971	Absolute number	18.507	13.896	32.403
	Per 100.000 population	264.00	188.30	225.18
1972	Absolute number	18.323	14.277	32.600
	Per 100.000 population	260.06	192.44	225.38
1973	Absolute number	18.732	14.124	32.856
	Per 100.000 population	264.12	189.13	225.66

Table 38

Mortality from Malignant Neoplasms in Czechoslovakia and its Administrative Regions, for the 1970 - 1972 Period

Countries Administrative Regions	1 9 7 0		1 9 7 1		1 9 7 2	
	Absolute number	per 100.000 population	Absolute number	per 100.000 population	Absolute number	per 100.000 population
Czechoslovakia /whole/	31.429	219.27	32.403	225.18	32.600	225.38
Czechoslovakia /whole/	24.487	249.74	25.167	256.01	25.237	255.74
Prague /Capital/	3.612	335.32	3.426	316.64	3.568	328.78
Middle Bohemia	3.571	299.39	3.799	319.36	3.598	302.56
Southern Bohemia	1.789	274.23	1.786	273.36	1.788	272.71
Western Bohemia	2.137	252.09	2.098	246.37	2.129	248.81
Northern Bohemia	2.459	223.32	2.623	237.48	2.693	242.82
Eastern Bohemia	3.089	256.91	3.242	269.55	3.216	266.70
Southern Moravian	4.335	223.84	4.494	231.87	4.564	234.62
Northern Moravian	3.495	194.71	3.699	204.51	3.681	201.98
SSR-/whole/	6.942	153.30	7.236	158.71	7.363	160.19
Bratislava /Capital/	483	171.33	580	137.53	585	185.74
Western Slovakian	2.868	179.79	2.995	188.96	2.954	185.28
Middle Slovakian	1.995	142.50	2.002	142.28	2.082	146.96
Eastern Slovakian	1.596	127.54	1.659	131.88	1.742	137.13

Table 39

Mortality from Malignant Neoplasms in Czechoslovakia by Age and Sex for 1970 and 1973

Age groups	1970				1973			
	Men		Women		Men		Women	
	Absolute number	per 100.000 population	Absolute number	per 100.000 population	Absolute number	per 100.000 population	Absolute number	per 100.000 population
Total	17.919	256.59	13.510	183.81	18.732	264.12	14.124	189.13
0-4	61	11.09	40	7.63	52	8.75	48	8.48
5-9	43	7.69	29	5.42	49	8.71	32	5.98
10-14	26	4.42	42	7.43	46	8.41	22	4.23
15-19	61	9.31	35	5.56	59	9.33	50	8.26
20-24	84	13.37	48	7.86	74	11.33	42	6.70
25-29	77	15.01	58	11.50	85	14.61	79	13.87
30-34	109	26.02	99	23.73	115	24.98	126	27.48
35-39	186	41.94	183	40.95	164	40.64	166	40.56
40-44	353	75.88	414	86.11	395	87.34	358	77.07
45-49	753	159.1	663	131.4	765	168.16	621	127.2
50-54	734	272.6	587	201.0	1.207	296.2	935	208.4
55-59	1.974	492.6	1.376	310.5	1.389	504.0	950	308.0
60-64	3.074	814.8	1.808	417.4	3.055	199.0	1.878	425.4
65-69	3.775	1.302	2.121	574.7	3.767	1.250	2.271	596.0
70-74	3.240	1.748	2.337	830.2	3.697	1.778	2.486	813.8
75-79	1.996	2.022	1.899	1.098	2.303	2.129	2.174	1.103
80-84	973	2.073	1.143	1.266	1.068	2.298	1.248	1.297
85+	400	1.884	623	1.377	442	2.139	638	1.359

Mortality from Malignant Neoplasms /Groups/ in Czechoslovakia
     / M e n /

Age groups	140-209 All sites		140-149 Oral cavity and pharyngeal cavity		150-159 Digestive organs and peritoneum		160-163 Respiratory organs	
	Absolute number	per 100.000 population	Absolute number	per 100.000 population	Absolute number	per 100.000 population	Absolute number	per 100.000 population
Total	18.732	264.12	302	4.26	7.164	101.01	6.606	93.14
0-4	52	8.75	-	-	2	-	-	-
5-9	49	8.71	-	-	-	-	-	-
10-14	46	8.41	-	-	-	-	-	-
15-19	59	9.33	-	-	6	-	1	-
20-24	74	11.33	2	-	4	-	2	-
25-29	85	14.61	2	-	15	2.58	2	-
30-34	115	24.98	-	-	27	5.87	17	-
35-39	164	40.64	7	-	48	11.89	44	10.90
40-44	395	87.34	15	3.32	116	25.65	126	27.86
45-49	765	168.16	14	3.08	251	55.17	294	64.63
50-54	1.207	296.2	29	7.12	403	98.90	459	112.6
55-59	1.389	504.0	25	9.07	503	182.5	564	204.7
60-64	3.055	799.0	47	12.29	1.136	297.1	1.233	322.5
65-69	3.767	1.250	49	16.26	1.469	287.4	1.477	490.1
70-74	3.697	1.778	50	24.05	1.458	701.2	1.376	661.8
75-79	2.303	2.129	26	24.04	1.008	931.8	708	654.5
80-84	1.068	2.298	25	53.79	509	1.095	228	490.6
85+	442	2.139	11	53.23	209	1.011	75	362.9

by Age and Sex for the year 1973

170-174 Bone, connective tissue, skin, breast		180-189 Urinary and genital organs		190-199 Other and unspecified sites		200-209 Lymphoid and haematopoietic tissues	
Absolute number	per 100.000 population	Absolute number	per 100.000 population	Absolute number	per 100.000 population	Absolute number	per 100.000 population
443	6.25	2.250	31.73	880	12.41	1.087	15.33
3	-	11	1.85	15	2.53	21	3.54
3	-	-	-	17	3.02	29	5.15
2	-	1	-	19	3.48	24	4.39
6	-	6	-	15	2.37	25	3.95
11	1.68	17	2.60	7	-	31	4.74
11	1.89	17	2.92	15	2.58	23	3.95
16	3.48	12	2.61	17	3.69	26	5.65
6	-	14	3.47	23	5.70	22	5.45
24	5.31	30	6.63	41	9.07	43	9.51
31	6.81	58	12.75	53	11.65	64	14.07
54	13.25	100	24.54	84	20.62	78	19.14
18	6.53	124	45.00	78	28.31	77	27.94
51	13.34	285	74.54	144	37.66	159	41.59
61	20.24	402	133.4	142	47.12	167	55.11
69	33.18	481	231.3	118	56.75	145	69.73
30	27.73	382	353.1	56	51.77	93	85.97
26	55.94	209	449.7	23	49.49	48	103.3
21	101.6	101	488.7	13	62.91	12	58.07

Table 40 /cont'd/   /Women/

Age groups	140-209 All sites		140-149 Oral cavity and pharyngeal cavity		150-159 Digestive organs and peritoneum		160-163 Respiratory organs	
	Absolute number	per 100.000 population	Absolute number	per 100.000 population	Absolute number	per 100.000 population	Absolute number	per 100.000 population
Total	14.124	189.13	83	1.11	6.748	86.74	788	10.55
0-4	48	8.48	-	-	4	-	4	-
5-9	32	5.98	-	-	-	-	-	-
10-14	22	4.23	-	-	-	-	-	-
15-19	50	8.26	-	-	3	-	2	-
20-24	42	6.70	-	-	2	-	2	-
25-29	79	13.87	1	-	13	2.28	3	-
30-34	126	27.48	2	-	26	5.67	6	-
35-39	166	40.56	-	-	26	6.35	8	-
40-44	358	77.07	4	-	82	17.65	20	-
45-49	621	172.2	4	-	151	30.94	34	6.97
50-54	935	208.4	1	-	281	62.64	56	12.48
55-59	950	308.0	2	-	354	114.8	56	18.15
60-64	1.878	425.4	10	2.27	809	183.3	114	25.82
65-69	2.271	596.0	9	-	1.071	281.1	134	35.17
70-74	2.486	813.8	22	7.20	1.306	427.5	147	48.12
75-79	2.174	1.103	10	5.08	1.241	629.9	120	60.91
80-84	1.248	1.297	6	-	728	756.7	61	63.41
85+	638	1.359	12	25.57	381	811.8	24	51.13

170-174 Bone, connective tissue, skin, breast		180-189 Urinary and genital organs		190-199 Other and unspecified sites		200-209 Lymphoid and hematopoietic tissues	
Absolute number	per 100.000 population	Absolute number	per 100.000 population	Absolute number	per 100.000 population	Absolute number	per 100.000 population
2.194	29.38	2.827	37.85	825	11.05	929	12.44
1	-	7	-	14	2.47	21	3.71
2	-	5	-	11	2.06	14	2.62
2	-	2	-	8	-	10	1.92
8	-	6	-	11	1.82	20	3.30
7	-	4	-	8	-	19	3.03
15	2.63	14	2.46	7	-	26	4.57
26	5.67	33	7.20	9	-	24	5.23
47	11.48	49	11.97	16	3.91	20	4.89
96	20.67	102	21.96	21	4.52	33	7.10
159	32.57	187	38.31	35	7.17	51	10.45
232	51.72	252	56.18	65	14.49	48	10.70
180	58.35	252	81.69	58	18.80	48	15.56
342	77.47	402	91.07	94	21.29	107	24.24
295	77.42	487	127.8	125	32.81	150	39.37
300	98.20	438	134.4	137	44.85	136	44.52
242	122.8	337	171.1	104	52.79	120	60.91
147	152.8	184	191.3	61	63.41	61	63.41
93	198.1	66	140.6	21	87.35	21	44.74

Table 41.1

Mortality from Malignant Neoplasms in Czechoslovakia by Selected Localizations and Sex for 1970 and 1973

Localization	ICD/8th rev. Code number	1970				1973			
		Men		Women		Men		Women	
		Absolute number	per 100.000 population	Absolute number	per 100.000 population	Absolute number	per 100.000 population	Absolute number	per 100.000 population
All malignant neoplasms	140-209	17.919	256.59	13.510	183.81	18.732	264.12	14.124	189.1
Oral and pharyngeal cavity	140-149	288	4.12	104	1.41	302	4.26	83	1.11
Lip	140	39	0.56	9		36	0.51	6	
Tongue	141	45	0.64	10	0.14	58	0.82	8	
Salivary gland	142	25	0.36	20	0.27	27	0.38	17	0.23
Other parts of oral cavity	143-145	75	1.00	32	0.34	84	1.10	26	0.19
Pharynx	146-149	103	1.47	44	0.48	97	1.37	26	0.19
Digestive organs and peritoneum	150-159	7.251	103.83	6.241	85.32	7.164	101.01	6.478	86.7
Esophagus	150	210	3.01	70	0.95	234	3.30	63	0.84
Stomach	151	3.339	47.81	2.370	32.34	3.107	43.81	2.294	30.7
Small intestine	152	50	0.72	39	0.53	49	0.69	40	0.54

Large intestine excluding rectum	153	707	10.12	783	10.65	879	12.39	928	12.43
Rectum and rectosigmoid junction	154	988	14.15	776	10.56	1.083	15.27	847	11.34
Liver	155	583	8.35	530	7.21	506	7.13	451	6.04
Gallbladder and bile ducts	156	230	3.29	621	8.45	261	3.68	734	9.83
Pancreas	157	671	9.61	466	6.34	637	8.98	547	7.32
Peritoneum and retro-peritoneal tissue and unspecified digestive organs	158–159	473	6.77	616	8.38	408	5.75	574	7.68
Respiratory organs	160–163	105	87.42	763	10.38	6.606	93.14	788	10.55
Nose, nasal cavities middle ear	160	30	0.43	21	0.29	25	0.35	23	0.31
Larynx	161	313	4.48	24	0.33	382	5.39	31	0.42
Trachea, bronchus and lung	162	5.599	80.18	659	8.97	5.861	82.64	650	8.70
Other and unspecified respiratory organs	163	163	2.33	59	0.80	338	4.77	84	1.12
Bone, connective tissue, skin and breast	170–174	384	5.50	54	27.94	443	6.25	2.194	29.38
Bone	170	151	2.16	132	1.80	148	2.09	107	1.43
Connective and other soft tissue	171	47	0.67	35	0.48	64	0.90	48	0.64
Melanoma of skin	172	97	1.39	90	1.22	125	1.76	93	1.25
Other skin	173	77	1.10	85	1.16	79	1.11	84	1.12

Table 41.2

Localization	ICD /8th rev. Code number	1970				1973			
		Men		Women		Men		Women	
		Absolute number	per 100.000 population	Absolute number	per 100.000 population	Absolute number	per 100.000 population	Absolute number	per 100.000 population
Breast	174	12	0.17	712	23.29	27	0.38	1.862	24.93
Genitourinary organs	180–189	2.009	28.77	720	37.01	2.250	31.73	2.827	37.85
Cervix uteri	180	–	–	553	7.52	–	–	550	7.36
Chorinoepithelioma	181	–	–	11	0.15	–	–	9	.
Other uterus	182	–	–	691	9.40	–	–	688	9.21
Ovary, fallopian tubes and broad ligament	183	–	–	788	10.72	–	–	840	11.25
Other and unspecified female genital organs	184	–	–	268	3.65	–	–	273	3.66
Prostate	185	848	12.14	–	–	955	13.47	–	–
Testis	186	79	1.13	–	–	76	1.07	–	–
Other and unspecified male genital organs	187	68	0.97	–	–	58	0.82	–	–
Urinary bladder	188	526	7.53	138	1.88	549	7.74	167	2.24
Other and unspecified uropoietic organs	189	488	6.99	271	3.69	612	8.63	300	4.02
Other and unspecified sites	190–199	757	10.84	805	10.95	880	12.41	825	11.05

Site	ICD	Count	%	Count	%	Count	%	Count	%
Eyes	190	19	0.27	21	0.29	24	0.34	17	0.23
Brain	191	293	4.20	264	3.59	313	4.41	186	2.49
Other parts of nervous system	192	55	0.79	47	0.64	76	1.07	46	0.62
Thyroid gland	193	37	0.53	106	1.44	48	0.68	126	1.69
Other endocrine glands	194	27	0.39	22	0.30	37	0.52	26	0.35
Ill defined sites	199	326	4.53	345	4.45	382	5.36	424	5.65
Lymphoid and haemato-poietic tissue	200-209	1.125	16.11	793	10.79	1.087	15.33	929	12.44
Lymphosarcoma and reti-culum-cell sarcoma	200	189	2.71	126	1.71	196	2.76	131	1.75
Hodgkin disease	201	241	3.45	133	1.81	183	2.58	141	1.89
Other lymphoid tissue	202	51	0.73	36	0.49	40	0.56	51	0.68
Multiplemyeloma	203	90	1.29	85	1.16	102	1.44	127	1.70
Lymphatic leukaemia, lymphoid leucosis, lymphadenosis	204	280	4.01	171	2.33	299	4.22	211	2.83
Myeloid leukaemia, myelo-sis, myeloleukaemia	205	153	2.19	155	2.11	160	2.26	174	2.33
Monocytic leukaemia, monocytic leucosis	206	5		6		4		5	
Other and unspecified leukaemia	207	91	1.30	66	0.90	79	1.11	71	0.95
Polycythemia vera and Myelofibrosis	208-209	25	0.36	15	0.16	24	0.34	18	0.17

225

REFERENCES

1. Jak dále v boji zhoubným nádorum. /How to continue the battle against malignant tumours./ Dvorák, V., Avicenum, Praha 1970, 1-123 p.

2. Organizace boje proti zhuobným nádorum. /Organization of fight against malignant tumours./ Dvorák, V. and Vadura, F., State Health Edit., Praha 1955, 1-73 p.

3. Komplexni ochrana před rakovinou děložního hrdla. /Complex protection against cancer of the uterine cervix./ Kaňka, J., Avicenum, Praha 1978, 1-257 p.

4. Náš boj proti rakovine. /Our battle against cancer./ Edit. Fremmer, J.E., Institute of Health Education, Bratislava 1974, 1-134 p.

5. Nádory dětského věku. /Tumours in childhood/. Koutecky, J., Avicenum, Praha 1978, 1-552 p.

6. Linická onkológia. /Clinical oncology./ Edit. Manka, I., Osveta. Martin 1979, 1-688 p.

7. Problémy klinickej a experimentalnej onkológie. /Problems of clinical and experimental oncology./ Edit. Thurzo, V., Publishing House of the Slovak Academy of Sciences, Bratislava 1962, 1-294 p.

CANCER CONTROL IN THE
GERMAN DEMOCRATIC REPUBLIC

H. Herold

GEOGRAPHICAL, ECONOMIC AND DEMOGRAPHIC
CHARACTERISTICS OF THE COUNTRY

The German Democratic Republic /GDR/ occupies an area of 108,174 sq. km, its population is about 17 million. The density of population is 150 persons per square kilometre on an average. The capital of the GDR, the city of Berlin, has over 1 million inhabitants. The population of the GDR is uniform by its national composition. There is a significant irregularity in the territorial distribution of population. The highest density of population is observed in industrial regions /the so-called zones of concentration/ such as Karl-Marx-Stadt, Dresden, Leipzig, Halle, and Berlin, the capital of the GDR; the lowest density of population is in the northern administrative areas /Neubrandenburg and Schwerin/; 73.2 % of the population live in small towns with the number of inhabitants over 2,000, of these 23 % reside in 14 big cities where population exceeds 100,000. The sex and age distribution of the population is deformed first of all as a result of the Second World War. Women account 53.9 %, men for 46.1 % of the population. 57.8 per cent of the population is in the working age. 19.5 % of the population are in the pensionable age and 22.6 % are children.

78.7 per cent of people in the working age work /without taking into account apprentices/; women amount to 48.3 % of the persons engaged in production. 74.8 per cent of women of working age work.

Two thirds of the territory of the GDR is occupied by a lowland situated in the north of the country adjoined by mountains of medium height in the south. The country is for the most part slightly broken or hilly, it has rather monotonous plains and wide lakes. A number of islands is located in the coastal region of the Baltic sea. The coastline is winding with numerous bays and regions of steep shore and extending to the east by a strip of sandy beach. In the south, a belt of intensive agriculture is stretching along the ridge of mountains of middle-height.

The region of mountains of middle-height includes the Harz, the Thüringer Wald, the Frankenwald, the Thüringian basin, the Erzgebirge, the sandy mountains along the Elbe and the Lausitz mountains.

Climate

The GDR is situated in the temperate zone and due to the influence of the Gulf Stream has a humid changeable climate intermediate between maritime and continental. It is manifested by the time of the setting in of spring: with the increase of latitude by 1 degree /from south to north/ or the height of the land by 100 metres the spring sets in 4 days later, while the increase of longitude by 1 degree /from west to east/ 1 day later.

In the eastern regions the climate is of the most pronounced continental character: the summer is warmer, the winter is colder. The winter temperatures decrease from the west toward the east in inverse relation to the summer temperatures.

A typical feature is the change of high pressure characteristic for all seasons when a warm dry air penetrates from the east and the southeast in summer, and a cold and dry air from the polar regions in winter; the rather frequent cyclones, together with depression moving to the east, bring masses of the Atlantic humid air causing a cool weather in summer and a relatively mild weather in winter, often with abundant rainfall. Precipitation falls in each season and amounts to approximately 600-700 mm /summer maximum/. The solid blanket of snow persists in winter only after the invasion of masses of cold air whereas at the height over 500 m it remains longer. The main temperature lowers with the increase in the relief height.

In winter this difference amounts to 0.3°C-0.5°C, in summer 0.5°C-0.7°C in every 100 metres.

Rainfall is most abundant on the western sides of mountains in the prevailing western winds at all seasons. Only some mountains exceed the height of 1,000 m.

The main rivers flowing along the territory of the GDR are the Elbe with its tributaries and the Oder. Dams are built on these rivers which serve the aims of providing drinking and technical water and also electric power. Navigable regions of the rivers are connected by canals /the Mid-German Canal, the canals Oder-Hafel and Oder-Spree/ with lowland lakes of glacial origin /the Mecklenburg lake region with the largest lake of Müritz having an area of 116.8 sq km and a depth of 33 m/. Mineral springs are at health resorts Elster, Liebenstein and Brambach, salt springs at health resorts Salzungen, Dürrenberg and Frankenhausen, and also at health resort Köthen. Soils are different both in minerals and fertility: the lowland has podzolic and marshy soils. Along the ridge of middle-height mountains a strip of fertile loessial soils stretches, on the middle-height mountains there are forests and stony soils. The initial forest area became reduced and at present occupies about 27 % of the whole territory of the country; these are mainly pine, spruce and deciduous forests, for the most part in monocultures. On middle-height mountains meadows are used as pasture lands. Waste lands and peat-bogs formed on the place of glacial sediment are for the most part cultivated.

The animal life has changed in favour of forest-steppe and steppe species such as hare, rabbit, hamster, which is related to the reduction of wooded areas and to industrialization; deer, roe, wild-boar, foxes and badgers were preserved. Water birds were ousted to the seashore and lakes. Fish considerably reduced in number.

The GDR is a state with a highly developed industry and a highly productive collectivized agriculture. The GDR holds the fifth place in Europe in the industrial output. The leading branches of industry are chemical industry, processing of crude oil, metal-working industry, electrotechnics, electronics,

229

mechanical engineering, production of apparatuses for research, electrical engineering, transport. Agriculture has been gradually transferred on an industrial basis /concerning organization and leadership/. Chemical industry accounts for 17.3 % of the total industrial production, of great importance are machinery, precision machines, optical instruments, production of electric apparatuses and textile industry. In the mining industry, lignite production plays a leading role, it constitutes 35 % of the world production. In addition to this there are deposits of rock salt and potash salt. Further, worth mining are deposits of iron ore, copper slate, non-ferrous metals, uranium, limestone, chalk, gypsum, and natural oilstone. 90 % of the power system management is based on brown coal. In addition, there are hydroelectric power plants and atomic power stations. Ships of various categories are built at shipyards.

Mainly rye, oats, wheat, barley, potatoe, sugar beet, vegetables and fruit are cultivated, with the areas alloted for grain crops being reduced in favour of fodder crops. Cattle is bred mainly in the north of the GDR, pig-breeding is developed in the central part of the country and in the south.

The transport system is characterized by a dense railway and road network. Navigable waterways amount to 2,519 km. The density of railways with the railway track being 14,658 km is 13.6 km per 10 sq. In the south the density of railways is much greater than in the north. There are more than 45,729 km of roads, of these motorways constitute 1,464 km and international highways 11,000 km.

The "Interflug" Airline Company has seven airports of which the central airport Berlin-Schönefeld is the biggest one.

Health service in the GDR

The system of public health and welfare of the GDR has a territorial structure. There are 224 regions in the GDR. The regional Council and the chief physician of the region who is a member of the regional Council are made responsible for the state of public health service in the region.

The methodological guidance is carried out by the chief physician of the administrative area /there are altogether 15

230

areas in the GDR/ who in his turn is subordinated to the Ministry of Health. As a rule, in every region there are one or two hospitals, several polyclinics and out-patient clinics. In addition, out-patient stations are set up at industrial enterprises; their tasks are to solve not only the problems of labour hygiene but to a certain extent the problems of medical service for the adjoining region as well. Special medical stations were set up at each large and middle industrial enterprises of the GDR. Altogether 81 large factory polyclinics and 212 factory out-patient clinics function, with 2,980 doctors, nurses and attendants. The personnel of these stations is responsible first of all for the organization of labour conditions in order to meet the requirements of hygiene, for a qualified first aid and for regular preventive examinations of the employees. They keep workers exposed to agents under constant medical supervision thus contributing to a considerable decrease in the rate of morbidity at enterprises.

In the public health system of the GDR a particular importance is attached to the preventive medical service of the rising generation of working people at enterprises as well as of elderly persons.

Among numerous measures, of particular significance are the regular preventive vaccinations against small pox, tuberculosis, diphtheria, pertussis, tetanus, poliomyelitis, measles and other infectious diseases. As a consequence poliomyelitis has been almost completely eliminated. Diphtheria has become a rare disease. Children and young people virtually do not die any longer from tuberculosis.

Systematic preventive examinations of the population play also an important part. They promote a timely diagnosis and treatment of such diseases as tuberculosis, cardiovascular diseases, diabetes, cancer, and others.

There are almost 2,000 pharmancies for providing the population with drugs. Some 330,000 courses of treatment, of these 200,000 sanatorium courses, are conducted at 192 sanatoriums and holiday homes; annually 5,500 patients undergo sanatorium treatment abroad, mainly in socialist countries.

There are 16 physicians, 4 dentists and 2 pharmacists per
10,000 inhabitants.

About 360,000 workers are engaged at the establishments
of the public health and welfare system. In every area there
is at least one regional hospital having specialized departments. University clinics are also highly specialized and solve
the problems of research and training.

A HISTORICAL REVIEW OF THE DEVELOPMENT OF CANCER CONTROL

In 1952 a special decree marked the beginning of the organization of the fight against cancer in the GDR. It was
followed by the decree of 1956 on the improvement of the treatment of oncological diseases and the system of information
about the cases of cancer. This decree covers the duties and
tasks of medical personnel with respect to oncological patients.

Not only the service of oncological patients had to be
improved, it was necessary for research purposes to develop
the system of registration of patients with primarily diagnosed
malignant tumours. Thus, the registration of malignant neoplasms
and some precancerous diseases became compulsory.

In all regions regional oncological consultation centres
were set up: in addition to basic work, the physician being in
charge of such an establishment has to consult the chief physician of the region on the organizational problems of cancer
control. The personnel of a regional consultation centre - dispensary nurses, nurses, office worker, typist /altogether 224
persons/ - is responsible for sending notices about primarily
deteched patients to the Cancer Register and performs dispensary measures, home visits of patients, medical examinations,
payment of allowances to patients, of subsidies for care if
necessary, and also rehabilitation measures. They also have to
organize medical examinations for oncological diseases at enterprises; during these examinations a particular importance

232

is attached to the detection of alterations of the urinary bladder, breast, rectum, prostate gland, and lungs /in cooperation with tuberculosis centres/.

The regional oncological consultation centres select 8,000 persons every year and send them to sanatoriums for convalescence. The duration of the course is usually 4 weeks.

Within an administrative area the regional consultation centres are headed by the physician responsible for the organization of oncological service in the area; he also consults the chief physician of the administrative area on the organizational problems of cancer control.

The heads of oncological service in the area are in their turn subordinated to the Ministry of Health and the leading institute on cancer control which is the Central Institute of Cancer Research of the Academy of Sciences of the GDR.

Diagnosis and treatment of malignant neoplasms are carried out by specialists at specialized departments and at surgical, internal, medical, radiological, and gynecological clinics. The percentage of oncological patients is particularly great at radiological clinics.

In Berlin there are two clinics where exclusively oncological patients are treated. These are the Robert Rössle Clinic of the Central Institute of Cancer Research of the Academy of Sciences of the GDR and the Charité Oncological Clinic of the Humboldt University. The latter one, in addition to the radiological department, has surgical, gynecological, and internal medical departments, as well as a department of experimental cancer research. The Central Institute of Cancer Research of the Academy of Sciences of the GDR is responsible for the coordination of investigations in the field of oncology and for a qualified guidance of cancer control. The Institute was founded in 1949 and since that time it has been continuously extended. It has departments of diagnosis, surgery, experimental and clinical X-ray therapy, experimental and clinical chemotherapy, endocrinology, experimental and clinical immunology, virology, chemical cancerogenesis, epidemiology /the National Canrer Register/, methodology and organization of cancer control. The heads of these departments are at the same time the heads of the corresponding joint researches on cancer control. There are 217 beds/at the Robert Rössle Clinic/ and over 600 workers at the Central Institute of Cancer Research.

THE SYSTEM OF REGISTRATION OF PATIENTS WITH
PRIMARILY DIAGNOSED MALIGNANT NEOPLASMS

The service of registration of oncological patients in the GDR was established in 1952. The registration system is based on the principle that no patient should be lost for follow-up starting from the establishment of a diagnosis suspecting an oncological disease up to the patient's recovery or death /irrespective of the cause of death/. Further, this method includes information on whether the diagnosis and treatment was delayed because of the negligence of the patient or of the doctor enabling the departments of public health to take appropriate measures.

The accepted system of registration provides almost a 100 % follow-up of patients with malignant tumours. According to the GDR legislation, a patient's registration is protected by medical secrecy.

All questionnaires are to be sent in duplicate by the physician, responsible for sending reports, to the address of the regional consultation centre according to the place of residence of the patient. The questionnaires as well as their copies are registered by the regional consultation centre by years. The year of registration is considered to be the year of establishing the diagnosis suspecting an oncological disease. If the diagnosis is not confirmed, the questionnaire is excluded from the Cancer Register.

Regional consultation centres continuously collate death certificates of all deceased /not only from cancer/ who lived in the given region with the list of the registered oncological patients.

There is a decree that all persons died from cancer should be subjected to autopsy if possible.

The first copies of the questionnaires are sent to the

234

National Cancer Registry for processing.

Owing to the issue of the decree charging physicians to inform within 14 days on all diagnoses suspecting an oncological disease, on new cases and cases of death of oncological patients, the Cancer Registry is an institution which has the most comprehensive information about the detection, diagnosis, treatment, and survival rate of oncological patients.

Annually over 60,000 new cases are registered and about 100,000 patients previously registered are kept under observation; 85 % of new cases are confirmed by histological examination and only 0.2 % of the cases registered only first after their death.

To facilitate the preparation of reports for the physician, special forms were elaborated in 1952. Several years later, /1956-1958/ when experience had been accumulated, these forms were revised. A physician had 5 different forms at his disposal:

1. Form of the diagnosis suspecting a malignant tumour.
2. Form of the disease and treatment.
3. Form of the additional treatment.
4. Form of the annually conducted control examination.
5. Form of the autopsy findings.

On account of a great number of the cases registered on the territory of the GDR /as early as in the first years more than 40,000 cases were registered; at present more than 60,000 new cases are registered annually/, registration and processing of the data could be carried out only by the method of punched cards.

A code was developed by means of which it would be possible to place as much information as possible on a punched card with 80 columns on every case of disease.

With the extension of the programme and the volume of information about an oncological patient it was established that 80-column punched cards were not up to the new tasks any more.

After a certain period of work by means of a conventional technique of punched cards in the Cancer Registry, employing different methods of processing, the experience of work with the use of computer was accumulated. At present the phase of transition to the use of computer and simultaneous change and expansion of the registration service may be considered to be completed.

For carrying out this transition, a number of complex problems had to be solved. It is not always easy to bring the requirements of physicians in the line with the requirements of computer specialists, and the main problem, the problem of preservation, continuity and comparability of the data available from the Registry with those to be processed in future, makes the affair even more complicated. A logical result of the requirement of concentration of efforts and of setting up a head institution for cancer control in the GDR was the joining of the Cancer Registry with the Central Institute of Cancer Research of the GDR Academy of Sciences on January 1, 1976 as the department called "National Cancer Register".

The basic principles of the work of the National Cancer Registry are as follows.

All inhabitants of the GDR have numbers that make possible to study, by means of a computer the state of health of every person and the detected alteration.

In addition, the number ensures the availability of the case record irrespective of the medical establishment where the patient was treated.

The introduction of computer required the revision of the code being used, so with regard to the foregoing the whole system of coding accepted in the Cancer Registry was revised.

Similarly in virtue of the use of computer, the research programme, as a whole, was extended. In connection with the extension of the research programme, all forms of registration of oncological morbidity were revised.

Before starting the elaboration of new forms for reports, a new system of coding and new possibilities of processing, it was necessary to solve some questions of principle. For instance, the system of direct coding by the physician who fills in the form has been tested particularly thoroughly. It appeared that it could be only partially realized since every physician had to have at his disposal a reference-book for coding which by its volume was approximately similar to the "International Classification of Diseases".

The expenditure of the physician's working time would thereby considerably increase. It has to be also taken into account that the percentage of mistakes during coding by unexperienced people is rather high. Therefore a decision was taken which under the present conditions is probably optimal. A direct coding is applied to form "B_1" /report on the history and epicrisis/ in order to obtain the information on the number of new cases as soon as possible. This form can be easily filled in by a physician /the heading of the form "B" is typed in advance/ and after the insertion of additional notes by the regional consultation centre it is put immediately into computer.

The advantages of filling in the form designed for the report on the history and epicrisis /form "B"/ using an uncoded text are that besides facilitating the task of filling in the form the text can find wider use.

Form "B" is coded in the Cancer Registry by a specially trained personnel.

The control forms and the report on the case of death /form "C"/ are composed to make possible an immediate perforation at the data processing centre.

If the autopsy report containing the necessary information is available, the pathologist does not have to fill in a special form.

For the registration of patients three forms are introduced; all the three forms have a similar section designed for the identification of the patient. Form "A" is filled in when a malignant neoplasm is detected or suspected. Its filling should provide a timely beginning of the treatment or, when a malignant tumour is suspected, precision of the diagnosis in the shortest possible time. In cases when the suspicion of a malignant tumour was not confirmed, the second part of form "A" is filled in. Further, the second part of form "A" is filled in when:

1/ the patient did not come to a hospital for the treatment;

2/ in cutaneous basaliomas.

Cutaneous basaliomas are known to fall into the category
of malignant neoplasms and account for over more than 10 % of
this category, which makes their registration compulsory. On
the other hand, the prognosis of cutaneous basaliomas is better
than that of many other skin diseases and the analysis of this
disease is of no particular interest for scientists.

Therefore an opinion has arisen that it would be quite
sufficient to consider these 6,000 cases per year only quantitatively, a detailed report on their history and epicrisis
is not necessary.

Thus, in the GDR patients with primarily diagnosed basalioma are registered but they are not subjected to a follow-up
observation.

In cases when the diagnosis of malignant neoplasm is confirmed, the patient is immediately sent for treatment. The
data on the history, epicrisis and treatment are recorded in
form "B".

Reports without confirmed diagnosis are accepted for the
purpose of comparison with subsequent reports but certainly
they are not entered in the Registry /i.e. they are not taken
into account in the Registry/.

On the first page of the questionnaire the character of
the treatment is indicated /primary, additional or repeated,
treatment for relapse or metastasis, etc./ as well as the
name and the address of the physician conducting the treatment,
and the address of the regional oncological consultation centre.

The personal data of the patient are entered by means of
a computer or, additional information is intended by the regional consultation centre.

For express information on the number of persons with
primarily diagnosed malignant neoplasm, the duplicates of the
first sheet of form "B" containing the information on the patient, the treatment employed, the address of the physician

and of the regional consultation centre /form B_1/ are put into computer.

On the back of the card there are additional instructions to fill in this part of form "B". The question "Which is the primary disease" is necessary for identifying the case so that in multiple tumours the data on the diagnosis and treatment could be compared with a similar case by the computer.

The patient's name is given uncoded in order to have the possibility to make correspondence by means of computer /if after a certain period of time the computer does not receive information about the patient, it sends an inquiry to the regional consultation centre/. It is for this reason that the number and the address of the corresponding regional consultation centre is indicated. /Changes are made using form "C"./

The information on the patient's address and the address of the medical establishment where the patient was first treated is necessary first of all for the regional consultation centre, for coding the address and the place of the patient's residence and for the possibility to ask for missing documents. An empty /free/ cell beside is left for archive marks in the Cancer Registry.

There are several new questions in the section "Anamnestic data":

1. Attendance at preventive examinations.
The question is introduced for studying the effectiveness of preventive examinations.

2. Use of contraceptives.
Up to the present a great variety of contradictory opinions and statements exists about the influence of contraceptives on tumour occurrence, however, these opinions are not supported by a sufficient number of convincing evidence.

3. Influence of occupation on the possibility of cancer occurrence.
It is considered all over the world that occupational hazards play a decisive role in the etiology of cancer.

To study this problem, four most common types of occupation were selected /with the indication of the enterprise or type of industry, period of work and the age of the patient at the beginning of working activity/. These data accumulated in the Cancer Register will serve as basis for studying the influence of occupational hazards on morbidity of malignant tumours.

4. Height, weight and blood pressure.

These parameters are assumed to be of importance also in the etiopathogenesis of malignant tumours, their diagnosis, treatment and survival. Since these data are recorded in a case history, their introduction into the Cancer Registry does not cause additional difficulties; this results only in the extension of the capacities of the Cancer Registry.

This additional information is aimed mainly at promoting the solution of the problem of "risk" group formation. In this connection the Cancer Registry makes it possible to intensify preventive measures, first of all to the decrease of mortality from oncological diseases.

The questions on diagnosis are directed at obtaining the most precise description possible of the primary tumour by its type, histology and localization. Besides, there are questions about metastases /if the primary tumour is unknown/ and the size of tumour. For the comparison of individual methods of treatment, the form has questions about the stage of the disease during various periods of observation and according to different classifications.

More recently the questions about blood type was included into the form. There is an opinion that for a wide variety of malignant tumours the patient's blood type is of certain significance. The accumulation of a sufficiently large material should help to clarify these questions.

The information on the diagnostic methods and the main concomitant diseases was transferred from the old forms. However, the structural arrangement was changed. The questions on the methods of treatment were systematized. Only the section on X-ray therapy was changed, due to the technological advance and the creation of new sources of radiation. The data of the medical establishment are additionally put into the coding and

decoding programme. This permits not only to study the therapeutic problems but also to detect the clinics having the optimal results of treatment.

This will make possible to recommend the most effective
methods of treatment to be introduced into practice which
results in improving the results of treatment.

Owing to the fact that the report form is an epicrisis,
it can be used for informing the physician who is to keep the
patient under a follow-up observation. In the new form a place
was assigned for the information and instructions as well as
for recommendations on further measures on the patient's dispensary examination. It is necessary to emphasize that form
"B" should not be used in the future if the epicrisis containing the answers to each question posed is available.

The new system raises the possibility to make form "B"
exclusively specialized. The experience will show which way
to choose. In any case, we assume that at present such a structure of epicrisis conforms much more to the ideas of a summarized review than the report individually made, without using
forms.

The "control report, the report on the stage of the disease,
on the treatment and the fatal out-come of an oncological disease subjected to compulsory registration" /form "C"/, serves
many purposes as it is shown by its name. This form is put
directly into computer as it is very easy to fill it in and
only few notions are coded by means of the code given on the
backside.

A personal number, a number of primary disease and the
year of registration are necessary for determining the place
of each case of disease in the card file.

A surname and name are also given in full form, this
provides and opportunity to identify the cases registered
before the introduction of new questionnaires. Since in case
of certain contradictions, mistakes, etc. the second inquiry
to the regional consultation centre should be sent directly
by computer, it is necessary to give the information on the
fact that a patient got into the scope of activity of another

regional consultation centre, in order to avoid excessive correspondence. The data on the courses of treatment for convalescent oncological patients are included into the reports of
the regional consultation centre. Such information is important
for conducting investigations in this field.

During control examinations which in the first 5 years
should be taken every year and in the subsequent period of
life less frequently, it is necessary to indicate the data
and results of the examinations.

In case of the patient's death, in addition to the date
of death the examination results, the cause of death and
indications for autopsy should be recorded. On the reception
of the report on death, the file is usually considered as
completed and is withdrawn from the "stock".

As earlier, the information collected is stored in the
Cancer Registry for scientific investigations. In case of
autopsy, the processing and coding of the autopsy protocol is
made in the Cancer Registry and the information is put into
the computer in the form of marked sheets /KK9/.

Since in our opinion in the near future it will be impossible to meet the need of devices for readout of documents
efficiently, we have to put the information into the computer
in the form of punched cards.

Six different punched cards /KK/ may be required for
every case:

KK1: Personal data according to card "B_1".

KK2: History data /marked sheet "A"/.

KK3: Diagnosis /marked sheet "D"/.

KK4: Treatment and observation /marked sheet "T"/.

KK8: Observation /Form "C"/.

KK9: Changes, additions /marked sheet "U"/.

Marked sheets are the working material in the Cancer
Registry; specially trained personnel transfers medical information on them in the language appropriate for computer processing.

The advantages of an individual form for every case as
compared with a marked sheet has been long discussed. In

242

comparison with the marked sheet, such a card has the advantage that every information on a patient is collected in one document, but it has also an essential disadvantage, namely that the possibility of conducting control measures is ruled out. Besides, a danger of losing data during their transfer to the computer centre increases. A marked questionnaire is more visual and easier to be looked over, besides it saves 50 % of paper. Of certain importance is the aspect that the personnel of the Cancer Registry got used to this method of coding and the transition to a new system is in itself sufficiently difficult.

The proposed plan of the flow of data and information in the system of cancer control and the relations between individual institution is shown in a diagram /Fig. 21/.

ORGANIZATION OF THE DETECTION AND EXAMINATION
OF ONCOLOGICAL PATIENTS

Every citizen of the GDR has the right to choose a physician at his own will. He is not compelled to go to a certain physician in his district or at work. As a rule, he goes to his "family doctor" who in most cases is an internist and works near the place of residence or work of the patient.

For the sake of long-standing and confidential relations between patient and physician the system of "family doctor" should be continuously improved. It quite often happens that a patient goes to a specialist who is in the treatment of certain diseases.

If a patient begins to suspect an oncological disease or, under the influence of health education, he wants to undergo a preventive examination, he often comes to the regional oncological consultation centre where either the diagnosis is made more precise or the patient is sent to the corresponding polyclinic or hospital. The right of a patient to a free choice of a physician is somewhat limited by the circumstance that payment of travelling expenses of a patient going to a physician working in an other area or region is provided only in cases when the necessity of the treatment in the other area

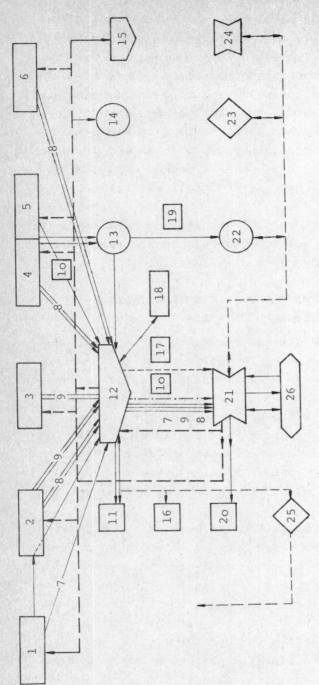

Fig.11. Information-retrieval system of registration of patients with malignant tumours.

1.Treating physician – 2.Medical institution establishing the diagnosis and providing treatment – 3.Medical institution providing additional treatment – 4.Office giving death certificate – 5.Pathological laboratory – 6.Sanatorium and rehabilitation – 7.Form MA – 8.Form MC – 9.Form MB – 10.Autopsy protocol – 11.District Council – 12.District oncological consultation – 13.Civil registry office – 14.People's district assistance – 15.Other dispensaries – 16.The Council of administrative region – 17.Questionnaire-report – 18.Patient – 19.Death certificate – 20.Ministry of Health – 21.Cancer Registry – 22.State Central Statistical Department – 23.Other forms of medical statistics – 24.Other cancer registries – 25. Group of information – 26. Centre for evaluation of data is confirmed by the physician. If the patient pays his travelling expenses himself, he can go to a physician in any distant region.

An early detection and timely beginning of treatment gives the patient a good chance of survival. Based on this consideration, regional oncological consultation centres began to conduct preventive examinations of the female genitalia, breast, rectum and prostate gland. In the course of the examinations of the female genitalia colposcopy and cytologic study are carried out.

In view of the fact that by means of preventive examinations it is impossible to examine every women, it is recommended that every gynecological examination should be simultaneously a preventive oncological examination. For this purpose a number of cytologic laboratories have been set up. The frequency of detection of cancer of the cervix uteri in the preclinical stage is at present different in various areas. On an average over one third of cases of cancer of cervix uteri in the country is detected in the stage of "carcinoma in situ". The studies conducted in the Cancer Registry showed that in case of breast cancer the distribution by stages did not change during the period of 1956-1974 despite the widely used preventive examinations.

The future will show whether preventive examinations in cancer of cervix uteri and cancer of some localizations contribute to a significant decrease in the mortality from these forms of cancer.

Regular periodical examinations of the lungs were first aimed at tuberculosis control. After a decrease in the rate of tuberculosis cases, the detection of bronchogenic carcinoma became their main task. Over 80 % of the population have undergone such radiological examinations.

In course of periodical radiological examinations about 40 % of the malignant tumours of the lungs and bronchi have been revealed. This concerns mainly peripherical tumours whereas central tumours are frequently not detected. The National Cancer Registry has showed that the survival rate in bronchogenic carcinoma detected by periodical radiological examinations is twice that in tumours detected by other methods.

The preventive examinations are organized at enterprises or at local medical establishments. It has appeared that only properly organized examinations have made in high percentage of population to participate in them. Persons called in for examination are persuaded by lectures and individual conversations. Research work includes the search for the best methods of examination. Thus, one of the task of these studies is the use of computer in this system. The computer prints invitation cards with the indication of the time and place of examination. The physician organizing the examination also receives a list of called patients from the computer; if a patient comes for examination the physician records the results in a special form and returns it to the computer. The findings of cytologic studies are also accumulated and processed by computer. At revealing a pathological finding, notification and call of patients for making the diagnosis more precise and for treatment is carried out the same way. With this form of organization a high attendance of the examinations was provided.

On the other hand, gynecological examinations were carried out using mobile out-patient stations. It has proved to be particularly important in rural regions.

As a rule, all physicians, polyclinics and clinics are required not to overlook such forms of cancer as of the uterus, breast, rectum,prostate gland, which are easily accessible for diagnosis, and to carry out the appropriate examinations. The criterion of the effectiveness of all these prophylactic measures is the increase in survival rate, and on evaluating the results it should be verified whether the success is not the result of carrying out some other measure, for instance, the improvement of methods of treatment. It is necessary to take into consideration relapse rate as far as possible in other forms and localizations of cancer. The studies based mainly on the mortality rate obtained from death certificates are unsatisfactory, and only the data of the observations of patients stored in the Cancer Registry throughout the course of

246

the disease make possible to draw objective conclusions.

ORGANIZATION OF HOSPITALIZATION AND RENDERING MEDICAL ASSISTANCE TO PATIENTS WITH MALIGNANT NEOPLASMS

Since a physician is obliged to inform on even a suspicion of oncological disease, the regional consultation centre always has the information on how many patients are referred for treatment. If a patient refuses treatment, the regional consultation centre must give him necessary explanations so that he understands that the treatment is in his interests and agrees to it.

The regional consultation centre must also observe that the time interval between the diagnosis, hospitalization and the beginning of treatment would not be impermissibly great.

Only then it is possible not to refer a patient to a hospital when in the diagnosis an incurable stage of a malignant neoplasm was established, the patient's condition allows not to hospitalize him and home care is guaranteed. Such a decision should be made not by a "family doctor" but by an oncologist working at an out-patient or in-patient departments.

As a rule, the patient is referred to the nearest hospital in his residential area or according to the tumour localization /if the patient has no particular requests concerning the hospital/. Patients with bronchogenic cancer are usually treated in the in-patient departments for patients with lung diseases or in oncological departments.

Oncological patients are usually directed to radiological departments by specialists working in polyclinics and hospitals rather than on request of "family doctors". In many clinics and hospitals special consultations are organized for oncological patients during which patients are examined by several specialists who collectively decide upon the most expedient treatment.

According to the recommendations of the Pediatric Society, the treatment of cancer in children which accounts for 1 % of all tumours is carried out in special children's hospitals. Such organizational form of treating children started first with the admission of children with leucoses.

Already many years ago the so-called "Central bulletins of therapeutic recommendations" had started to be published. These recommendations had been elaborated by the commission of specialists /oncologists/ and coordinated with oncological societies. They also contain instructions on the diagnostics of tumours. Naturally, such therapeutic recommendations are periodically revised in order to coordinate them with the up-to-date international scientific level. Nevertheless, the strict adherence to these therapeutic recommendations in every case is not required of a physician. On the other hand, if a physician is reproached with doing harm to his patient by the treatment, the reason why he did not observe these recommendations /as a result of negligence or on purpose/ is thoroughly checked.

DISPENSARIZATION OF PATIENTS WITH MALIGNANT NEOPLASMS

As stated above, the treatment of oncological patients may be carried out in all hospitals and clinics. The law and the system of registration of oncological patients have established that all oncological patients are kept under the observation of a medical institution for five years. After five years the observation of the patient is discontinued only when he is considered cured. The treating physician is obliged to give information on the control examinations through the system of registration of oncological patients at least once a year.

The Cancer Registry, in cooperation with the regional consultation centres, is keeping the patient under observation until his death. The substitution of the attending physician for a special oncological therapeutic establishment in the observation of the patient seems inexpedient as the physician is better informed about the treatment employed and is interested in a careful analysis of results.

The search for the ways of improving coordination is conducted in cooperation with the medical administration of the regional consultation centre. In many clinics consulting hours of oncologists are established particularly for patients who have undergone surgical and X-ray treatment.

Usually, it is the duty of the physician making primary treatment to send control reports, however, by agreement these functions may be transferred to the physician continuing the treatment. Oncological patients with operable forms of tumours are admitted to a hospital or to an adequately specialized department. Inoperable patients are referred to radiological departments and to hospitals for treatment or consultation. The number of bed of the radiological departments is limited, therefore many patients are accommodated in other surgical departments of the hospital or in other hospitals and they are brought for treatment to an X-ray therapy department. Patients with leucosés, for example, are admitted to specialized therapeutic departments. Regional hospitals and hospitals at higher educational establishments usually have a special haematological department where patients with malignant neoplasms of the haemopoietic and lymphatic tissues are also treated. In some hospitals haematological departments have been transformed into oncological ones, that is, the haematological department deals with the chemotherapy of solid tumours.

In the operable forms of cancer the priority of surgical methods of treatment is universally acknowledged. In some forms and stages of the disease surgical intervention and X-ray therapy are considered to be of equal value. In these cases the combination of the two methods of treatment for finding an optimal method for every patient has proved to be expedient. This method helps to exclude a subjective aspect when the question about the necessity of additional X-ray treatment and chemotherapy for the given patient depends exclusively on the decision and competence of the physician making primary treatment. Such form of cooperation is also useful because there is no uniform opinion of the role and importance of additional treatment of patients following operation and X-ray therapy. An increasing attention is paid to combined treatment. The opinion that X-ray therapy is a method of treatment of mainly palliative character, which has settled from the earliest times, is undoubtedly incorrect

and can be changed most likely as a result of cooperative investigations. The present situation, is which the assistance of
a radiologist is sought only if there is much evidence that the
disease is in the advanced stage or if the patient cannot be
operated on because of concomitant diseases or because of old
age, is wrong and should be revised.

On the basis of its work, the National Cancer Registry
has put forward the requirement that elderly patients should
also be operated on for cancer of the stomach and lungs. This
requirement has been satisfying in the above forms of cancer
and the survival rate of elderly persons has proved to be far
better than expected by surgeons.

During subsequent service of oncological patients who
have undergone treatment, hospitals work in close contact with
their polyclinics, physicians of general medical establishments,
specialized out-patient stations and regional oncological consultation centres.

THE STUDY OF THE EFFECTIVENESS OF THE TREATMENT OF
ONCOLOGICAL PATIENTS

The National Cancer Registry plays an important role in
the study of the effectiveness of treatment of patients. It
can compare the results obtained in the country with respect
to various localizations, stages, types of tumours, age groups,
etc. with the international results, draw conclusions and
elaborate recommendations on the cooperation of experts. It can
also reveal differences between the results obtained in certain
hospitals and draw appropriate conclusions. An important
evidence of the success of the treatment is the survival of
patients in the years following the treatment.

The determination of the percentage of survived patients
five years after treatment plays a particularly important role.
Both the total mortality rate in selected age groups, and the
relative survival rate which shows the ratio of the number of
the survived patients to the number of the patients treated by
a certain method has to be defined. Only on the basis of a such
method it is possible to draw comparisons on an international

scale, since every country uses its own method of analysis. The method based on the comparison of the data on the number of new cases and cases of deaths from cancer according to death certificates cannot be considered accurate and it should inevitably lead to wrong conclusions. Unfortunately, this method is still used in some countries. Admittedly, it should be noted that in countries where efficiently working registries are missing it is uncertain that other possibilities exist. Hospital registries cover a certain group of patients and often have much more favourable survival rate than national registries giving information on the total number of cases with certain forms of cancer. It is of particular importance if in a particular hospital a precise criterion is necessary for the selection of patients and for the exclusion of the risk group, that is, the patients with concomitant diseases or the patients too old.

Already several years ago the National Cancer Registry has made an analysis and shown that in cancer of the esophagus the results of treatment in the GDR are unsatisfactory as compared with other countries. The final analysis made by experts has shown that during the preparation for operation in this localization the necessity of preoperative care of the patient which would assist him to survive the operation and its concomitant burdens was not taken into consideration in our country.

The right tendency to subject a patient to radical treatment as soon as possible is unacceptable with respect to patients with cancer of the esophagus who are often already in the state of cachexia. The significance of various methods of treatment is studied by different collectives of investigators by means of consecutive testing.

ORGANIZATION OF MEDICAL DETERMINATION OF DISABLEMENT AND REHABILITATION OF ONCOLOGICAL PATIENTS

In case of diseases disablement is determined by the attending physician. He gives the patient a sick-leave certificate which entitles the patient to receive payment. In our country every working person paying insurance dues has the right to receive payment accounting for 90 % of the amount of his average wage up to 6 weeks per year. During the period of disablement, exceeding six weeks the patient receives 50 % of his average total wage.

If the patient remains disabled longer than 35 days, the physician is obliged to send him to a medical commission. On the basis of the conclusion of the attending physician and the examination by the members of the commission, the commission decides upon further measures. It has the right to require further measures for making diagnosis more precise, to refer the patient to a hospital for this purpose or in agreement with the attending physician, to extend or discontinue the period of disablement.

The period of disablement can be prolonged up to 52 weeks if the patient cannot be considered capable of working. As for many oncological patients, it becomes clear already before the expiration of this term that one should not expect the restoration of the ability to work. In this case the patient will be considered invalid. If the patient is treated in a hospital, the medical establishment can send, simultaneously with the medical conclusion, an application for disability certificate to the address of the expert of the region where the hospital is located.

If the patient gets treatment in out-patient conditions, the physician who makes out the medical certificate gives another conclusion in case of prolonged disablement or at the request of the enterprise or of the medical commission. In case of oncological patients, the regional expert, as a rule, gets in touch with the medical administration of the regional onco- logical consultation centre and decides upon whether to consider the patient invalid, or to ask the attending physician or a more competent physician of the field to give the necessary conclusion.

If the patient's disablement persists longer than for 52 weeks, but despite this a complete restoration of the ability to work cannot be excluded the patient is sent to the rehabili- tation commission. Such a commission consists of physicians, representatives of social insurance bodies /in our country these functions are performed by the Independent German Trade Union/, and of the representatives of social organizations. In the presence of the patient the commission discusses the possibilities of rehabilitation. There are various means of rehabilitation, for instance, occupational re-education, transfer to lighter work at the same enterprise, temporary transfer to lighter work, reduced working day for a certain period, sending to a sanatorium for treatment and the implementation of other measures of medical rehabilitative character. Naturally, the rehabilitation commission can draw a conclusion that the status of disablement is the most beneficial way out for the patient. The period of disablement is determined individually and it is rarely less than one year. The period can be unlimited from the very beginning in case of an irreversible persistent lesion. If the period is limited, it is necessary to carry out a medical examination before its expiration in order to decide whether the signs of improvement have appeared. If such signs are not detected, the disablement pension can be neither cancelled nor reduced. If the patient does not agree to the commission's decision, he has the right to appeal to higher bodies and to require an additional expertise or a meeting of the Higher Expert Commission. The payment of the disability pension depends on the medical conclusion about the presence of disability and on the certificate about the right to social security.

The disability status signifies that the patient cannot earn more than one third of his average wage. The right disability allowance within the framework of social insurance depends on the length of service, that is, on the duration of the period of paying social insurance dues. However, there is a statement about the financial support of uninsured patients /children and adolescents who have not begun their working activities yet/. In these cases a minimum allowance is paid. Along with the assistance from health service bodies, in other words, along with health service and social security /sick benefit, disability pension, payment of auxiliary means such as prostheses, etc./ working people are rendered assist-

ance by enterprises and trade unions of enterprises and non-
-working people who are in need of assistance - from welfare
organizations. If the patient needs to be taken care of, he can
be allowed a certain sum of money the amount of which depends
on the degree of care and the severity of the patient's condition. This sum makes possible for the patient to pay for the
services of the person taking care of him. Besides, the members
of the patient's family also have the right to be paid for
taking care of the sick person. Further privileges can be
granted depending on the degree of the severity of the disease.
Thus, persons working at enterprises have the right to an additional leave and they pay reduced taxes. In case of necessity,
on presentation of a special document in public transport, a
patient can take a seat assigned to invalids, he also has the
right to service out of turn in shops, in social organizations
and in state institutions. Owing to the four-week courses of
treatment oncological patients usually have additional opportunities for recuperation in one of the eleven sanatoriums for
convalescent patients.

In many administrative areas of the country, special
centres for after-treatment of oncological patients immediately
following radical treatment were set up. They proved to be an
excellent means of the restoration of psychic and somatic
state of the patient.

In our country a versatile and differentiated system of
social welfare and rehabilitation has been organized providing
the implementation of all measures along with the possibilities
of medical rehabilitation in order to achieve the return of
convalescent patients in the society.

The social and political programme of the IXth Congress
of the German Socialist Unity Party further developed by the
decisions of the VIIIth Congress of the Party significantly
expanded the material means and legal guarantees for the support of patients and rehabilitation of the convalescent.

ORGANIZATION OF MEDICAL ASSISTANCE TO PATIENTS WITH
ADVANCED TUMOUR .

Unfortunetely, a great part of malignant neoplasms are revealed or can be revealed in the locally advanced stage or even after the appearance of metastases.

Many oncological patients who have undergone a radical operation or X-ray therapy have shown relapses and metastases later. The service of the patient and psychological work on him and on the members of his family are often not an easy task for the regional oncological consultation centres, especially for the physician and the dispensary nurse who must work in close contact with the family doctor and out-patient and in-patient institutions of the patient's residence, as well as with the hospitals if such exist. If home service is provided or can be organized, medical service is primarily supplied by the family doctor in agreement with the hospital the patient is discharged from and the family doctor is instructed on the further treatment. Nurses of the community are entrusted with the care of the patient at request of and according to the instructions of the family doctor. Dispensary nurses from regional oncological consultation centres visit patients at their homes and help to solve the problems of social welfare. They frequently resort to the assistance of such social organizations as "The People's Solidarity" and "The Democratic Women's Union".

The patients who are in need of care can be admitted to a local hospital or to a home for invalids. In spite of the fact that the number of homes for invalids constantly increases it is still limited at present. For this reason it is not always possible to avoid a long stay of incurable oncological patients in oncological departments or specialized hospitals. If the service and treatment of incurable oncological patients with advanced forms of cancer were carried out in special in--patient institutions, the danger would exist that such thera-peutic establishment would get the reputation among the popu-lation of being "houses for the dying" though there is no doubt that medical treatment and personnel's experience in this special field would be certainly more perfect and technical equipment could be particularly purposeful. There is only one specialized establishment of this type for incurable oncological patients. In general, to set up such in-patient institutions is considered to be inexpedient.

For incurable patients it is particularly urgent to maintain the "quality of life" as long as possible. Even in the incurable stage of a number of localizations and forms of cancer it is possible to use methods of treatment which contribute to the inhibition of the tumour's growth for a long time. In such cases treatment in a specialized hospital may prove to be useful. If the patient's state has deteriorated to such an extent that only symptomatic treatment and care remained to be possible, such a patient should stay in the family circle as long as possible or should be admitted to a hospital in his residential area.

TEACHING OF ONCOLOGY, TRAINING OF ONCOLOGISTS AND MIDDLE-LEVEL MEDICAL PERSONNEL FOR ONCOLOGICAL ESTABLISHMENTS

In the medical universities students receive first /introductory/ information on general oncology in the third year of their studies included in pathology and general semiology. Special problems of oncology are elucidated at lectures, seminars and practical studies in the 4th and 5th years by lecturers of various disciplines /surgery, internal medicine, radiology, gynecology, urology, etc./. In the 5th year the curriculum is terminated by the so-called "Interdisciplinary complex" which is taught by lecturers of many disciplines. Such an organization of teaching contributes to the integration of the material delivered at the studies on general disciplines and is aimed at the strengthening of basic knowledge on oncology and at the preparation for practical activities. The latter begin in the 6th year when a student works for 4 months each at medical and surgical departments of an in-patient establishment and for 4 months in a chosen branch of medicine.

This is followed by a 4-year course of training of the physician in a chosen speciality. The requirements of the training of specialists elaborated on the basis of the recommendations of the scientific and medical societies of the Academy of Postgraduate Training of Physicians envisage the sufficient knowledge on the treatment of oncological patients necessary for the particular medical specialty.

Until recently, specialization on oncology as an independent branch or as a subspecialization has not existed in our country. However, at present, discussions are being held on the expediency of the introduction of additional specialization of specialists, for instance internists, radiologists, surgeons, on oncology.

Only radiotherapists could call themselves oncologists as they have to deal exclusively with oncological patients. A special training of a radiologist on X-ray therapy lasts only for one year. This period is obviously insufficient in duration for the preparation for independent activities on X-ray treatment of oncological patients. Those who are going to devote themselves to this work can study X-ray therapy for one more year and on receiving the diploma of a specialist improve their knowledge and skills in a department or in a clinic of radiotherapy.

The training course of a specialist is ended with taking examinations. Oncology is not included at present. As oncology overlaps with many clinical sciences, the higher education of students should have the continuation in the organization of additional measures on the advanced oncological training of physicians of various specialities. The Academy of Postgraduate Training of Physicians of the GDR under the Ministry of Health is made responsible for this.

At postgraduate training courses the special problems are within the competence of the leading organization dealing with cancer control, the Central Institute of Cancer Research of the Academy of Sciences. It organizes the activities of other societies such as the Society of Surgeons, the Society of Gynecologists, as well as other postgraduate training courses particularly for head physicians in co-operation with the Society of Cancer Control.

Similar courses of postgraduate training of about one

week's duration are held twice a year at the Central Institute of Cancer Research. The postgraduate training on all specialities compulsory for every physician is organized according to the territorial principle. The Academy of Postgraduate Training of Physicians annually drafts a programme containing a number of topics compulsory for the persons working in the system of higher medical education /these are physicians, stomatologists, pharmacists, biologists and the representatives of natural sciences/. In addition to this a list of topics is offered from which the head physician of a region can select those which are of particular interest for him. As a rule many of them deal with the problems of oncology. For the authors delivering lectures in regions within the framework of the system of postgraduate training of physicians, the Academy publishes materials in the form of summaries or other reviews in the Journal for Postgraduate Training.

When selecting topics for the preparation of written material the Academy of Postgraduate Training of Physicians proceeds from the recommendations of medical societies on the appropriate disciplines /in the present case first of all of the Council of the "Society of Cancer Control of the GDR" and also of the Central Institute of Cancer Research/.

Once in two years the congresses of the Society of Cancer Control are held. At these congresses particular emphasis is placed on the popularization of specific knowledge on oncology and on the postgraduate training on oncology of physicians and middle-level personnel working in regional oncological consultation centres. According to the structure of cancer control in our country, problems of oncology are also dealt with at postgraduate training courses for physicians of various specialities, at the meetings of the other medical societies and in the medical press as well.

Furthermore, higher educational establishments, local societies of physicians, hospitals, regional physicians responsible for fight against cancer and regional oncological consultation centres often hold special "days of advanced training" or meetings on a smaller scale on their own initiative.

At present a uniform programme of postgraduate training of physicians is being prepared in order to help the medical management of regional oncological consultation centres in accomplishing the set tasks, and physicians in the work in the regional oncological clinics.

The responsibility for improving the qualifications of medium-level personnel is placed on a special institute of the Ministry of Health in Postdam. It publishes educational materials, organizes courses and test exams as an individual method of improving the qualifications. At present a special programme of training and improvement of qualifications for middle-level personnel particularly at oncological therapeutic establishments is in the stage of elaboration.

HEALTH EDUCATION OF THE POPULATION

The principles of health education and propaganda among the population of the GDR are determined by the instructions of the Ministry of Health. The German Museum of Hygiene of the GDR in Dresden is subordinated to the Ministry of Health; the Museum includes the Central Institute of Health Education. The National Committee on Health Education works as a central consultative body. When considering questions related to oncology it is the right of the Central Institute of Cancer Research to decide. The German Red Cross Society also contributes to this work using educational measures for this purpose. Concerning the questions of health education of women, the Democratic Women's Union actively supports educational work especially in relation to preventive oncological examinations. There is a variety of forms of health educational work. The Museum of Hygiene publishes lists of instructions, booklets, posters and series of slides which are purchased by local bodies of health service and welfare and are subsequently distributed by them among the population. These publications are especially often used for the propagation of preventive examinations and in the struggle against bad habits. The guidance and organization of these activities are the duties of the head physician of the area who has a study for these purposes.

On the regional level the coordination of health educational work is carried out by a physician who combines this
job with his main one. He works in the closest cooperation with
"Urania", /a popular scientific society/ which also publishes
written materials for lecturers.

In many daily and weekly newspapers articles on health
education regularly appear, among these are the articles on oncological topics. The central organ of health education and
propaganda is the newspaper "Your health" which comes out once
a month and is highly popular. The television and radio of the
GDR also organize telecasts and broadcasts on health education
and propaganda. For example, a film about breast cancer made
at the Central Institute of Cancer Research was shown on TV
several times. Similar telecasts from the friendly socialist
countries are also shown. Health education should be used for
suppressing a useless fear of cancer and for the prevention and
early detection of cancer by using expedient and tactically
founded methods. On getting cancer, the person informed in the
field of oncology would be more susceptible to therapeutic
measures than the person having vague ideas of cancer or the
person who has got wrong and exaggerated ideas of his disease
due to sensational reports. Such a well-informed patient will
understand the physician's explanations about his disease
quite in a different way. Nowadays the knowledge of cancer
presents a problem, namely that the population knows about
quite a great number of people who died of cancer both among
their relatives and acquaintances. The population knows much
less about persons cured of cancer. The reason in not only
that most oncological patients unfortunately cannot be cured
yet; this impression is strengthened due to the fact that
quite a number of physicians inform the relatives of oncological
patients with unfavourable prognosis that in the patient in-
question apparently a disease is detected in the early stage
and with a good prognosis or the physicians do not talk
about the diagnosis of "cancerous disease" at all as if
ostensibly not wishing to cause an emotional shock. Thus,
sometimes cured patients and their relatives cannot let other

people know about the successful treatment as they are not informed about the diagnosis. The extent to which a physician explains the diagnosis undoubtedly depends on his personal point of view as well as on the particular circumstances of the case.

In can be understood that a physician avoids revealing the merciless truth about the condition of an obviously incurable patient. In cases of an oncological disease in the early stages, especially of localizations which have a good prognosis of survival, the patient should be informed about the diagnosis. The best propagator of the opinion that cancer in the early stage can be cured is the cured patient himself.

COORDINATION OF RESEARCH WORK ON THE PROBLEM "SCIENTIFIC BASIS OF THE ORGANIZATION OF CANCER CONTROL"

In the GDR the coordination of research work on oncology is carried out by the Central Institute of Cancer Research of the Academy of Sciences of the GDR. The participating institutions are united into a Research Union headed by the Central Institute of Cancer Research. The Director of the Central Institute of Cancer Research is simultaneously the head of this Union and the chairman of the Scientific Council of the Union. The heads of the departments of the Central Institute of Cancer Research are responsible heads of the corresponding subjects elaborated within the framework of the Research Union. Thus the collective of the institutions participating in the research work on oncology subordinated to the Academy, higher educational establishments, the State Health Service and other organizations, irrespective of their administrative subordination, are under professional guidance. The complex of subjects of investigations is divided into 9 parts following the example of the programme on oncology within the framework of the CMEA. From these the problem "Scientific principles of the organization of cancer control" is elaborated by the treatment of methods and organization of cancer control of the Central Institute of Cancer Research which cooperates particularly closely with the department of the National Cancer Register and Oncological Statistics responsible for the problem "Epidemiology of malignant tumours".

Such a close cooperation is necessary, since the principles of the scientific organization of cancer control are developed on the basis of the analysis of the Cancer Register's material and on that of the studies of analytical and epidemiological character.

The most urgent tasks for the present and for the nearest future are related to investigations dealing with the analysis of the importance of mass prophylactic examinations first of all in frequently occurring visible forms of cancer the diagnosis of which is not particularly difficult and also with the formation and detection of risk groups in various forms of cancer.

Much attention is being given now to occupational forms of cancer as the occupation of the person is an essential criterion characterizing the environment. First of all, the possible relations between cancer in animals and in people are taken into consideration, though it was found that there are no connections between the place of the occurrence of cattle leucosis and the place of residence of the persons who contracted leucosis. Apparently, the studies mentioned above should be always preceded by the analysis of the state of cancer control. A great variety of institutions with different administrative subordination participate in such investigations. The institutions subordinated to the Academy of Sciences closely cooperate with higher educational establishments and institutions in the system of the state health service. For instance, the Central Institute of Occupational Medicine of the Ministry of Health works in close cooperation with the National Cancer Registry on the problem of occupational cancer which is registered separately in the new system of registration of oncological diseases.

PROSPECTS FOR THE IMPROVEMENT OF THE ORGANIZATION OF ONCOLOGICAL ASSISTANCE

According to the agreement between the Minister of Health and the President of the Academy of Sciences, the Central Institute of Cancer Research of the Academy of Sciences of the

GDR has been recently entrusted with the task to consult the
Ministry of Health and the bodies of the state health service
subordinated to it on the problems of cancer control. Thereby
the Central Institute of Cancer Research has also assumed responsibility for the practical aspects of cancer control in the
country. The top-level officials of the Central Institute of
Cancer Research have draught a long-term plan of the further
development of cancer control.

Knowledge of the etiopathogenesis of cancer which has become very extensive in the recent years will make possible to
find the methods of prevention of cancer. Particularly important
are here the epidemiological studies which make possible to
collect a large number of facts about the causes of cancer development; at the same time not only the knowledge of the
causes of tumour development is necessary for prevention but
also that of the ways for their elimination.

Taking into account that the ways of cancer prevention
will remain limited as before, the measures of secondary
prevention /early diagnosis and treatment of cancer/ are of
great importance. With respect to the early detection of
tumours the situation in the GDR undoubtedly cannot be considered satisfactory yet, but, on the other hand, it is for this
reason that it offers wide possibilities for taking constructive
measures on the improvement of cancer control.

Comparative studies of the materials of the National Cancer Registry and the data of the national statistics have shown
that the results obtained in the GDR are in accordance with
the international standards; despite this it is necessary to
continue working on their improvement. An essential prere-
quisite of the further improvement of tumour prevention is the
centralization of the special treatment of tumours at well-
equipped in-patient therapeutic establishments having multidisciplinary clinical oncology. In this case the term "multidisciplinary clinical oncology" implies a systematic interaction of oncosurgery, oncoradiology and chemotherapy of cancer. Without departing from the principles of the development
of clinical oncology, we should find the ways of providing a

263

high level of special diagnostics and therapy of oncological patients by using national and economical means.

A particular and ever increasing attention should be given to the purposeful observation and rehabilitation of oncological patients; it concerns patients who have real chances of recovery after primary treatment; on the other hand, it concerns patients who have undergone not a therapeutic but only a palliative course of treatment and for whom systematical additional treatment can essentially improve the "quality of the remaining life".

The rehabilitation of oncological patients means both physical and psychological rehabilitation. Owing to the more purposeful treatment in sanatoriums for convalescent oncological patients, the effectiveness of rehabilitation of oncological patients significantly increases. The introduction of prolonged therapy after primary treatment - which is an increasingly urgent requirement - is also more effective following treatment in the sanatorium.

The care of incurable patients cannot be a final goal of cancer control; however, the reality of our days shows that this complex of tasks should receive more emphasis. All available and newly produced facilities particularly for X-ray therapy must fully serve these aims. In the GDR there is a network of regional oncological consultation centres, there are oncologists-consultants in areas and regions which creates a certain advantage in accomplishing the above tasks. Nevertheless, the character of the work of these consultation centres should be changed: it has to proceed from the activities of the care and observation to an active therapeutic activities of greater extent. Considerable attention should be given to solving the problems of clinical oncology. With regard to our manpower and material possibilities we must set up special oncological, diagnostic and therapeutic establishments in every area in the near future, if necessary, by changing the profiles of the available establishments.

The training and postgraduate training of physicians in oncology need efficient organizational forms as well as forms of cooperation of the physicians participating in the prevention of malignant tumours.

In some cases this undoubtedly purposeful orientation and investments for increasing the effectiveness of cancer control and achieving maximum benefit for oncological patients; in a number of cases many years' efforts will be required in this direction. The necessity of systematic effective coordination of all types of activities in the field of cancer control is obvious. Medical societies, especially the Cancer Control Society, must put the strategy of cancer control into practice according to a well-considered plan. The accomplishment of all basic tasks of cancer control requires a systematic training and improvement of qualifications of the personnel having sufficient special knowledge on oncology. First of all it concerns all workers of regional oncological consultation centres as well as the physicians and nurses working at therapeutic and diagnostic oncological establishments. It is necessary to concentrate efforts in the future at the attainment of greater specialization and at the increase in the qualifications of a relatively limited number of medical workers who deal mainly with oncological problems. It is necessary to take into consideration that while planning research work on cancer control one should put forward basic tasks which are to be accomplished in the first place. It seems obvious that at present the final goal of specialized and highly specialized oncological assistance to the population is to set up regional oncological clinics in all the 15 administrative areas of the GDR.

Part I should be filled in by the physician and typed in duplicate! The first copy should be immediately sent to the regional oncological consultation centre of the patient's residence, the second copy should be sent to the medical establishment where the patient is admitted in order to make the diagnosis more precise /oncologist, hospital/.

Part 2 should be filled in at the institution where the patient's diagnosis is made more precise and sent urgently to the appropriate regional oncological consultation centre. See additional instructions on the back side!

The Council of Ministers
of the German Democratic Republic
The Ministry of Health
The Academy of Sciences of the GDR
The Central Institute of Cancer
Research, the National Cancer Registry, 1197, Berlin

A

According to the resolution of the Central Statistical Office the questionnaire does not require a special permission the decree of
2. 10. 1958.

To the regional oncological consultation centre

....
/region/

/Stamp of the regional oncological consultation centre/

The information about oncological disease or case suspected of it

Date of reception ...
....
No. of diary ....

I   Patient's number
/according to the passport/

Date of birth

Which is the primarily diagnosed disease?

Year of diagnosis /date of the establishment of the first diagnosis suspecting an oncological disease/:

....
/Maiden name/

Surname:

266

Name: [ ] ..... male /   /   female /   /

Address: ....
/ZIP code - community - region - street - No.of house/

Type/localization of tumour .:...................................

No. of diagnosis /ac-
cording to the Inter-
national Classification   State before the
of Diseases/ ....beginning of treatment ....

Referred ....
          when?   where?

....
/Stamp with the address   /Date/   Signature of the phy-
of the establishment   sian /also in type-
sending the questionnaire/   written form/

II To be filled in by the institution where the patient is
   referred to make the diagnosis more precise, if a detailed
   history and epicrisis are not required/

The above-mentioned oncological disease /type/localization/
/stage/ is confirmed - not confirmed - remained suspected

Method of establishing the diagnosis: clinical - roentgenologic
- endoscopic - cytological - histological - other methods.
What other methods? ....

Histological findings ....

On changing the diagnosis: /Type/localization/stage/ ....

In cutaneous basaliomas: Method of treatment ....ˌ.

Patient has not come despite repeated calls.

Reception - Referral to another institution - Return of notice
....

When?............... Where? .... Why? ....

....
/Stamp with the address   /Date/   Signature of the phy-
of the establishment   sician /also in type-
where the diagnosis was   written form/
verified, No. of insti-
tution and its name/

Filled in and typed in duplicate by the therapeutic establishment; not later than 14 days after the completion of treatment
it should be sent to the regional consultation centre of the
patient's residence! See additional instructions on filling in
on the back side of the card.

The Council of Ministers
of the German Democratic Republic
The Ministry of Health
The Academy of Sciences of the GDR
The Central Institute of Cancer
Research, the National Cancer
Registry, 1197, Berlin

According to the deci-
sion of the Central
Statistical Office the
present form does not
require a special per-
mission according to
the order of 2.10.1958.

To

B

Report on case history
and epicrisis of onco-
logical patient

Basic course of treat-
ment

Primary treatment - Ad-
ditional treatment -
Treatment of relapse -
Treatment of metastases

Date of admission:.....

No. of diary: ....

/Stamp of regional oncological consultation centre/

KK Patient's number /according to the passport/

KK   Date of birth

Which is
the pri-
mary
disease?

Date of
the es-
tablish-
ing the
first diagnosis
suspecting on-
cological dis-
ease:

1   2   13   14   15   16

Sur-
name   ..../..........   male
                                        /Maiden name/   female
17   31

268

Name:

Family status:
/unmarried=0,
.... married=1,
widowed=2,
divorced=3,
separated=4,
unknown=9/

| | | | | | | | | | | | | | |

32   46

47

/Day/Month/Year/

| Date of the beginning of treatment | Diagnosis /No. according to the International Classification of Diseases/ | Does the patient has /only/ cutaneous basalioma? /yes = 1/ | Is there pregnancy? /yes=1/ |

| | | | |

48   53

| | | |

54   57

58

59

Additional information provided by regional consultation centre

. . . .

/Area/region/community/

No. of the regional consultation centre

Place of patient's residence /according to the list of communities and local administrative division/

Timely reception of forms?
/form "A" = 1,
form "B" = 2,
form "A"+
+form "B" =3/

| | | |

60   63

| | | | | |

64   69

70

See additional instructions on the back side of the cover!

Address of patient: . . . .
. . . .

Therapeutic establishment where primary treatment was carried out: . . . . .
. . . .

Anamnestic data:

Date of the appearance of the first symptoms of oncological disease . . . . Date of the first medical consultation . . . .

Date of establishing the first diagnosis with suspicion of malignanos . . . . where, by whom? . . . .

Was the diagnosis established as a result of preventive examination? yes   no

Did the patient regularly undergo prophylactic examinations of the corresponding localization? yes   no, date of the last prophylactic examination: ....

Any previous diseases of this organ? ....

Previous oncological and precancerous diseases /type/localization/year/ ....

Oncological diseases among members of the family: /in whom?/ /localization/ ....

Does the patient smoke? yes   no   does not smoke any longer since .... cigarettes   - cigars   - pipe   - other .... Average alcohol consumption .... - no   - no longer since .... beer   - wine   - spirits

On an average regular consumption of alcohol for .... years

Beginning of the monthly period at .... years of age.
At what age did menopause occur? ....

Number of pregnancies ...... Age at the first pregnancy ....

Delivery: live birth........ stillbirth .... miscarriage .... abortion ....

Occupation practised for the longest time: /what?/name, type, enterprise/duration/.

	What occupation?:	Enterprise?:	from - to
1	....	....	19... - 19.....
2	....	....	19... - 19.....
3	....	....	19... - 19.....
4	....	....	19... - 19.....

Occupational or other influences which could be the cause of oncological disease /indicate also the date and duration:/ ....

DIAGNOSIS:

Localization of primary tumour: ....
/As detailed as possible!/   ....
                                 Size of tumour........cm in
                                                    diameter

Localization of metastases: ....

Type /histology of oncological disease: /with regard for the
morphological code according to ICD-O/ ....
.... ICD-O No: M..............

Stage: before treatment: carcinoma in situ - I - II - III
- IV - systemic disease - it is impossible to give information

After operation or after treatment: carcinoma in situ - I -
II - III - IV - systemic disease - it is impossible to
give information

According to the TNM system: T..... N..... M..... P..... O.....

Method of diagnosis: /indicate all diagnostic methods employed!/

Concomitant diseases

Now   Before

Clinical only   Histological   Tuberculosis
Cytological   Palliative   Diabetes
Colposcopy   interven-   Syphilis
Endoscopy   tion   Other
Roentgen   curettage   venereal
    diagnosis   When? ....   diseases
Other methods   Other
                       Puncture   serious
                       When? ....   diseases
                                            What
                       Laparoscopy,   diseases? ....
                       trepanbiopsy   ....
                       When? ....

                       Immediate observa-
                       tion /during oper-
                       ation/
When? ....   Examination of
                       surgical
                       preparation

Height: ...... cm / Weight .... kg /Blood pressure ....

Blood group .... Rhesus factor ....

TREATMENT: Date of the beginning
                                    of the treatment men-
                                    tioned here: ....
Surgical intervention? yes - no

Date of surgery .... Method of surgical intervention ...
....

Character of surgical intervention: radical   - palliative

- exploratory operation - it is impossible to give information

X-ray therapy?   yes   - no

Was X-ray therapy of radical
                    palliative   character?

Discontinuation of X-ray therapy?   yes   - no   - why? ....

                                     Dosage   from   to

Deep penetrating - mid-penetrating
     roentgenotherapy - close-
     focus roentgen radiation
     Method: ....

High-voltage irradiation - what
     kind? ....
     Method: ....

Isotopes - what kind? ....
     Method: ....

Other ionizing irradiation -
     what kind? ....
     Method: ....

Irradiation of regional lymph
     nodes? ....

Chemotherapy: yes   - no
     Preparations: ....
     ....
     ....
     Method: ....

Hormonotherapy?   yes   - no   -
     what kind?.................. ....
     Preparations: ....
     ....
     ....
     ablative   additive
     ....

Other adjuvant tumour therapy:
     yes   no   what ....
     ....

Functional blocking of endocrine glands? yes   - no   - what
glands? ....
     Method: ....

Other additional types of specific treatment? yes   - no   -
what kind? ....
....
....

If only symptomatic treatment was employed? yes why? ....
no

If no treatment was employed:

If patient refused treatment, from what one?...................

Complications following treatment: yes   - no   - what? ....
....
....
....

Report on case history and epicrisis

Patient' number   Which is the   Date of estab-
                                primary dis-   lishing of the
        Date of birth   ease?   first diagnosis
                                                    suspecting an
    ☐☐☐☐☐☐☐☐☐☐☐☐   ☐   oncological   ☐☐
                                                    disease:

Surname:☐☐☐☐☐☐☐☐☐☐☐☐☐☐....../Name: ☐☐☐☐☐☐☐☐☐☐☐☐☐☐☐☐

Final results:
/Including general/
/local results of
clinical examina-
tions/

Roentgenologic/ra-
dioisotope diag-
nosis:

Haematology: Clinical chemistry: Hb ..... % Hematocrite ..... %
Platelets ...../mm^3 Reticulocytes ..... %ooo Leukocytes ....mm^3
/juvenile forms ..... %; rod nuclei .... %; segmented nuclei ..
.. %. Eosinophils .... % Basophils .... % Lymphocytes .... %/
Total protein g % ..... Creatinine mg % ..... Total bilirubin .
.... mg % Serum asparate-amino-transferase - IU. Alanine-amino
-transferase - IU. Aldolase - IU. Alkaline phosphatase - IU.
Acid phosphatase - IU. Lactate dehydrognase - IU. Blood sugar
....

Other tests:

Results of treatment after primary treatment:

Absence of tumour symptoms   Obvious regression
           No change   Progress of disease

Recommendations on the
continuation of treatment:

Recommendation for the regional
consultation centre:

Disabled since ....   Capable of work approximately
Disability   - no   since ....
Change of place of work
    yes   no   Transferral to lighter work
Disability certificate   yes   no
    yes   no   Category of disability: mild,
Provision of allowance for   moderate, sever /with/without
    care of patient   provision of "seat"/
    yes   no
                        Category of allowance:
                        I - II - III - higher

What information did the patient get on his disease? ....
....
....

Date of discharge .... Referred to ....
                              When?   Where?
Date of first visit .... Where? ....

In case of death:

Date of death: .... Was the death caused by oncological
disease subjected to registration?   yes   no

Cause of death /according to the death certificate/: ....
....

Cause of death with   or without   mentioning oncological
                                   disease
Was autopsy performed? yes   - no   - why not?.................
Only partial autopsy: why? ....
Histological examination was not performed: why?............
Name of medical institution where autopsy was performed ....
.... autopsy No ....

....
/Stamp with the address of   /Date/   Signature of the phy-
the institution sending this   sician /also in a
form, no.of the institution   typewritten form/
and name of the department/

Filled in by the patient
Please fill in thoroughly

/Office stamp/

Name: .... First name: ....

Personal No /by passport, page 2/ ....

Address: ....
            /ZIP code - community - district - street - house No/

Family states: unmarried, married   - widowed   - divorced
                     - separated

Did you undergo treatment? Yes   No

Where? On what occasion? ....

Have you been already operated on? Yes   No

When, where, on what occasion? ....
....

Do /or did/ you suffer from diabetes, tuberculosis, oncological
or venereal diseases?..
Which? .... from - to ....
Which? .... from - to ....

Does /did/ anybody of your family suffer from one or the above
diseases?

Diabetes   who?
Tuberculosis   who?
Oncological disease   who? which organ?
Venereal diseases   who?

Do you think that your disease is related to occupational or
other influences to which you were subjected? /If yes, please
indicate the type of influence, date and duration/ ....
....

Do you smoke? Yes   - No   - Rarely
Did you smoke earlier? Yes   - No   from .... to ......

What do you smoke /smoked/? How many pieces a day?

Cigarettes   - yes   - no

Cigars   - yes   - no

Cigarillos   - yes   - no

Pipe   - yes   - no

Do you take alcoholic drinks? Yes   - No   - Rarely

If you do not take drinks any more put down: have not taken alcohol since 19 ....

What do /did/ you drink? ....

How much did you drink a day, as a rule? ....

Beer

Wine

Spirits .... other drinks ....

What professional activity have you been engaged in? ....
....

Professional activity	Enterprise /address/	Time period
1.	....	from ... to ....
2.	....	from ... to ....
3.	....	form ... to ....
4.	....	from ... to ....
5.	....	from ... to ....

Date ....

Signature ....

Filled in by the therapeutic institution in block letters and not later than 14 days after the completion of treatment should be sent in duplicate to the regional oncological centre of the patient's residence! Instructions on filling in are on the back side!

According to the decision of the Central Statistical Office the present form does not require a special permission in line with the degree of 2. 10. 58.

The Council of Ministers
of the German Democratic Republic

The Ministry of Health
of the Academy of Sciences of the GDR

The Central Institute of Cancer
Research, the National Cancer Registry,
1197, Berlin

Case history of oncological patient and
epicrisis of oncological disease
Card for computer

Basic course of treatment

B₁ $\quad$ B₁

Primary treatment   – Additional treatment – Treatment of relapse   –
Treatment of metastases

Date of admission ....
No. of diary ....

To

/Stamp of the regional oncological consultation centre/

Patient's number /according to the passport/

/Date of birth/

Which is the   Year of diagnosis /date of establish-
primarily   ing the diagnosis with the suspicion
disease?   of oncological disease/:

KK

1   2   13   14   15 16

Surname:

⬚⬚⬚⬚⬚⬚⬚⬚⬚⬚⬚⬚⬚⬚⬚
17   31

....
                                /Maiden name/

Name:

⬚⬚⬚⬚⬚⬚⬚⬚⬚⬚⬚⬚⬚⬚
32   46

male

female ⬚
        47

.........../

Family status:
/unmarried = 0, married = 1,
widowed = 2, divorced = 3,
separated = 4, unknown = 9/

/Day/month/Year/

Date of the
beginning
of treat-
ment

⬚⬚ ⬚⬚ ⬚⬚⬚
48   53

Diagnosis /No.
according to
the International
Classification of
Diseases/

⬚⬚⬚⬚
54   57

Does the patient
has /only/ cuta-
neous basalioma?
/yes = 1/

⬚
58

Is there
pregnan-
cy?
/yes = 1/

⬚
59

Additional notes of the regional consultation centre .... /Area/region/community/

No. of the
regional
consultation
centre

⬚⬚⬚
60   63

Place of the patient's
residence /according to
the list of communities
and local administrative
division/

⬚⬚⬚⬚⬚
64   69

Timely reception
of forms:
/"A" = 1; "B" = 2;
"A" + "B" = 3/

⬚
70

See additional instructions on the back side:

Instructions on filling in:

Carbon copies can be made while filling in the card for computer /detailed case history –
epicrisis – final report /form "B"/, as this part is similar to the upper half of the page.
Nevertheless, a clear, legible writing is required for computer processing /first copy/.

Put a cross /x/ in the circle   in case of agreement.

278

The card is filled in from left to right. Only one letter, mark or figure can be typed in every box, written if necessary. Dates should be completed by "0", if necessary /e.g.03.05.07/.

What is primary disease? 1 = primary disease   4 = fourth disease
                          2 = secondary disease   5 = primary multiple disease
                          3 = third disease   6 = secondary multiple disease

Precancerous diseases /for example, carcinoma in situ/ for technical reasons should be considered malignant neoplasms.

Date of establishing the diagnosis, that is, the year when the diagnosis suspecting and oncological disease was primarily established.

Surname: If the surname consists of more than 15 letters /including marks/, it is permitted to go out of the limits of the assigned boxes; only 15 letters will be put into the computer but ambiguity will be excluded. Prefixes of surnames /for instance "von"/ are not included into the surname but are added to the name by hyphen.

Diagnosis is coded according to the International Classification of Diseases of the last revision /in four digits/. If the fourth place is not envisaged then box 57 is left empty.

Cutaneous basaliomas: In case of cutaneous basaliomas, a detailed conclusion is not required. However for A is attached to the card for computer as the necessary data will not be otherwise covered /for example, address/.

No. of the regional oncological consultation centre is given by the National Cancer Registry.

Place of patient's residence is made more precise according to the available "List of communities and local administrative division of the GDR". The Cancer Registry informs regional oncological consultation centres which lists cover the years in question.

Timely reception of forms /according to the legislative decrees/
    1 = form A before the beginning of treatment is in the regional consultation centre
    2 = form B is mailed from the hospital not later than 14 days after the completion of
        treatment
    3 = Both form A and form B were received in time by the regional consultation centres

279

Filled in by typewriter in duplicate and sent to the regional oncological centre of the patient's residence. Please observe the limits of boxes as this document is to be proccessed in a computer.

The Council of Ministers of the German Democratic Republic The Ministry of Health The Academy of Sciences of the GDR The Central Institute of Cancer Research, the National Cancer Registry, 1197, Berlin

According to the resolution of the Central Statistical Office the present form does not require a special permission according to the degree of 2. 10. 58.

C

To the regional consultation centre

Control card
Card of neglected case
Card with the information on the death from the oncological disease subjected to compulsory registration.

Date of admission ......
No. of diary ....

/Stamp of the regional consultation centre/

Patient's number
/according to the passport/

/Date of birth/

KK

Which is the primary disease?

Year of admission /date of the establishment of the first diagnosis with suspicion/

1   2   13   14   15   16

Sur-
name: ....

17   31

On changing the address it is filled by the regional consultation centre!
No. of the appropriate regional consultation centre

Name: ....

32   46

47   50

Address: ....
        /ZIP code - community - region - street - No. of house/

Immediate mailing promotes avoiding repeated questions

280

Former address ....
　　　　　　　　/according to the data of the patient's case
　　　　　　　　record - filled in only if the address has
　　　　　　　　changed/

Type/localization of tumour ....

Treatment of convalescents from .... to .... □
　　　　　　　/which course of treatment of convalescent oncolo-　51
　　　　　gical patients/

Control examination:　Date of repeated　/day/month/year/
　　　　　　　　　　　　　examination　　　┌─┬─┬─┬─┬─┐
　　　　　　　　　　　　　　　　　　　　　└─┴─┴─┴─┴─┘
　　　　　　　　　　　　　　　　　52　　　　　　　57

Results of examination: /code on the backside/　　　　□
In case of relapse/metastases: localization 58

Was histological confirmation obtained?　　　　yes　　　　no

It is impossible to carry out control examination since ....

Information on death:
　　　　　　　　　　　　　　　　　　/day/month/year/
　　　　　　Date of death　　　　┌─┬─┬─┬─┬─┐
　　　　　　　　　　　　　59　　└─┴─┴─┴─┴─┘　64
Result of examination /code on the backside/　　□
　　　　　　　　　　　　　　　　　　　　　　　　65

Cause of death: /code on the backside/　　　　□
　　　　　　　　　　　　　　　　　　　　　　66

Data of the death certificate: ....

Autopsy: /code on the backside/　　　　　□
　　　　　　　　　　　　　　　　　　　67

If autopsy was not performed, then why?.......................
Autopsy No .... Pathology: ....

....　　.........　......................
/Stamp　with the address of　　/Date/　Signature of physi-
the institution sending　　　　　　　cian /also in type-
this form, No. of the insti-　　　　written form/
tution and name of the
department/

Individual primary diseases are numbered; for technical reasons
precancerous diseases /for example, carcinoma in situ/ are
considered to be malignant tumours. The number given here

281

should correspond to the data on the card for computer processing of the data of anamnesis and epicrisis.

That also concerns the date of diagnosis. That date is indicated
when the oncological disease subjected to compulsory registration
was primarily suspected. If, in exceptional cases, the surname
comprises moure than 15 letters it is permitted to go out the
limits of the boxes. But it is necessary to begin always from the
first box on the left!

Report on treatment:
1=first course of treatment in
  a sanatorium for convalescents
2=second course of treatment
  in a sanatorium for convalescents
3=third course of treatment in
  a sanatorium for conva-
  lescent
4=fourth course of treatment
  in a sanatorium for
  convalescents
5=stay in a sanatorium for
  reconvaléscents
6=stay in a sanatorium for re-
  convalescents plus one or
  more courses of treatment in
  a sanatorium for convalescents

Control examination:
Result of the examination:
1=absence of tumour symptoms
2=relapse   after
3=regional   radical
  metastases   treat-
4=distant   ment
  metastases
5=malignant transformation
  of precancerous disease
6=progressive growth of
  tumour
7=latter was not confirmed
8=patient did not come for
  repeated examination however
  it is known from the inquiry
  sent to the patient's address that he is alive /the
  date of the inquiry is indicated instead of the date of
  repeated examination/

Information about death:
Result
A=death from intercurrent disease
B=death due to relapse   after
  of tumour   radical
C=death due to regional   treatment
  metastases
D=death due to distant metastases
E=death from the oncological dis-
  ease developed as a result of
  malignant transformation of
  precancerous disease
F=death at progressive growth of
  tumour
G=it is impossible to indicate
  any of the points A-E

Cause of death:
1=death from oncological disease
2=other cause of death in the presence of oncological disease
3=other cause of death in the absence of oncological disease
4=death from complication after
  treatment
5=it is impossible to indicate
  any of the points 1-4

Autopsy:
0=autopsy was not performed
1=autopsy with histological
  examination
2=partial autopsy with histological examination
3=autopsy without histological
  examination
4=partial autopsy without histological examination
5=autopsy was performed but it
  is impossible to indicate any
  of the points
6=it is unknown whether autopsy
  was performed

The Central Institute of Cancer Research of the GDR
The National Cancer Registry and Cancer Statistics
    1197 Berlin-Joachimsthal, Sterndamm, 13

Personal data

	Date of birth			male/female	current No.		patient's No.	primary, secondary, etc.disease	year of diagnosis
	day	month	year						
boxes			01					02	03
columns 1	2	3	4	5	6	7	8	9	10	11	12	13	14	15	16
1															
1															
1															
1˙															
1															
1															
1															
1															
1															
1															
1	2	3	4	5	6	7	8	9	10	11	12	13	14	15	16
1															
1															
1															
1															
1															
1															
1															
1															
1	2	3	4	5	6	7	8	9	10	11	12	13	14	15	16
1															

283

Surname

	10														
17	18	19	20	21	22	23	24	25	26	27	28	29	30	31	
17	18	19	20	21	22	23	24	25	26	27	28	29	30	31	
17	18	19	20	21	22	23	24	25	26	27	28	29	30	31	

Name

family status

11														12
32	33	34	35	36	37	38	39	40	41	42	43	44	45	46	47
32	33	34	35	36	37	38	39	40	41	42	43	44	45	46	47
32	33	34	35	36	37	38	39	40	41	42	43	44	45	46	47

Date of the beginning of primary treatment					No. according to the International Classification of Diseases					cutaneous basalioma	pregnancy	No. of regional consultation centre, area, region			
day		month		year											
		13					14			15	16			17	
48	49	50	51	52	53	54	55	56	57	58	59	60	61	62	63
48	49	50	51	52	53	54	55	56	57	58	59	60	61	62	63
48	49	50	51	52	53	54	55	56	57	58	59	60	61	62	63

Date: ....

Personal data according
to form B_1

Place of residence						timely admission of patient	class of patient's residence										
		18				19	1A										
64	65	66	67	68	69	70	71	72	73	74	75	76	77	78	79	80	
																	1
																	2
																	3
																	4
																	5
																	6
																	7
																	8
																	9
																	1o
64	65	66	67	68	69	70	71	72	73	74	75	76	77	78	79	80	11
																	12
																	13
																	14
																	15
																	16
																	17
																	18
																	19
																	20
																	21
64	65	66	67	68	69	70	71	72	73	74	75	76	77	78	79	80	22

The Central Institute of Cancer Research of the GDR
The National Cancer Registry and Cancer Statistics
1197, Berlin-Joachimsthal, Sterndamm, 13

Personal data

| | | Date of birth | | | male/female | Current No. | | | | patient's No. | primary, secondary, etc. treatment | year of diagnosis | |
		day	month	year									
boxes				01							02	03	
columns 1	2	3	4	5	6	7	8	9	10	11	12	13	14	15	16
2															
2															
2															
2															
2															
2															
2															
2															
2															
2															
1	2	3	4	5	6	7	8	9	10	11	12	13	14	15	16
2															
2															
2															
2															
2															
2															
2															
2															
2															
2															
1	2	3	4	5	6	7	8	9	10	11	12	13	14	15	16
2															

diagnosis was made /by whom?/	preventive examination	month when suspicion arose	delayed diagnosis		time in months	t o t a l	previous disease	cancer in the family	what?	smoking	for how long?
			patient	physician						how many?	
20	21	22	23		24		25	26		27	
17	18	19	20	21	22	23	24	25	26	27	28
17	18	19	20	21	22	23	24	25	26	27	28
17	18	19	20	21	22	23	24	25	26	27	28

/cont'd/

what?	how much?	for how long?	what?	since when?	for how long?	live birth	still-birth	miscarriage	pensioner; housewife
alcohol consumption			contra-ceptives			delivery			
28			29				2A		2B
29	30	31	32	33	34	35	36	37	38
29	30	31	32	33	34	35	36	37	38
29	30	31	32	33	34	35	36	37	38

1st place of work   2nd place of work

from ..... to   from ..... to

<table>
<tr><td colspan="11" align="center">2 C</td><td colspan="7" align="center">2 D</td></tr>
<tr><td>39</td><td>40</td><td>41</td><td>42</td><td>43</td><td>44</td><td>45</td><td>46</td><td>47</td><td>48</td><td>49</td><td>50</td><td>51</td><td>52</td><td>53</td><td>54</td><td>55</td><td>56</td></tr>
<tr><td></td><td></td><td></td><td></td><td></td><td></td><td></td><td></td><td></td><td></td><td></td><td></td><td></td><td></td><td></td><td></td><td></td><td></td></tr>
<tr><td></td><td></td><td></td><td></td><td></td><td></td><td></td><td></td><td></td><td></td><td></td><td></td><td></td><td></td><td></td><td></td><td></td><td></td></tr>
<tr><td></td><td></td><td></td><td></td><td></td><td></td><td></td><td></td><td></td><td></td><td></td><td></td><td></td><td></td><td></td><td></td><td></td><td></td></tr>
<tr><td></td><td></td><td></td><td></td><td></td><td></td><td></td><td></td><td></td><td></td><td></td><td></td><td></td><td></td><td></td><td></td><td></td><td></td></tr>
<tr><td>39</td><td>40</td><td>41</td><td>42</td><td>43</td><td>44</td><td>45</td><td>46</td><td>47</td><td>48</td><td>49</td><td>50</td><td>51</td><td>52</td><td>53</td><td>54</td><td>55</td><td>56</td></tr>
<tr><td></td><td></td><td></td><td></td><td></td><td></td><td></td><td></td><td></td><td></td><td></td><td></td><td></td><td></td><td></td><td></td><td></td><td></td></tr>
<tr><td></td><td></td><td></td><td></td><td></td><td></td><td></td><td></td><td></td><td></td><td></td><td></td><td></td><td></td><td></td><td></td><td></td><td></td></tr>
<tr><td></td><td></td><td></td><td></td><td></td><td></td><td></td><td></td><td></td><td></td><td></td><td></td><td></td><td></td><td></td><td></td><td></td><td></td></tr>
<tr><td>39</td><td>40</td><td>41</td><td>42</td><td>43</td><td>44</td><td>45</td><td>46</td><td>47</td><td>48</td><td>49</td><td>50</td><td>51</td><td>52</td><td>53</td><td>54</td><td>55</td><td>56</td></tr>
</table>

3rd place of work   4th place of work

from .....   to   from .....   to

						2 E							2 F						
57	58	59	60	61	62	63	64	65	66	67	68	69	70	71	72	73	74	75	76
57	58	59	60	61	62	63	64	65	66	67	68	69	70	71	72	73	74	75	76
57	58	59	60	61	62	63	64	65	66	67	68	69	70	71	72	73	74	75	76

surname

name

04

77	78	79	80	
				1
				2
				3
				4
				5
				6
				7
				8
				9
				10
77	78	79	80	11
				12
				13
				14
				15
				16
				17
				18
				19
				20
				21
77	78	79	80	22

The Central Institute of Cancer Research of the GDR
The National Cancer Registry and Cancer Statistics
1197 Berlin-Joachimsthal, Sterndamm, 13

Personal data

		Date of birth					male/female		current No.			patient's No.	primary,secondary etc.disease	year of diagnosis	establishment
		day		month		year									
boxes					01								02		03	
columns	1	2	3	4	5	6	7	8	9	10	11	12	13	14	15	16
	3															
	3															
	3															
	3															
	3															
	3															
	3															
	3															
	3															
	3															
	1	2	3	4	5	6	7	8	9	10	11	12	13	14	15	16
	3															
	3															
	3															
	3															
	3															
	3															
	3															
	3															
	3															
	3															
	1	2	3	4	5	6	7	8	9	10	11	12	13	14	15	16

	localization	regional lymph nodes		tumour size	morphology					
	30	31		32	33					
17	18	19	20	21	22	23	24	25	26	27
17	18	19	20	21	22	23	24	25	26	27
17	18	19	20	21	22	23	24	25	26	27

/cont'd/

	stage											blood type	Method of diagnosis		
before treatment	final												roentgen diagnosis	endoscopy	needle biopsy
34	35				36				27	38				39	
28	29	30	31	32	33	34	35	36	37	38	39	40	41	42	43	44
28	29	30	31	32	33	34	35	36	37	38	39	40	41	42	43	44
28	29	30	31	32	33	34	35	36	37	38	39	40	41	42	43	44

concomitant diseases								height		weight			blood pressure								No. according to the International Classification of Diseases	
No. according to the International Classification of Diseases		" - -																					
3A			3B				3C			3D				3E								3F	
45	46	47	48	49	50	51	52	53	54	55	56	57	58	59	60	61	62	63	64	65	66		
45	46	47	48	49	50	51	52	53	54	55	56	57	58	59	60	61	62	63	64	65	66		
45	46	47	48	49	50	51	52	53	54	55	56	57	58	59	60	61	62	63	64	65	66		

Date: ....

D

topography			type		histology					surname			name	
3G			3H		3K					O4				
67	68	69	70	71	72	73	74	75	76	77	78	79	80	
														1
														2
														3
														4
														5
														6
														7
														8
														9
														10
67	68	69	70	71	72	73	74	75	76	77	78	79	80	11
														12
														13
														14
														15
														16
														17
														18
														19
														20
														21
67	68	69	70	71	72	73	74	75	76	77	78	79	80	22

The Central Institute of Cancer Research of the GDR
The National Cancer Registry and Cancer Statistics
1197 Berlin-Joachimsthal, Sterndamm, 13

Personal data

	Date of birth			male/female	current No.				patient's No.	primary, secondary etc. disease	year of diagnosis
	day	month	year								
boxes	01								02	03	
columns 1	2	3	4	5	6	7	8	9	10	11	12	13	14	15	16
4															
4															
4															
4															
4															
4															
4															
4															
4															
4															
1	2	3	4	5	6	7	8	9	10	11	12	13	14	15	16
4															
4															
4															
4															
4															
4															
4															
4															
4															
4															
1	2	3	4	5	6	7	8	9	10	11	12	13	14	15	16
4															

surgery		chemotherapy	hormonotherapy	unspecific symp- tomatic treatment	no treatment	patient refused treatment	treatment of convalescents	medical establishment I /lines 40-44/										staff number
40		41	42	43	44	45						46						47
17	18	19	20	21	22	23	24	25	26	27	28	29	30	31	32	33		34
17	18	19	20	21	22	23	24	25	26	27	28	29	30	31	32	33		34
17	18	19	20	21	22	23	24	25	26	27	28	29	30	31	32	33		34

| | radiation | | | | | | isotopes | | | | |
| type | lymph nodes | dosage | | | time | what? | | dosage? | | time | |

			48			49		4A		4B	
35	36	37	38	39	40	41	42	43	44	45	46	47
35	36	37	38	39	40	41	42	43	44	45	46	47
35	36	37	38	39	40	41	42	43	44	45	46	47

medical establishment II /lines 48-49/										staff number	duration of of stay in hospital		day	month	year
						4C				4D	4E			4F	
48	49	5O	51	52	53	54	55	56	57	58	59	6O	61	62	63	64	65	66	67
48	49	5O	51	52	53	54	55	56	57	58	59	6O	61	62	63	64	65	66	67
48	49	5O	51	52	53	54	55	56	57	58	59	6O	61	62	63	64	65	66	67

Date of last examination or date of death

Date: ....

T

results of examination	first relapse	regional metastases	distant metastases	death	autopsy	year of death				surname		name
4G	4H	4K	4L	4M		4N				04		
68	69	70	71	72	73	74	75	76	77	78	79	80	
													1
													2
													3
													4
													5
													6
													7
													8
													9
													10
68	69	70	71	72	73	74	75	76	77	78	79	80	11
													12
													13
													14
													15
													16
													17
													18
													19
													20
													21
68	69	70	71	72	73	74	75	76	77	78	79	80	22

The Central Institute of Cancer Research of the GDR
The National Cancer Registry and Cancer Statistics
1197, Berlin-Joachimsthal, Sterndamm, 13

Personal data

		Date of birth			male/female	current No.			patient's No.	primary, secondary, etc. disease	year of diagnosis	establishment
		day	month	year								
boxes						01				02	03	
columns	1	2	3	4	5	6	7	8	9	10	11	12	13	14	15	16
	9															
	9															
	9															
	9															
	9															
	9															
	9															
	9															
	9															
	9															
	1	2	3	4	5	6	7	8	9	10	11	12	13	14	15	16
	9															
	9															
	9															
	9															
	9															
	9															
	9															
	9															
	9															
	9															
	1	2	3	4	5	6	7	8	9	10	11	12	13	14	15	16
	9															

17	18	19	20	21	22	23	24	25	26	27	28	29	30	31	32	33	34	35	36	37	38

17	18	19	20	21	22	23	24	25	26	27	28	29	30	31	32	33	34	35	36	37	38

17	18	19	20	21	22	23	24	25	26	27	28	29	30	31	32	33	34	35	36	37	38

39	40	41	42	43	44	45	46	47	48	49	50	51	52	53	54	55	56	57	58	59
39	40	41	42	43	44	45	46	47	48	49	50	51	52	53	54	55	56	57	58	59
39	40	41	42	43	44	45	46	47	48	49	50	51	52	53	54	55	56	57	58	59

Date: ....

V

surname

name

04

60	61	62	63	64	65	66	67	68	69	70	71	72	73	74	75	76	77	78	79	80	
																					1
																					2
																					3
																					4
																					5
																					6
																					7
																					8
																					9
																					10
60	61	62	63	64	65	66	67	68	69	70	71	72	73	74	75	76	77	78	79	80	11
																					12
																					13
																					14
																					15
																					16
																					17
																					18
																					19
																					20
																					21
60	61	62	63	64	65	66	67	68	69	70	71	72	73	74	75	76	77	78	79	80	22

Table 42

Age-Sex Structure of the Population of the German Democratic
Republic on 30. June, 1971

Age in years	Total population	Men	Women
0 - 1	234.686	120.287	114.399
1 - 4	967.600	496.263	471.337
5 - 9	1.412.034	723.680	688.354
10-14	1.340.900	686.609	654.291
15-19	1.312.087	673.301	638.786
20-24	1.035.582	530.629	504.953
25-29	1.026.129	514.795	511.334
30-34	1.347.561	677.969	669.592
35-39	1.101.118	554.335	546.783
40-44	1.014.181	481.146	533.035
45-49	888.871	347.447	541.424
50-54	694.245	262.355	431.890
55-59	912.111	343.657	568.454
60-64	1.085.224	428.173	657.051
65-69	1.012.700	421.203	591.497
70-74	776.994	296.758	480.236
75-79	497.592	169.541	328.051
80-84	269.145	91.699	177.446
85-89	96.606	33.099	63.507
90-	24.278	8.126	16.152
Total	17.049.644	7.861.072	9.188.572

Table 43

Number and Incidence of Malignant Neoplasms in the GDR in the
1970-1974 Period

	1970	1971	1972	1973	1974
Absolute number	58.645	58.479	59.113	59.762	60.017
Incidence per 100.000 population	343.8	348.9	346.8	352.0	355.5

Table 44

Absolute Number and Incidence of Malignant Neoplasms in the Population of the GDR and its Administrative-Economic Districts in 1970, 1973 and 1974

Administrative economic districts	Absolute number Total population			Incidence per 100.000 population		
	1 9 7 0	1 9 7 3	1 9 7 4	1 9 7 0	1 9 7 3	1 9 7 4
Berlin	4.403	4.431	4.282	406.3	407.0	392.9
Cottbus	2.597	2.705	2.683	302.5	310.7	307.7
Dresden	6.949	7.043	7.194	370.7	378.8	388.6
Erfurt	3.854	3.974	4.046	307.1	317.3	323.9
Frankfurt	2.289	2.248	2.167	337.4	326.7	314.4
Gera	2.530	2.857	2.827	343.0	385.8	382.3
Halle	6.253	6.152	6.375	324.3	322.4	336.1
Karl-Marx-Stadt	8.047	8.168	8.098	392.3	405.1	404.5
Leipzig	5.693	5.799	5.771	381.2	394.1	394.4
Magdeburg	4.233	4.547	4.690	321.0	347.6	360.3
Neubrandenburg	1.826	1.841	1.845	285.9	290.9	292.9
Potsdam	3.780	3.665	3.705	333.7	324.4	328.8
Rostock	2.548	2.575	2.620	297.1	297.4	301.9
Schwerin	1.826	1.889	1.885	305.9	317.4	317.6
Suhl	1.817	1.868	1.829	328.6	338.3	331.7
Total	58.645	59.672	60.017	343.8	352.0	354.6

	All locali-zations	Oral and pharynge-al cavi-ties /140-149/	Lips /140/	Esophagus /150/	Stomach /151/	Rectum /154/
Absolu-te num-ber						Total
1970	58.645	1.004	551	438	7.183	2.953
1971	59.479	1.048	522	412	7.143	2.948
1972	59.113	986	518	451	6.940	2.953
1973	59.762	1.044	532	474	6.810	3.205
1974	60.017	1.001	527	462	6.572	3.186
Incidence per 100.000 population						
1970	343.8	5.9	3.2	2.6	42.1	17.3
1971	348.9	6.1	3.1	2.4	42.1	17.3
1972	346.8	5.8	3.0	2.6	40.7	17.3
1973	352.0	6.1	3.1	2.8	40.1	18.9
1974	354.6	5.9	3.1	2.7	38.8	18.8

45

GDR by Tumour Localization in 1970-1974

Larynx /161/	Trachea, bronchi and lungs /162/	Skin /173/	Breast /174/	Cervix uteri /180/	Other organs	Lymphatic haemato- poietic tissues /200-209/
population						
534	7.371	7.651	5.156	3.895	18.878	3.031
533	7.594	8.091	5.184	3.790	19.179	3.005
558	7.374	8.034	5.012	3.727	19.567	2.993
593	7.409	8.161	5.030	3.554	19.929	3.021
558	7.349	8.392	5.367	3.527	20.082	2.994
3.2	43.3	44.9	30.2	22.8	110.1	17.8
3.1	44.6	47.4	30.4	22.2	112.5	17.6
3.3	43.3	47.2	29.4	21.9	114.8	17.6
3.5	43.7	48.0	29.6	20.9	117.4	17.8
3.3	43.4	49.6	31.7	20.9	118.7	17.7

Absolute Number and Incidence of Malignant Tumours of Different

tive-Economic Districts

	Lips /140/		Esophagus /150/		Stomach /151/		Trachea bronchi, lungs /162/	
	A	B	A	B	A	B	A	B
1970								
Berlin	12	1.1	28	2.6	430	39.7	650	60.0
Cottbus	34	4.0	24	2.8	309	36.0	373	43.4
Dresden	59	3.1	68	3.6	923	49.2	898	47.9
Erfurt	31	2.5	18	1.4	435	34.7	374	29.8
Frankfurt	18	2.7	19	2.8	276	40.7	288	42.4
Gera	24	3.3	11	1.5	304	41.2	287	38.9
Halle	75	3.9	47	2.4	758	39.3	795	41.2
Karl-Marx-Stadt	52	2.5	70	3.4	1.161	56.6	948	46.2
Leipzig	48	3.2	34	2.3	680	45.5	685	45.9
Magdeburg	37	2.8	22	1.7	452	34.3	563	42.7
Neubrandenburg	39	6.1	18	2.8	227	35.5	257	40.2
Potsdam	37	3.3	36	3.2	438	38.7	552	48.7
Rostock	39	4.5	19	2.2	286	33.3	318	37.1
Schwerin	29	4.9	15	2.5	264	44.2	188	31.5
Suhl	17	3.1	9	1.6	240	43.4	195	35.3
Total	551	3.2	438	2.6	7.183	42.1	7.371	43.3

A = Absolute number
B = per 100.000 population

46

Localizations in the Population of the GDR and its Administra-
in 1970 and 1974

Skin /173/		Breast /174/		Cervix uteri /180/		Lymphatic and haematopoietic tissues /200-209	
A	B	A	B	A	B	A	B
438	40.4	443	40.9	305	28.1	216	19.9
342	39.8	212	24.7	160	18.6	141	16.4
896	47.8	556	29.7	424	22.6	349	18.6
548	43.7	363	28.9	315	25.1	206	16.4
271	39.9	209	30.8	171	25.2	119	17.5
400	54.2	210	28.4	149	20.2	118	15.9
873	45.3	567	29.4	481	24.9	333	17.3
1.190	58.0	672	32.8	390	19.0	345	16.8
660	44.2	515	34.5	379	25.4	306	20.5
516	39.1	380	28.8	336	25.5	243	18.4
235	36.8	154	24.1	104	16.3	101	15.8
445	39.3	359	31.7	246	21.7	199	17.6
310	36.1	243	28.3	180	21.0	158	18.4
225	37.7	144	24.1	144	24.1	94	15.7
302	54.6	129	23.3	111	20.8	103	19.4
7.651	44.9	5.156	30.2	3.895	22.8	3.031	17.8

Table 46 /cont'd/

	Lips /140/		Esophagus /150/		Stomach /151/		Trachea bronchi, lungs /162/	
	A	B	A	B	A	B	A	B
1974								
Berlin	15	1.4	32	2.9	352	32.6	592	54.3
Cottbus	32	3.7	2.7	3.1	280	32.1	388	44.5
Dresden	48	2.6	56	3.0	812	43.9	877	47.4
Erfurt	31	2.5	24	1.9	394	31.5	394	31.5
Frankfurt	16	2.3	17	2.5	230	33.4	257	37.3
Gera	19	2.6	21	2.8	344	46.5	291	39.4
Halle	61	3.2	32	1.7	712	37.5	773	40.8
Karl-Marx-Stadt	57	2.8	64	3.2	1.017	50.8	991	49.5
Leipzig	41	2.8	43	2.9	613	41.9	690	47.2
Magdeburg	47	3.6	37	2.8	482	37.0	632	48.5
Neubrandenburg	38	6.0	25	4.0	224	35.6	245	38.9
Potsdam	38	3.4	35	3.1	371	32.9	497	36.1
Rostock	32	3.7	26	3.0	284	32.7	328	37.8
Schwerin	32	5.4	14	2.4	216	36.4	198	33.4
Suhl	20	3.6	9	1.6	241	43.7	196	35.5
Total	527	3.1	462	2.7	6.572	38.8	7.349	43.4

Skin /173/		Breast /174/		Cervix uteri /180/		Lymphatic and haematopoietic tissues /200-209/	
A	B	A	B	A	B	A	B
466	42.8	443	40.6	318	29.2	194	17.8
381	43.7	245	28.1	139	15.9	122	14.0
1.016	54.9	610	32.9	353	19.1	378	20.4
612	49.0	379	30.3	312	25.0	198	15.8
258	37.4	189	27.4	196	28.4	115	16.7
457	61.8	243	32.9	149	20.2	129	17.4
933	49.2	558	29.4	367	19.3	339	17.9
1.220	60.9	700	35.0	369	18.4	348	17.4
720	49.2	511	34.9	364	24.9	289	19.7
690	53.0	422	32.4	279	21.4	257	19.7
234	37.1	163	25.9	100	15.9	96	15.2
494	43.8	344	30.5	230	20.4	182	16.2
358	41.3	221	25.5	167	19.2	143	16.5
294	49.5	175	29.5	89	15.0	123	20.7
259	47.0	164	29.7	95	17.2	81	14.7
8.392	49.6	5.367	31.7	3.527	20.8	2.994	17.7

Incidence of Malignant Tumours of the Population of the

M a l e s   Incidence per 100.000

Localizations	ICD /8/ Code Number	Total abso-lute number	Age in year Total per 100.000	0-	5-	10-	15-	20-
All malignant tumours	140-209	95.690	243.5	9.2	8.5	5.5	9.8	12.8
Lips	140	103	0.3	-	-	-	-	-
Tongue	141	200	0.5	-	-	-	-	-
Salivary glands	142	169	0.4	-	-	-	-	-
Other parts of oral cavity and naso-pharynx	143-147	519	1.3	-	0.1	0.1	-	-
Other and non-speci-fied parts of the pharynx	148-149	168	0.4	-	-	-	-	-
Oral and pharyngeal cavities	140-149	1.159	2.9	-	0.1	0.1	-	0.1
Esophagus	150	1.712	4.4	-	-	-	-	-
Stomach	151	18.398	46.8	0.1	-	-	-	0.2
Small intestine	152	235	0.6	-	-	-	-	0.1
Large intestine	153	4.489	11.4	-	0.1	-	-	0.3
Rectum,rectosigmoid section	154	5.583	14.2	-	-	0.1	-	0.2
Liver	155	1.550	3.9	0.2	0.1	-	0.1	0.1
Gallbladder	156	2.001	5.1	-	-	-	-	-
Pancreas	157	3.518	9.0	-	-	-	-	-
Other and non-speci-fied digestive organs	158-159	442	1.1	-	-	-	0.2	0.1
Digestive and peri-toneal organs	150-159	37.928	96.5	0.4	0.3	0.2	0.5	1.2
Nose and nasal cavities	160	197	0.5	0.1	-	-	0.1	0.1
Larynx	161	1.158	2.9	-	-	-	-	-
Trachea,bronchi,lungs	162	29.119	74.1	-	0.1	-	0.1	0.2
Other and non-speci-fied respiratory organs cont'd	163	721	1.8	-	0.1	-	0.1	0.1

47

GDR in 1970-1974, by Localizations, Age and Sex

population

25-	30-	35-	4C-	45-	50-	55-	60-	65-	70-	75-	80-
18.0	22.3	37.7	70.2	129.6	237.1	428.8	683.9	1.031.3	1.337.1	1.605.3	1.220.1
-	-	0.1	-	0.1	0.1	0.1	0.5	0.1	1.8	1.9	3.0
-	0.1	0.1	0.2	0.4	0.3	0.5	1.7	1.6	2.3	4.3	3.8
-	-	0.1	0.2	0.4	0.5	0.7	1.0	1.4	1.6	3.4	4.9
0.1	0.2	0.3	0.7	1.0	1.2	2.8	4.0	4.5	6.4	8.1	9.1
-	-	0.2	-	0.2	0.4	0.7	1.1	2.3	2.1	2.3	2.3
0.2	0.4	0.8	1.1	2.1	2.5	4.8	8.3	10.8	14.2	20.0	23.1
-	0.1	0.2	0.8	2.0	4.3	7.7	12.1	18.1	25.8	30.0	29.7
0.7	1.5	4.6	10.2	20.3	37.9	74.7	124.4	189.1	276.1	359.9	326.7
-	0.1	0.1	0.2	0.2	0.8	1.1	1.7	2.9	2.8	4.2	2.7
0.3	0.9	2.0	3.5	7.0	9.6	15.8	26.0	43.4	64.5	90.1	92.1
0.5	0.8	1.6	3.5	6.4	13.0	18.7	33.6	57.5	82.8	107.3	115.1
0.3	0.2	0.6	1.5	2.3	4.9	9.9	13.3	17.0	18.7	20.4	18.4
-	0.1	0.3	0.7	1.8	3.2	7.3	12.9	19.1	30.8	41.6	45.4
0.2	0.8	1.3	2.9	5.4	10.8	19.5	25.7	38.3	47.8	56.6	45.2
0.2	0.1	0.2	0.4	0.9	1.4	1.9	3.2	3.8	5.9	7.5	5.8
2.3	4.6	10.9	23.7	46.4	86.0	156.5	252.9	389.2	555.2	717.5	681.2
-	0.1	0.1	0.3	0.3	0.7	1.2	2.0	1.9	2.1	1.7	2.4
0.1	0.1	0.3	1.0	2.0	3.4	5.8	9.4	11.7	15.5	20.4	15.4
0.5	1.5	6.2	20.1	38.6	80.6	150.7	254.1	382.4	458.3	421.5	83.9
0.2	0.2	0.5	0.7	1.3	2.1	3.2	5.4	8.5	10.0	10.9	4.6

Table 47 /cont'd/

Localizations	ICD /8/ Code number	Total abso-lute number	Age in years Total per 100.000	0-	5-	10-	15-	20-
Respiratory organs	160-163	31.195	79.4	0.2	0.2	-	0.3	0.4
Bones	170	549	1.4	0.1	0.3	0.5	1.0	0.8
Connective tissue and other soft tissues	171	315	0.8	0.2	0.1	0.1	0.3	0.4
Skin melanoma	172	554	1.4	-	-	-	0.1	0.2
Other malignant tumours of the skin	173	363	0.9	-	-	-	-	-
Breast	174	112	0.3	-	-	-	-	-
Bones, connective tissue the skin and breast	170-174	1.893	4.8	0.3	0.4	0.6	1.4	1.4
Prostate	185	6.408	16.3	-	-	-	0.1	-
Testicle	186	684	1.7	0.1	0.1	0.1	1.4	3.1
Other and non-specified male genital organs	187	220	0.6	-	-	-	-	-
Bladder	188	4.071	10.4	0.1	-	-	-	-
Other and non-specified uropoietic organs	189	2.199	5.6	0.7	0.2	-	-	-
Male genital and uropoietic organs	185-189	13.582	34.6	0.9	0.3	0.1	1.7	3.3
Eyes	190	111	0.3	0.1	0.1	-	-	-
Brain	191	1.427	3.6	1.6	1.8	1.1	1.1	0.9
Other parts of the nervous system	192	200	0.5	0.9	0.3	0.5	0.2	0.3
Thyroid gland	193	248	0.6	-	-	-	-	-
Other endocrine glands	194	139	0.4	0.3	0.1	-	0.1	-
Non-exactly specified secondary and with licalization not indicated	195-199	2.058	5.2	0.2	0.3	0.1	0.2	0.5
Lymphosarcoma and reticulum cell sarcoma cont'd	200	953	2.4	0.5	0.8	0.9	0.7	0.8

population

25-	30-	35-	40-	45-	50-	55-	60-	65-	70-	75-	80-
0.8	1.9	7.2	22.1	42.3	86.8	160.9	270.9	404.5	485.9	454.5	106.3
0.4	0.5	0.4	0.8	0.9	1.6	1.9	3.6	4.2	4.9	6.6	6.4
0.2	0.4	0.4	0.3	0.8	0.8	0.9	1.6	2.3	3.1	5.0	5.8
0.7	0.9	1.6	1.6	2.1	2.9	4.4	3.2	3.0	3.9	4.5	5.8
-	0.1	0.1	-	0.4	0.8	1.0	1.6	2.5	3.4	8.2	17.5
-	-	0.1	0.1	0.3	0.3	0.7	0.6	0.9	1.5	2.0	2.6
1.3	1.9	2.6	2.8	4.6	6.5	8.9	10.6	12.9	16.8	26.3	38.1
-	-	0.2	0.3	1.1	3.4	10.0	26.7	58.1	111.2	174.8	187.3
5.0	4.2	2.7	2.0	1.1	0.6	1.1	0.7	1.5	1.6	1.9	2.9
-											
-	0.1	0.3	0.1	0.3	0.6	1.0	0.8	2.2	2.3	4.3	6.2
-	0.1	0.4	0.7	2.7	6.6	14.8	26.8	46.4	65.9	79.9	72.3
0.2	0.6	1.0	1.8	4.4	9.7	15.6	19.8	21.5	26.7	26.3	18.3
5.2	5.0	4.6	4.9	9.6	21.0	42.4	74.8	129.8	207.7	287.1	287.0
-	0.1	-	0.1	0.2	0.4	0.7	0.8	1.2	0.9	1.2	2.1
1.7	2.6	2.8	4.3	7.1	10.1	12.3	10.4	6.3	3.9	3.1	2.0
0.2	0.1	0.5	0.3	0.4	0.5	1.1	1.0	1.2	0.7	0.8	1.2
-	0.1	0.1	0.3	0.3	0.5	1.9	1.3	2.5	4.5	3.5	2.4
0.1	0.1	0.2	0.2	0.3	0.6	0.7	1.1	1.3	1.2	1.0	0.6
0.5	0.5	0.9	2.1	3.9	5.0	10.1	15.7	22.7	26.4	27.8	28.0
0.9	0.9	1.2	1.5	2.5	3.2	4.6	5.4	8.0	8.9	9.9	8.1

Incidence per 100.000

Localizations	ICD /8/ Code Number	Total absolute number	Age in years Total per 100.000	0-	5-	10-	15-	20-
Hodgkin's disease	201	944	2.4	0.1	0.2	0.3	0.9	1.6
Other neoplastic diseases of the lymphoid tissues	202	290	0.7	0.3	0.2	0.1	0.1	0.1
Multiple myeloma	203	652	1.7	-	-	-	-	-
Lymphatic leukemia, lymphoid leukemia, lymphadenosis	204	1.069	2.7	0.9	1.0	0.7	0.1	0.1
Myeloid and mono-cytic leukemia, leukemiae	205-206	1.275	3.2	1.2	1.2	0.7	1.5	1.4
Other and non-speci-fied leukaemiae, leukoses	207	572	1.5	1.1	1.3	0.5	0.9	0.7
Neoplasms of the lymphoid and haemato-poietic tissues	200-207	5.755	14.6	4.1	4.5	3.2	4.2	4.7
Other neoplasms of the lymphoid and haema-topoietic tissues	208-209*	35	0.4	-	-	0.2	0.2	-

* Since the data on localizations 208-209 are available only for 1973 they are given separately and not included into total indices /absolute and relative

F e m a l e s								
All malignant tumours	140-209	96.124	210.0	6.8	4.9	10.6	6.5	7.7
Lips	140	18	-	-	-	-	-	-
Tongue	141	100	0.2	-	-	-	-	-
Salivary glands	142	152	0.3	-	-	-	-	-
Other parts of oral cavity and nasopharynx	143-147	265	0.6	-	0.1	-	0.1	-
Other and non speci-f fied parts of the pharynx	148-149	46	0.1	-	-	-	-	-
Oral and pharyngel cavities	140-149	581	1.3	-	0.1	-	0.1	-

population

25-	30-	35-	40-	45 -	50-	55-	60-	65-	70-	75-	80-
'2.5	2.1	2.1	2.8	3.7	3.2	5.0	6.0	6.5	5.7	4.4	2.6
0.1	0.2	0.4	0.4	0.7	1.0	1.3	2.0	2.8	2.8	3.9	1.8
-	-	0.4	0.4	1.5	2.1	3.8	5.1	7.8	8.3	9.0	7.0
0.2	0.2	0.1	0.5	0.9	1.8	4.6	6.6	10.1	14.8	18.2	17.2
1.3	1.5	2.1	2.2	2.5	4.5	7.0	7.9	9.7	10.7	10.7	8.2
0.5	0.5	0.9	0.5	0.9	1.4	2.1	3.0	3.9	4.5	6.4	3.2
5.5	5.4	7.1	8.3	12.6	17.2	28.3	36.0	48.9	55.8	62.5	48.1
0.2	-	1.2	0.5	0.3	2.0	0.8	1.5	2.5	0.6	-	--

15.0	28.7	46.1	85.5	144.9	209.7	309.1	400.8	548.4	720.1	890.1	981.5
-	-	-	-	-	-	-	-	0.1	0.1	0.2	0.7
0.1	-	-	-	0.3	0.2	0.3	0.4	0.8	0.5	0.8	1.2
-	-	0.1	0.1	0.2	0.1	0.4	0.3	0.7	1.0	1.6	3.4
-	-	0.1	02.	0.4	0.6	0.8	1.1	1.3	1.8	2.2	4.1
-	-	-	-	-	0.1	0.1	0.2	0.4	0.3	0.5	0.5
0.2	-	0.2	0.3	0.8	1.0	1.5	2.0	3.4	3.7	5.4	9.8

Table 47 /cont'd/

Localizations	ICD /8/ Code Number	Total absolute number	Age in year Total per 100.000	0-	5-	10-	15-	20-
Esophagus	150	663	1.4	-	-	-	-	-
Stomach	151	14.916	32.6	0.1	-	-	-	0.4
Small Intestine	152	267	0.6	-	-	-	-	-
Large intestine	153	7.411	16.2	-	-	-	0.1	0.2
Rectum and rectosigmoid section	154	6.500	14.2	-	-	-	-	0.2
Liver	155	1.415	3.1	0.1	-	-	0.2	0.1
Gallbladder	156	7.053	15.4	0.1	-	-	0.1	-
Pancreas	157	3.616	7.9	-	-	-	-	0.1
Other and non-specified digestive organs	158-159	686	1.5	0.1	-	-	-	-
Digestive and peritoneal organs	150-159	42.527	92.9	0.4	0.1	-	0.3	1.0
Nose, nasal cavities	160	132	0.3	-	0.1	-	0.1	-
Larynx	161	93	0.2	-	-	-	-	-
Trachea, bronchi, lungs	162	3.922	8.6	-	-	-	-	-
Other and non-specified respiratory organs	163	422	0.9	0.1	-	0.1	0.1	0.1
Respiratory organs	160-163	4.569	10.0	0.1	0.1	0.1	0.2	0.1
Bones	170	521	1.1	0.1	0.2	0.4	0.8	0.3
Connective tissues and other soft tissues	171	379	0.8	0.1	-	0.1	0.1	0.2
Skin melanoma	172	692	1.5	-	-	-	0.1	0.2
Other neoplasms of the skin	173	461	1.0	-	-	-	-	-
Breast	174	11.893	26.0	-	-	-	-	0.1
Bones, connective tissue, skin and breast	170-174	13.946	30.5	0.3	0.3	0.6	1.0	0.8
Cervix uteri	180	7.411	16.2	-	-	-	-	0.4
Chorionepithelioma	181	140	0.3	-	-	-	-	0.3
Other malignant tumours of the uterus	182	3.969	8.7	-	-	-	-	-
Ovary, fallopian tubes and the broad ligament	183	7.043	15.4	-	-	0.1	0.5	0.4

25-	30-	35-	40-	45-	50-	55-	60-	65-	70-	75-	80-
-	-	0.1	0.1	0.3	0.8	1.7	2.3	3.5	5.4	7.4	11.3
0.1	1.8	3.2	7.0	10.4	16.0	30.4	47.6	84.2	134.4	192.0	200.4
-	-	0.1	0.2	0.4	0.4	0.8	1.1	1.8	1.8	2.5	3.4
0.3	0.8	1.8	2.6	5.1	10.3	18.0	25.8	41.6	64.0	87.0	102.8
0.5	0.9	1.8	3.1	6.1	10.2	18.7	25.1	41.0	54.7	67.8	73.6
0.4	0.1	0.2	0.6	1.6	2.9	4.6	6.2	7.8	12.7	13.7	13.3
-	0.2	0.7	1.9	5.5	8.7	16.2	27.6	43.4	62.5	82.9	86.7
0.2	0.2	0.2	1.6	2.6	5.2	10.3	15.8	23.7	32.1	37.1	37.9
0.1	0.1	0.2	0.3	0.8	0.8	1.7	2.8	4.3	6.2	7.0	7.0
2.6	4.0	8.3	17.5	32.8	55.3	102.5	154.4	251.3	374.1	497.4	536.4
0.1	0.1	0.1	0.1	0.1	0.3	0.4	0.3	0.6	1.2	1.1	1.7
-	-	0.1	-	0.2	0.3	0.3	0.4	0.4	0.6	0.9	1.1
0.3	0.5	1.3	2.6	4.9	9.2	13.4	20.7	28.3	31.5	31.7	23.5
0.1	0.1	0.3	0.5	0.6	0.7	1.3	2.3	2.5	3.1	3.5	2.5
0.5	0.7	1.8	3.1	5.9	10.5	15.4	23.8	31.9	36.4	37.2	28.7
0.4	0.2	0.2	0.5	0.5	1.3	1.7	2.1	2.9	2.8	4.0	4.0
0.2	0.3	0.3	0.4	0.7	0.7	1.4	1.6	2.0	2.1	2.4	4.4
0.6	0.5	1.3	1.1	1.8	2.3	2.6	2.7	2.9	3.6	5.0	5.7
-	0.1	0.1	0.1	0.1	0.3	0.4	0.7	1.5	3.1	4.7	16.1
1.1	3.6	8.4	18.3	31.2	40.1	50.9	55.7	58.8	68.5	82.8	105.4
2.3	4.8	10.2	20.4	34.3	44.5	57.0	62.8	68.0	80.1	98.8	135.6
2.3	5.6	11.3	18.4	24.8	32.1	33.5	34.7	36.4	36.9	35.5	30.8
0.1	0.1	0.1	-	0.2	0.3	0.2	0.4	0.8	1.2	1.1	1.4
0.2	0.5	1.5	2.6	5.5	9.8	15.6	19.4	25.4	29.6	33.6	30.8
0.9	1.3	3.0	8.5	16.9	22.1	31.5	37.7	41.3	48.4	47.4	36.3

Table 47 /cont'd/

Localizations	ICD /8/ Code Number	Total Abso- lute Number	Age in year Total per 100.000	0-	5-	10-	15-	20-
Other and non-speci- fied female genital organs	184	1.517	3.3	0.1	-	-	-	0.1
Urinary bladder	188	1.313	2.9	-	-	-	-	-
Other and non-speci- fied uropoietic organs	189	1.913	4.2	0.6	0.2	0.1	0.1	-
Urogenital organs	180-189	23.306	50.9	0.7	0.2	0.2	0.7	1.1
Eyes	190	148	0.3	0.2	-	0.1	-	-
Brain	191	1.313	2.9	1.3	1.6	1.3	0.8	0.5
Other parts of the nervous system	192	423	0.9	0.6	0.3	6.1	0.1	0.3
Thyroid gland	193	678	1.5	-	-	-	-	-
Other endocrine glands	194	139	0.3	0.1	-	-	0.2	-
Non-exactly specified secondary and with localization not indi- cated	195-199	3.056	6.7	0.1	0.1	0.1	0.3	0.2
Other and non-speci- fied localizations	190-199	5.757	12.6	2.4	2.0	7.7	1.3	1.0
Lymphosarcoma and reticulum cell sarcoma	200	917	2.0	0.1	0.2	0.2	0.4	0.4
Hodgkin's disease	201	720	1.6	-	-	0.2	0.8	1.2
Other neoplastic diseases of the lymphoid tissues	202	229	0.5	0.2	-	0.1	0.1	0.1
Multiple myeloma	203	796	1.7	-	-	-	-	-
Lymphatic leukemia, lymphoid leukosis, lymphadenosis	204	745	1.6	0.5	0.5	0.4	0.1	0.1
Myeloid, and mono- cytic leukemia, leukoses	205-206	1.468	3.2	1.1	0.4	0.5	1.0	1.4
Other and non-speci- fied leukaemiae, leukoses	207	563	1.2	1.0	1.0	0.5	0.5	0.4
Neoplasms of the lymphoid and hemato- poietic tissues	200-207	5.438	11.9	3.0	2.2	2.0	2.8	3.5
Other neoplasms of the lymphatic and hematopoietic tissues	208-209	53	0.5	-	-	-	-	0.2

25–	30–	35–	40–	45–	50–	55–	60–	65–	70–	75–	80–
–	0.1	0.2	0.9	1.4	2.0	2.6	5.7	8.6	12.9	17.7	21.6
–	–	0.1	0.2	0.9	1.3	3.2	5.2	7.6	11.3	16.3	17.6
0.1	0.3	0.6	1.2	2.6	4.1	7.3	10.0	13.4	14.0	16.1	11.3
3.7	7.9	16.8	31.8	52.3	71.6	94.1	113.1	133.6	154.1	167.7	150.0
–	–	–	0.1	0.2	0.2	0.6	0.7	0.8	1.0	1.3	1.5
1.4	1.5	2.5	2.9	4.7	5.7	8.0	5.8	5.1	2.1	2.0	1.4
0.1	0.1	0.3	0.3	0.4	0.8	0.7	1.0	1.1	1.2	0.6	0.8
0.1	–	0.1	0.3	0.7	1.2	2.0	3.2	4.1	5.2	7.5	6.7
0.1	–	0.1	0.1	0.4	0.4	0.7	0.5	0.7	0.8	0.5	1.4
0.4	0.5	1.1	2.7	4.4	5.8	9.7	12.8	18.1	24.3	30.1	28.2
2.1	2.1	4.2	6.3	10.8	14.0	21.6	23.9	29.9	35.0	41.9	40.1
0.2	0.5	0.7	0.9	1.0	2.0	2.7	3.8	5.6	6.8	6.6	7.9
1.7	1.6	1.3	1.1	1.4	1.7	2.2	2.3	3.5	3.5	4.0	2.7
0.1	0.1	0.1	0.3	0.4	0.9	0.8	0.7	1.2	1.8	1.6	1.6
–	0.1	0.1	0.2	0.6	1.8	3.5	3.3	6.7	6.3	7.9	3.4
0.1	0.1	–	0.3	0.5	0.5	1.5	2.5	4.0	7.2	8.4	8.2
1.1	1.3	1.7	2.6	3.1	4.4	5.0	6.1	7.1	8.3	9.7	4.8
0.5	0.5	0.6	0.7	0.8	1.3	1.4	2.1	2.3	3.1	3.5	2.5
3.7	4.2	4.7	6.1	7.9	12.7	17.1	20.8	30.4	36.9	41.7	30.8
–	0.5	0.4	0.6	1.1	1.2	1.6	1.8	1.6	1.6	1.2	–

Table 48

Highest Morbidity of Malignant Neoplasms by Localization,
Age and Sex in 1973

Code number according to the international Classification of Diseases 8th revision /ICD-8/	Localization	Average age /years/
M a l e s		
140-149	Oral and pharyngeal cavities	66.8
150	Esophagus	69.3
151	Stomach	68.9
154	Rectum	69.5
162	Trachea, bronchi, and lungs	66.9
172-173	Skin	67.6
200-209	Lymphatic and haemato-poietic tissues	66.8
F e m a l e s		
140-149	Oral and pharyngeal cavities	67.2
150	Esophagus	71.3
151	Stomach	70.3
154	Rectum	68.1
162	Trachea, bronchi and lungs	68.0
172-173	Skin	69.1
174	Breast	62.0
180	Cervix uteri	53.5
200-209	Lymphatic and haemato-poietic tissues	67.2

Table 49

Incidence of Malignant Neoplasms of the Population of the GDR by Administrative Districts Age and Sex in 1973

Administrative districts	M a l e s		F e m a l e s	
	All malignant tumours per 100.000 population	Standardized index	All malignant tumours per 100.000 population	Standardized index
Rostock	292.1	357.5	300.2	354.9
Schwerin	320.7	349.5	314.6	341.3
Neubrandenburg	289.8	336.3	291.0	333.0
Potsdam	312.7	337.0	333.6	344.7
Frankfurt	309.9	350.9	342.8	373.7
Cottbus	309.6	341.4	311.3	334.5
Magdeburg	340.7	343.2	353.8	357.2
Halle	323.8	324.7	321.8	326.5
Erfurt	301.7	311.8	331.2	347.3
Gera	377.9	375.6	392.5	394.9
Suhl	336.7	334.4	339.7	398.3
Dresden	385.5	350.6	373.4	340.7
Leipzig	396.0	367.8	392.3	368.8
Karl-Marx-Stadt	420.9	363.6	391.9	349.9
Berlin	392.9	408.0	418.9	407.8
Total	349.6	349.6	353.9	353.9

Table 50.1

Number of Deaths and Mortality from Malignant Tumours in the GDR by Sex in 1970-1974

Localization	ICD /8th rev./ Code Number	Absolute number	per 100.000	Standard indices by Segi	Absolute number	per 100.000	Standard indices by Segi
All malignant tumours	140-207	95.690	241.3	163.3	96.124	157.9	109.4
Lips	140	103	0.2	0.2	18	0.04	0.02
Tongue	141	200	0.5	0.3	100	0.2	0.1
Salivary glands	142	169	0.4	0.3	152	0.2	0.2
Oral and pharyngeal cavities	143-147	519	1.3	0.9	265	0.4	0.3
Other and non-specified parts of the pharynx	148-149	168	0.4	0.3	46	0.1	0.05
Oral and pharyngeal cavities	140-149	1.159	2.8	2.0	581	0.9	0.7
Esophagus	150	1.712	4.3	2.8	663	1.0	0.6
Stomach	151	18.393	45.6	29.8	14.916	22.2	14.5
Small intestine	152	235	0.6	0.4	267	0.4	0.3
Large Intestine	153	4.489	11.2	7.4	7.411	11.2	7.3
Rectum and rectosigmoid	154	5.583	13.9	9.1	6.500	10.1	6.7
Liver	155	1.550	4.0	2.7	1.415	2.3	1.5
Gallbladder	156	2.001	4.9	3.2	7.053	10.6	6.9

Pancreas	157	3.518	9.0	6.0	3.616	5.5	3.6
Other non-specified digestive organs	158–159	442	1.1	0.8	686	1.1	0.7
Digestive and peritoneal organs	150–159	37.923	94.6	62.2	42.527	64.4	42.1
Intestine	152–154	10.307	25.7	16.9	14.178	21.7	14.3
Liver, gallbladder, pancreas	155–157	7.069	17.9	11.9	12.084	18.4	12.0
Nose and nasal cavities	160	197	0.5	0.4	132	0.2	0.2
Larynx	161	1.158	3.0	2.0	93	0.2	0.1
Trachea, bronchi and lungs	162	29.119	74.3	50.0	3.922	6.3	4.3
Other and non-specified respiratory organs	163	721	1.8	1.2	422	0.7	0.5
Respiratory organs	160–163	31.195	79.6	53.6	4.569	7.4	5.1
Bones	170	549	1.4	1.1	521	0.9	0.7
Connective tissue and other soft tissues	171	315	0.8	0.6	379	0.7	0.5
Skin melanoma	172	554	1.6	1.2	692	1.3	0.9
Other neoplasms of the skin	173	363	1.0	0.6	461	0.7	0.4
Breast	174	112	0.3	0.2	11.893	21.2	14.9
Bones, connective tissue, skin and breast	170–174	1.893	5.1	3.7	13.946	24.8	17.4

Table 50.2

Localization	ICD /8th rev./ Code number	Absolute number	per 100.000	Standard indices by Segi	Absolute number	per 100.000	Standard indices by Segi
Cervix uteri	180	-	-	-	7.411	14.3	10.5
Chorionepithelioma	181	-	-	-	140	0.2	0.2
Other neoplasms of the uterus	182	-	-	-	3.969	6.5	4.4
Ovary, fallopian tubes and broad ligament	183	-	-	-	7.043	12.3	8.6
Other and non-specified female genital organs	184	-	-	-	1.517	2.3	1.5
Prostate	185	6.408	15.2	9.4	-	-	-
Testicle	186	684	1.7	1.7	-	-	-
Other and non-specified male genital organs	187	220	0.6	0.4	-	-	-
Bladder	138	4.071	9.8	6.4	1.313	2.0	1.3
Other and non-specified uropoietic organs	189	2.199	5.8	4.1	1.913	3.1	2.2
Urino-genital organs	180-189	13.582	33.1	22.0	23.306	40.7	28.7
Female genital organs	180-184	-	-	-	20.080	35.6	25.2
Male genital and uro-poietic organs	185-187	7.312	17.5	11.5	-	-	-

Malignant tumours of the urinary bladder, other and non-specified uropoietic organs	188–189	6.720	15.6	10.5	3.226	5.1	3.5
Eyes	190	111	0.3	0.2	148	0.2	0.2
Brain	191	1427	4.2	3.5	1.313	2.8	2.4
Other sections of the nervous system	192	200	0.5	0.5	423	0.9	0.9
Thyroid gland	193	248	0.6	0.4	678	1.1	0.7
Other endocrine glands	194	139	0.4	0.3	139	0.3	0.2
Other and non-specified localizations	190–199	4.183	11.2	8.5	5.757	10.2	7.8
Eyes, brain and other sections of the nervous system	190–192	1.738	5.0	4.2	1.884	3.9	3.5
Thyroid gland and other endocrine glands	193–194	387	1.0	0.7	817	1.4	0.9
Non-exactly specified secondary and with not indicated localizations	195–199	2.058	5.2	3.6	3.056	4.9	3.4
Lymphosarcoma and reticulum cell sarcoma	200	953	2.5	1.9	917	1.5	1.1
Hodgkin's disease	201	944	2.5	2.1	720	1.4	1.1
Other neoplasms of the lymphatic tissue	202	290	0.7	0.6	229	0.4	0.3
Multiple myeloma	203	652	1.7	1.1	796	1.3	8.9

cont'd

Table 50.3

Localization	ICD /8th rev./ Code number	Absolute number	per 100.000	Standard indices by Segi	Absolute number	per 100.000	Standard indices by Segi
Lymphoid leukaemia, lympholeukosis, lymphadenosis	204	1.069	2.6	1.9	745	1.2	0.9
Myeloid and mono-cytic leukaemia and leukoses	205-206	1.275	3.3	2.7	1.468	2.8	2.2
Other and non-specified leukaemia, leukoses	207	572	1.4	1.2	563	1.1	0.9
Neoplasms of the lymphoid and haematopoietic tissues	200-207	5.755	14.7	11.5	5.438	9.6	7.4
Lymphomas	200-203	2.839	7.4	5.7	2.662	4.6	3.4
Leukoses, leukaemiae	204-207	2.916	7.3	5.8	2.776	5.0	4.0
Other neoplasms of the lymphoid and haemato-poietic tissues	208-209	No data					

REFERENCES

1. Textbook of special pathology. 3rd edition /von Kettler/
   Chapter "Morbidity and survival rates in malignant neoplasms
   in the GDR 1960, 1965 and 1970."
   VEB Gustav-Fischer-Verlag Jena, 1976
2. Supplement Cancer control in "Oncological Care System in
   the GDR" /Duties of nurses of oncological out-patient
   clinics by oncological patients./
   Potsdam 1970, Vol. II, p. 61-73
3. Problems of epidemiology in oncology
   Zeitschrift für die gesamte Hygiene und ihre Grenzgebiete,
   1967. Vol. 13. no. 2.
4-17. Supplement Cancer in "Health care of the GDR"
   Vol. 1-14. Berlin 1965-1979.
18. Oncology.
   /Eds: Gläser and Herold/ VEB Verlag Volk und Gesundheit,
   Berlin 1980. 2nd Edition
19-23. Statistical annuals of the GDR Vol. 3-7, VEB Deutscher
   Zentralverlag Berlin, 1957-1962.
24-40. Statistical annuals of the GDR Vol. 8-24, Staatsverlag
   der DDR, Berlin 1963-1979.

CANCER CONTROL IN HUNGARY

Z. Péter

GEOGRAPHICAL, ECONOMIC AND DEMOGRAPHIC CHARACTERISTICS
OF THE COUNTRY, HISTORICAL SURVEY OF CANCER CONTROL

Hungary lies between the latitudes $45^O45'$ and $48^O35'$ north
and longitudes $16^O5'$ and $22^O55'$ east in the central part of the
Carpathian basin encircled by the Alps, Carpathians and Dinaric
Alps along the middle course of the rivers Danube and Tisza.
The area of Hungary is 93,032 km^2. The largest part of its
surface is a plain located at a height of 200 m above sea level. The mountains are of medium height with the highest point
at Kékestető /1015 m/; the lowest point of the country is along
the Tisza near the town Szeged /77 m/. The country has hardly
any mineral resources; the most considerable of them are the
oil and natural gas discovered in the last few years. The
country is rich in thermal springs.

The geological basis of the country's territory is an
ancient massif formed of crystalline schist and granite. In the
flat part of the country the shifting sands, dunes and hills
formed by alluvia give place to large loessial territories.

The rivers flowing through Hungary belong to the catch-
ment area of the Danube, the biggest river in Central Europe.
The largest of its tributaries is the Tisza. The country is
covered by a net of smaller tributaries, which provide it with
natural irrigation. /On the average the Danube and its tributaries give 114 thousand million m^3 of water annually, whereas
the amount of precipitation is 58 m^3/. The system of canals
built along the river ensures even distribution of the water
resources. The largest lake of the country is Balaton, which
is also the biggest one in Central and Western Europe. Besides

Lake Balaton there are a few smaller lakes. Over a long period
of its geographical history large areas of marshland were
found in the country which have been drained in the last few
decades.

The climate of the country is determined by its height
above sea level and also by its equal distance from the North
Pole and the Equator. Moreover, the climate is influenced by
the winds blowing from the Atlantic Ocean and also by the
factors resulting from Hungary's location at the beginning of
the expanding continental trunk of Europe and causing the
country's temperate-continental climate. Due to the variable
continental, Mediterranean and oceanic influences the weather
is rather changeable in the country: frosty in winter /the
average temperature in January is -1 - -3°C/, and hot in summer /the average temperature in July is +20 - +26°C/. The
highest temperature measured in Hungary has been +43.3^{o}C, the
lowest -34.5^{o}C. As a result of the temperature oceanic influence the country's average temperature is +9 - +11°C. The number of sunny days per year is quite high, making up a minimum
of 1500 hours and maximum of 2500 hours. May and June are
marked by the heaviest rainfall, while in the middle of the
country there may be drought for several years running.

Hungary is an industrial-agrarian country. Before the
liberation in 1945 it was an agricultural country with a back-
ward industry. The development of its industry began in 1940-
-1950s.

At present the gross national product is distributed as
follows: industry - 61.9 per cent and agriculture - 32.1 per
cent. In spite of the fact that the country is poor in mineral
resources, it is rapidly becoming industrialized owing mainly
to the cooperation with the socialist countries.

The country is relatively poor in sources of power, particularly in waterpower; this shortage is compensated to a
certain extent by the oil and natural gas deposits. Apart from
the chemical and heavy industry, great progress has been made
in the food and pharmaceutical industries. The most important
product of the mining industry is bauxite; the country is

sixth in the world's bauxite production.

Administratively the country is divided into the capital and 19 independent administrative units, i.e. counties /Fig.12/. Besides, five big cities /with a population of more than 100,000/ are independent units as well. The counties are divided into towns and villages. The governmental decisions are implemented by the governing body of the regional councils. To each county and city council belongs a health department which is administratively subordinated to the executive committee of the council. The scientific and methodological supervision of the health departments is carried out by the Ministry of Health. The medical institutions located in the cities and counties are administratively subordinated to local councils. Their work is directly controlled by the health departments of the councils and, on a higher level, by the Ministry of Health directly or indirectly, through state health establishments.

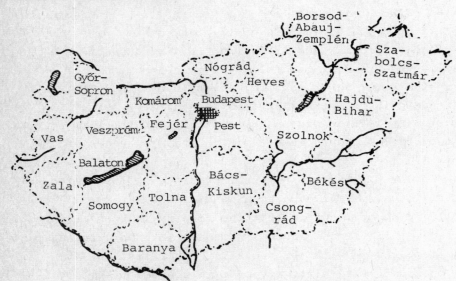

Fig. 12 Population number in the administrative regions of the Hungarian People's Republic
/for January 1, 1975, thous./

The number of inhabitants of Hungary was 10,508,956 /5,097,229 men and 5,411,727 women/ by January 1, 1975

336

/Table 51, Fig. 13/. 19.6 % of the population live in Budapest.

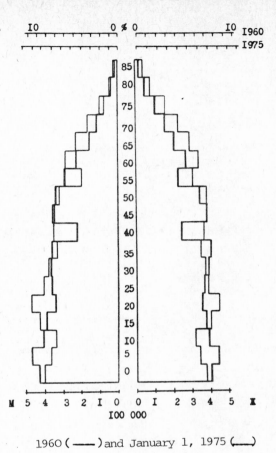

1960 (——) and January 1, 1975 (___)

Fig. 13 Age-sex structure of the population of the Hungarian
People's Republic

The size of the administrative regions and their population vary. In the largest administrative region the population numbers 934,000, and in the smallest 235,000. The capital with 2,055,646 inhabitants is an independent administrative
unit.

Table 52 presents the proportion of young and elderly
people in the country's overall population structure /21.1 %
and 17.1 % respectively/. The age structure of the population

tends to include more elderly people.

Table 51

Population Figures for Hungary

	1960	1965	1970	1.1. 1975
Total population:				
Men	4,804,043	4.896,837	5,003,651	5,097,229
Women	5,157,001	5,238,653	5,318,448	5,411,727
Total	9,961,044	10,135,490	10,322,099	10,508,956
Population of the capital:				
Men	856,859	902,547	946,830	972,887
Women	987,084	1,032,984	1,054,253	1,082,759
Total	1,843,943	1,935,531	2,001,083	2,055,646
Population of the capital in per cent of the total population	18.5	19.1	19.4	19.6

Before 1960 the index of natural population growth was
7.5, today it has fallen to 3.5-3.6. In ten years there were
14 live births per 1000 population and only in the past five
years has the number increased to 15 after the law on family
protection was passed. The death rate of 10.3/1000 population
of the fifties increased to 11.7/1000 in the first half of
the seventies /Table 53, Fig. 14/. There are fewer and fewer
large families. In 1955-1959, third and subsequent child
births made up almost 30 % of all the live births. At present
the percentage has fallen to 17.3.

The country's industrialization and the construction of
industrial complexes have resulted in an increased migration
of the population within the country. In the seventies the
migration gradually began to slacken off. While in 1966 the
constant migration was 31.1 per 1000 population and the temporary 30.3, in 1974 the figures were 23.6 and 23.2, respectively.

Table 52

Percentage of Young and Elderly People in Relation to the
Total Population in Hungary

Age	1960	1965	1970	1975
0-15	25.4	23.5	21.1	20.2
15-60	60.8	61.0	61.8	61.4
60 -	13.8	15.5	17.1	18.4
Total	100.0	100.0	100.0	100.0

Table 53

Basic Demographic Indices of Hungary

Years	Live births	Death rate	Natural population growth
1955-59	17.8	10.3	7.5
1960-64	13.6	10.1	3.5
1965-69	14.3	10.8	3.5
1970-74	15.3	11.7	3.6

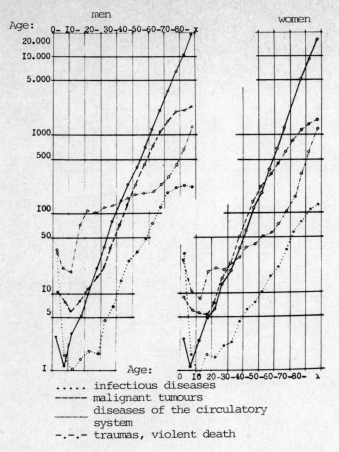

Fig. 14 Age-sex rates of mortality among HPR population
         according to the basic groups of death causes
                        for 1970-1974

                    /per 100,000 population/

..... infectious diseases
----- malignant tumours
_____ diseases of the circulatory system
-.-.- traumas, violent death

It should be pointed out that among the main causes of
death and the increase in mortality the first place is taken
by diseases of the circulatory system /International Classification of Diseases, 8th revision/. The second place is occupied
by malignant tumours, followed by injuries, poisoning and
violent death together; in the fourth place come infectious
and parasitic diseases, whose share in the statistics for
causes of death is gradually decreasing.

In 1955-1959, 34.5 % of the causes of death in men consisted of the diseases of the circulatory system. In 1970-74 the index rose to 49.2 %.

A significant increase in the mortality caused by malignant tumours is observed: in 1955-1959 the average was 14.5 %, whereas in 1970-1974 it had increased to 19.7 %. The group of causes of death "injuries, poisoning, violent death" made up 8.8 % of the total mortality in men in 1955-59, while in 1970-74 it was 10.4 %. The frequency of infectious diseases as causes of death decreased from 5.6 to 2.5 per cent. In 1970-75 these four groups of causes of death in men made up 81.8 % of the total mortality structure /Table 54/.

The diseases of the circulatory system made up 43 % of all the causes of death in women in 1955-59; in the past five years the figure has increased to 57.9 per cent. The proportion of malignant tumours among the causes of death has significantly increased, from 15.7 % in 1955-1959 to 19.7 % in 1970-74. A slight increase in the indices is also observed in the group of traumas as causes of death in women, i.e. from 3.8 % to 5.7 %. The significance of infectious diseases in the statistics of causes of death in women has fallen from 3.4 to 1.4 %. These four groups of causes of death in women make up 83.8 % of total mortality. With the present age structure of the population, in 1974 the number of deaths caused by the diseases of the circulatory system was 621.5 in men and 636.1 in women per 100,000 population; the number of deaths from malignant tumours was 265.7 in men and 215.2 in women /Tables 55 and 56/. After the standardization of death indices /Segi standard of world population/, it turned out that during the past 18 years the total mortality in men remainded roughly at the same level, but the index of the death rate caused by malignant tumours rose by 26.6 % /Table 57/. In women the index of total mortality fell by 12.9 %. However, the index of the death rate caused by malignant tumours increased by 6.9 %. A comparison of the age indices of death rate shows that in men the indices of deaths caused by malignant tumours were invariable in each five year group under the age of 30 in 1960-

341

Table 54

Main Causes of Death in Hungary
/average percentage for 5 years/

Men	1955-59	1960-64	1965-69	1970-74
Diseases of the circulatory system	34.5	43.8	47.8	49.2
Malignant tumours	14.5	17.4	18.9	19.7
Traumas, poisonings, violent death	8.8	8.6	9.2	10.4
Infectious and parasitic diseases	5.6	4.6	3.5	2.5

Women				
Diseases of the circulatory system	43.0	52.5	56.9	57.9
Malignant tumours	15.7	17.7	18.3	18.8
Traumas, poisonings, violent death	3.8	3.8	5.0	5.7
Infectious and parasitic diseases	3.4	2.9	1.6	1.4

Both sexes				
Diseases of the circulatory system	38.6	48.0	52.2	53.4
Malignant tumours	15.1	17.5	18.6	19.3
Traumas, poisonings, violent death	6.3	6.4	7.1	8.2
Infectious and parasitic diseases	4.5	3.5	2.6	2.0

Table 55

Total Mortality and Mortality from Malignant Tumours in Hungary
/average number for three year
periods/

| Years | Number of deaths per 100.000 population | | | | |
| | Men | | Women | | |
	Total mortality	Mortality from malignant tumours	Total mortality	Mortality from malignant tumours	
1957-59	1.061.97	166.89	973.02	156.74	
1960-62	1.076.	181.44	963.91	165.24	
1963-65	1.081.99	197.11	956.78	173.91	
1966-68	1.136.16	218.29	1.000.60	184.80	
1969-71	1.249.06	237.40	1.077.51	196.47	
1972-74	1.260.61	253.80	1.096.06	209.86	

-1974; above the age of thirty years the indices increased
significantly in almost every age group. In women from 0 to
14 years of age a slight increase in the death rate caused by
malignant tumours is observed. At the age group of 15-19 years
the index somewhat decreases. In the age groups from 20 to 70
years the death rate is steadily increasing /Table 58, Fig.
15/.

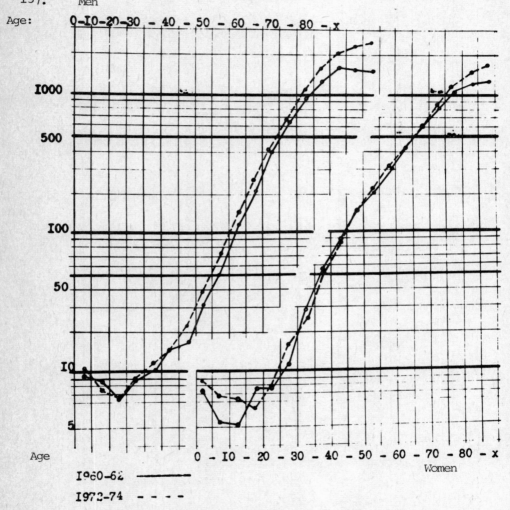

Fig. 15 Age-sex rates of mortality from malignant tumours
         on the average for 1960-1962 and 1972-1974

         /per 100,000 population of the corresponding age/

The study of the death rate caused by malignant tumours of different localizations reveals that in men the first place is taken by the tumours of the trachea, bronchi and lungs, the second by malignant tumours of the stomach and the third by that of the prostate; in women the first place is taken by the malignant tumours of the stomach, the second by those of the mammary gland and the third by malignant tumours of the uterus /cervix and corpus uteri/. If these two localizations are considered separately, the third place is occupied by malignant tumours of the small and large intestine /Fig. 16, 17/.

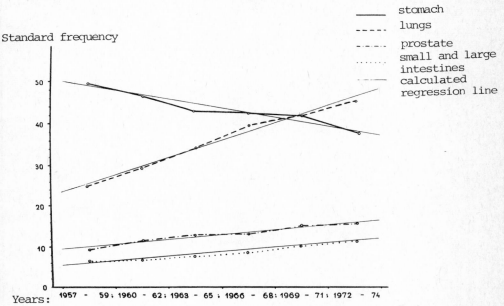

Fig. 16 Dynamics of mortality of men from malignant tumours of the basic localizations

With regard to the studies of the incidence and death rate of the population, it should be pointed out that in Hungary the beginning of cancer control dates back to the beginning of the 20th century; it was marked by data collection on cancer statistics by I. Farkas in 1901. With the support of the Society of Physicians and under the guidance of Dr. Gy. Dollinger the work was continued in 1904 and statistics

Table 56

Mortality in Hungary /per 100,000 population/

	Men	Women
Total mortality	1,288.7	1,117.8
Diseases of the circulatory system	621.5	636.1
Malignant tumours	265.7	215.2
Traumas, poisonings, violent death	136.7	68.7
Infectious and parasitic diseases	28.4	13.1

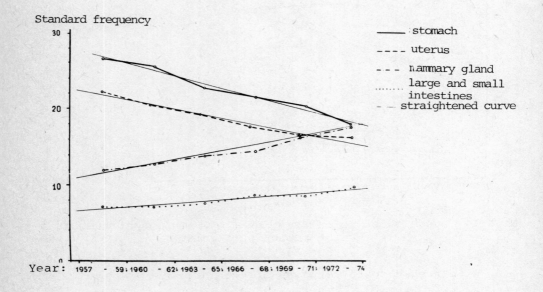

Standard frequency

—— stomach
---- uterus
--- mammary gland
.... large and small intestines
-- straightened curve

Year: 1957 - 59; 1960 - 62; 1963 - 65; 1966 - 68; 1969 - 71; 1972 - 74

Fig. 17 Dynamics of mortality of women from malignant tumours of the basic localizations

on oncology diseases in the country were collected. This study is often referred to in the literature, for it has played an

Table 57

Total Mortality of the Population of Hungary and Mortality from Malignant
Tumours /average number for a three-year period, standardized indices[x]/

Years	Men		Women	
	Total mortality	Mortality from malignant tumours	Total mortality	Mortality from malignant tumours
1957-1959	1.021.70	145.73	778.74	117.44
1960-62	1.016.03	151.47	760.48	118.51
1963-65	984.07	157.19	714.53	118.55
1966-68	988.42	166.96	702.14	119.85
1969-71	1.040.96	176.23	701.16	121.96
1972-74	1.022.42	184.48	678.45	125.53

x Segi's standard

Table 58

Mortality from Malignant Tumours among the population Hungary by age and sex /averaged for three years/

Number of deaths per 100.000 population of the corresponding sex and age

Age groups	Men					Women				
	1960-62	1963-65	1966-68	1969-71	1972-74	1960-62	1963-65	1966-68	1969-71	1972-74
0-4	9.7	9.9	11.2	9.8	10.6	7.4	7.4	8.4	8.6	8.6
5-9	8.6	7.2	6.6	8.2	7.4	4.8	6.0	6.5	5.5	6.6
10-14	6.3	6.7	7.6	6.5	6.6	4.0	4.8	6.2	5.6	6.1
15-19	8.8	7.7	9.0	8.7	8.9	7.4	6.2	6.1	5.3	5.3
20-24	10.4	10.8	13.6	10.9	11.7	7.1	7.3	7.4	7.5	7.5
25-29	15.0	13.8	15.7	15.3	14.9	11.7	12.9	14.1	14.0	15.1
30-34	17.5	19.4	21.6	20.9	21.5	28.0	21.8	25.0	23.3	24.6
35-39	31.0	33.7	35.7	37.5	33.0	56.5	50.8	45.9	48.4	51.7
40-44	50.5	57.1	60.1	69.2	72.7	87.7	90.6	84.2	86.1	85.2
45-49	113.4	109.7	107.1	124.9	139.0	143.4	148.1	141.0	144.8	141.6
50-54	214.5	210.5	213.5	208.6	251.0	207.2	194.6	203.3	214.5	218.0
55-59	389.0	398.4	387.5	393.9	416.1	297.3	283.3	293.4	305.1	322.0
60-64	682.0	652.7	680.3	683.0	680.2	422.6	421.1	405.0	413.4	427.7
65-69	985.0	986.8	1060.2	1091.5	1108.0	604.7	608.3	607.1	603.9	608.8
70-74	1231.1	1298.9	1408.6	1522.9	1547.9	826.0	855.9	858.7	859.0	878.8
75-79	1567.0	1611.2	1730.5	1928.9	2062.9	1087.4	1098.1	1129.2	1156.4	1189.6
80-84	1572.5	1787.7	1951.9	2286.6	2101.7	1228.5	1282,9	1368.8	1361.7	1477.5
85-	1519.8	1670.1	1944.8	2394.6	2521.3	1238.5	1417.8	1486.8	1575.9	1701.7

important part in the history of Hungarian medicine. Today
these data have no practical significance, but at that time
their importance was undeniable for the whole of Europe. The
attempts of the Cancer Committee organized by the Society of
Physicians of that time to attract the attention of the public
to the serious problem of providing cancer patients with medical treatment were important in themselves. At that time in
Hungary progress was almost impossible in this field. Only in
1930 was the country's first oncological department set up in
a metropolitan hospital. In 1936, the Eötvös Loránd Radium-
-Röntgen Institute was founded with 100 hospital beds /the
predecessor of the present National Institute of Oncology/.
The two establishments, however, could not meet the need of
all the cancer patients in the country for radiotherapy. A
number of university clinics gradually began to acquire radiological equipment.

The undertakings were interrupted by the Second World War.
Most radiation sources were destroyed. After the war radiologists and gynecologists joined their efforts in setting up
the foundations of a cancer control service to meet the demands
of Hungarian socialist public health. The new movement was
largely supported by Professor B. V. Petrovsky, at that time
working in Hungary, who shared the experience of cancer control
in the Soviet Union with B. Wald, leader and organizer of this
movement in Hungary. As a result of the invaluable support
rendered by Professor B. V. Petrovsky the National Institute
of Oncology acquired new premises with 300 hospital beds on
January 1, 1953. The valuable experience gained by the Eötvös
Loránd Radium-Röntgen Institute was made use of in the activities of the Institution. As early as before the war the Institute already had a consultative system of examination and
therapy for cancer patients. Each patient was sent to the
consultative committee that decided on further therapy on the
basis of examination data. It can be stated that the consultative method of work at that time reached the level of the
present team work.

The second method that has become widespread was the

organization of control and home nursing of cancer patients
treated at the Institute. The physicians of the Institute had
been convinced that the control of patients discharged from
the Radium-Röntgen Institute was the responsibility of the
Institute itself. Hence, it may be concluded that, even from
a modern point of view, the work of the predecessor of the
Institute of Oncology was based on progressive principles.

The advice of Professor B. V. Petrovsky and the experience
of the Hungarian gynecologists gave the idea of organizing
screenings aimed at the active detection of malignant diseases
since this was the only way of detecting the disease in the
early stages and thus of providing greater hope of permanent
recovery. Thus, the work of the National Institute of Oncology
and the movement to organize oncologic screening for women
began practically at the same time. It was then that the
departments of radiology, surgery, gynecology and urology were
set up at the Institute of Oncology; later they were completed
by the department of chemotherapy. The department of urology
was subsequently replaced by the oncodermetological, isotope
and ENT departments. In 1954 the department of pathology
attached to the Institute was reorganized into a Research Institute of Oncopathology where histological studies and
autopsies are combined with large-scale research work. An out-
patient department has been also organized at the National Institute of Oncology. The radiation sources of the Institute
are constantly being replenished; at present, apart from the
two cobalt units, there is also a betatron.

Together with the expansion of the National Institute of
Oncology the establishment of oncoradiological centres in
Hungary began. Oncoradiological departments were organized at
hospitals in Szombathely, Miskolc and later in Győr and Deb-
recen.

Independent X-ray and radiological departments with
modern equipment for diagnosis and therapy of cancer patients
have gradually been set up at the universities. In the general
hospitals the diagnostic equipment as well as the X-ray
therapeutic equipment for external irradiation has been

considerably improved.

The order of the Minister of Health issued in 1954 envisaged the establishment of a network of oncological out-patient clinics, and determined their tasks. The order substantiated the development of a network of oncological outpatient clinics that would provide oncological screening and treatment for oncological patients all over the country. The scientific-methodological guidance of the oncologic network is provided by the National Institute of Oncology, whereas administratively the oncological centres are subordinated to local councils.

In 1955-1959 the number of these outpatient clinics forming the basis of oncologic network in Budapest was 12, in other parts of the country 21 /totalling 33 in the country as a whole/ until 1975 the number increased considerably, i.e. to 21 in Budapest and to 50 in the other parts of the country /altogether 71 oncological outpatient clinics/. The initial period of the functioning of the oncological network was characterized by the organization of temporary oncological screening stations. In 1955, the number of such stations in the country was 615, later they were used as bases for organizing permanent oncological clinics. Thus, in 1960, there were only 349 temporary screening stations but 88 oncological outpatient clinics providing oncological screening for women.

The number of patients annually attending oncologic clinics in 1955-59 had been barely 195,000 by 1975 this increased to 400,000 /Table 59/. In accordance with the tasks of oncological clinics, this number depends on many factors. The main task of the clinics is to organize and provide preventive oncological examinations for women from 30-69 years of age. The clinics advise patients and take an active part in the examination of persons suspected of suffering from malignant tumours, at the place of their residence and work. They provide treatment for patients with pre malignant diseases and register cancer patients as well. According to different tasks of the oncological outpatient clinics, the distribution of their patients was gradually transformed /Table 60/. In

Table 59

Annual Indices of Patients Attending Oncologic Centres in Hungary

/averaged for five years/

	1955-59	1960-64	1965-69	1970-74
In Budapest	89.474	118.872	126.105	112.718
In other regions of the country	105.706	172.763	231.436	282.072
Total for the country	195.180	291.635	357.541	394.790

Table 60

Indices of the Activities of Oncologic Centres in Hungary /average number for
five years periods/.

	Number of visits	Screenings in centres	Consultations	Control of on-cological patients	Control of pre-tumourous patients	Follow-up of cancer patients
1955-1959	195.180	52.894	29.277	52.113	20.494	40.402
1960-1964	291.635	84.883	39.284	65.897	26.856	74.715
1965-1969	357.541	122.435	42.471	80.159	25.980	86.496
1970-1974	394.790	148.406	37.737	92.790	29.791	86.066

1955-1959, 27.1 % of the total annual number of patients attending the centres were women undergoing screenings; 10 % were patients receiving treatment for pre-malignant diseases, and 20.7 % of patients treated for cancer. In 1975, 34 % of the total number of patients underwent screenings, 23 % received treatment for malignant tumours, and 8 % treatment for pre-malignant diseases.

The regulation introduced by the order of the Minister of Health for the National Institute of Oncology and the oncological network have involved the compulsory registration of cancer cases. Apart from data collection on cancer statistics, the organizational and methodological department set up at the National Institute of Oncology is assigned to collect and systematically evaluate the data characterizing the work of the oncological network. Furthermore, it is the task of this department to exercise control and guidance by advising the workers of the oncological network in their organizational work; in other words, the department is a link between the oncological network and the National Institute of Oncology as a scientific, methodological and consulting centre of oncology.

In the Hungarian public health system the general practitioners providing patients with basic treatment, the outpatient clinics, specialized medical establishments and general hospitals are administratively subordinated to the local councils. In their activities the local councils are guided by the law on public health as well as by the orders and instructions of the Minister of Health. Each special field of activities is supervised by the national establishment subordinated directly to the Ministry of Health. The main task of such national establishments is to test modern methods of diagnosis and therapy and introduce them in the medical institutions of the country. The latter are scientific-methodological and consulting bodies of the Ministry of Health and exercise control over the work of the local medical institutions. The budget and staff of hospitals and outpatient clinics subordinated to the local councils, as well as their equipment, depend on the distribution of the budget of the local councils. Thus, the methodological letters of state establishments are just recommendations, the fulfilment of which depends on the decisions of local councils. In solving problems of nationwide importance the state establishments can apply to the Ministry of Health, particularly if the order of the Minister of Health is required for their country-wide realization. These orders and instructions are also carried out in the organization and work of the oncological network. The oncological clinics and centres, as well as regional radiologic centres are attached to local hospitals. This means that, apart from the National Institute of Oncology, there are no other independent oncologic establishments in the country. In the Hungarian public health system cancer patients receive treatment within the general medical network. Thus, the surgical, gynecological, therapeutic and other departments of every hospital also provide treatment for cancer patients. In some departments of the large regional hospitals there is a tendency toward oncological specialization; for example, one of the general medical departments specializes mainly in gastroenterologic diagnosis, and another in the treatment of patients with leukemia and chemotherapy in general. Hospital beds for cancer patients are available only in oncoradiological centres and radiological departments of medical universities, but their number is very limited. Thus, cancer patients treated with radiotherapy are mainly kept in surgical, gynecological and other departments and from there they are transferred to the X-ray therapeutic department of the hospital. In such hospitals the X-ray therapy and X-ray diagnosis are carried out in the same department /Fig. 18/.

In each region of the country there is a regional oncological centre, attached to the main regional hospital, and an outpatient department. The head of the centre /an oncologist, as a rule/ is the scientifico-methodological supervisor of the regional centres and oncological clinics and acts as the chief oncologist of the region. The oncological clinics provide only preventive oncological screenings; the centres also furnish consultations with regard to the

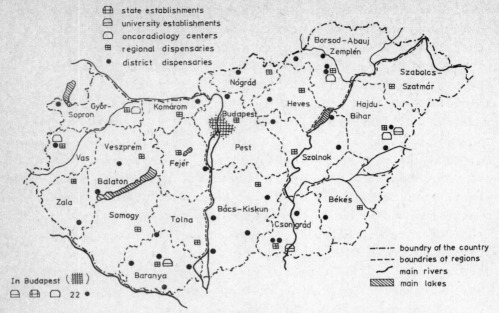

Fig. 18 Distribution of radiology establishments, district
oncoradiology centres and oncology, dispensaries on
the territory of the Hungarian People's Republic

diagnosis of malignant tumours, as well as to the treatment of
precancerous and cancer patients. Their organizing activities and the work on statistical processing of estimates and
observation data are also significant. Within the region the
chief oncologist is responsible for the organization of
screenings for women with the partial participation of regional
gynecologists. The regions do not have hospital beds for cancer
patients.

The head of the oncological centre works as chief physician, and the physicians of the oncologic clinics work as
specialists of the outpatient departments. As a rule their consulting units consist of one or two rooms. They have one to
three nurses. The equipment is similar to that of a medium
gynecological outpatient clinic including the colposcope and
electric coagulator.

In the capital there are district oncological outpatient
clinics with a chief oncologist in almost every district. They
are subordinated to the chief physician of the general district

outpatient clinic and they cooperate with the Department of Oncoradiology of the capital that has hospital beds and is the radiological centre serving the oncological patients of the capital. The system is supervised by the National Institute of Oncology.

In 1974, the number of oncoradiological hospital beds in Hungary was 732 /7.0 per 100,000 population/. In Budapest there are 427 oncologic beds /including 300 at the National Institute of Oncology/. In other regions of the country there are 305 hospital beds in nine towns, including 234 in departments with facilities for intracavitary radiotherapy /3 medical universities and four large county hospitals/; the remainder are in institutions with X-ray therapeutic units /Table 61/.

Table 61

The Number of Oncological Beds in Hungary

	1960	1965	1970	1974
Actual number of oncoradiological beds	592	581	643	732
per 100,000 population	5.9	5.8	6.2	7.0

It is obvious from the above-said that in Hungary the solution of the complex problem of providing treatment for cancer patients rests mainly on the network of general public health; hence it seems expedient to give a few details about it. By the end of 1974 there were 4014 organized medical districts and further 822 districts for children below the age of 14 years. The average number of the population per district was 2,613. In 1974, the number of patient visits was 50,200,000. At the end of 1974, the number of special outpatient departments was 197, including 150 with not less than seven clinics providing basic medical treatment.

In 1974 there were 172 medical establishments in Hungary for inpatient services /five medical universities, 101 general hospitals, 55 specialized hospitals, eight sanatoria and three establishments for courses of additional treatment/. Out of the total number of hospitals 142 were administratively sub-

ordinated to local councils /regional or town/, from which 27
were in the capital and 115 in other regions of the country.
By the end of 1974, the number of hospital beds was 87,251,
i.e. 83.2 beds per 10,000 population. The number of general
hospital beds per 10,000 population was 58.7. The hospital beds
were distributed as follows: internal diseases - 17.5 %,
surgery - 13.1 %, gynecology and obstetrics - 9.9 %, pediatrics
- 9.9 %, oncoradiology 0.9 %. At the end of 1974, the number of
physicians reached 23,095 /220.2 per 100,000 population/ including full-time oncologists, 0.79 per 100,000 population and
0.4 per cent of all the physicians.

When setting up the oncological network, great efforts
were made by the workers of the organizational methodological
department of the National Institute of Oncology in Budapest
to systematize all the required data and statistic materials.

REGISTRATION OF PATIENTS WITH PRIMARILY DIAGNOSED
MALIGNANT NEOPLASMS

In 1951, by the order of the Council of Ministers, the
compulsory registration of cancer incidence and mortality
caused by it was introduced. In addition, the hospitals and
medical establishments responsible for the notification of
each case of treatment or examination of cancer patients are
enumerated in detail in the above order of the Ministry of
Health. The heads of the above establishments must report on
the diagnosis of malignant tumours, on the treatment of the
patient and on the patient's death on special forms. The head
of the medical establishment may charge the heads of the departments with this duty. The form consisting of three parts
/notification of the cancer patient/ contains the patient's
personal data, the date of the patient's visit to the doctor
and that of the diagnosis, the exact diagnosis /localization
of the primary tumour, stage, metastases/, type and date of
therapy, method used for the confirmation of the diagnosis
/X-ray, endoscopy, biopsy, laboratory methods/, as well as
information on the patient's admission for treatment or assignment to another place /Supplement 13/. Initially the

The notification is filled in only by the institutions dealing with outpatients. /The notification of patients detected at screenings is drawn up by the oncological centres/. The notification is sent in two copies with a certificate in a closed envelope to the National Institute of Oncology.

NOTIFICATION OF THE CANCER PATIENT[x]/

Name:	Diagnosis-stage-localization of the primary tumour:
Maiden name:	
	Metastases:
Mother's name:	
Permanent place of residence:	When and what treatment was received in connection with the tumourous disease?
	Did the patient have the tumour at the time of compiling the notification?
	Yes...... No........
Place of work:	Has the diagnosis been confirmed?
Occupation:	X-ray: Yes.... No.....
Spouse's occupation:	Endoscopy: Yes.... No....
Day....... month..... year... Date of visit to doctor	Lab. tests: Yes.... No....
	Biopsy: Yes.... No....
Sex: male, female, Year of birth:	
	Has any treatment been prescribed? If not, where was the patient sent?

| Is the notification drawn up on the basis of the screening form sent to the oncological centre:

yes..... no.....

/This question is answered only by the oncological centre/ | Any other important comments:

Date of compiling the notification:

Name and address of the institution that has drawn up the notification:

Physician's signature: |

CONTROL FORM OF THE NOTIFICATION OF THE
CANCER PATIENT

Patient's name: ....

Mother's name: ....

Place of residence: ....

Diagnosis: ....

Date of compiling
the notification: ....

Filled in by the author
of the notification

Organizing-methodological
Department of the Na-
tional Institute of
Oncology

---

x/Name and address of the establishment that has drawn up
the notification

notification had to be sent to the organizational-methodological department of the National Institute of Oncology, where its receipt was acknowledged by sending a control check to the notifier. /The control check must be attached to the hospital documentation of the patient/. A part of the notification was sent to the local oncological centre in the patient's place of residence. Finally, the last part of the notification was sent to the archives. The form entitled "Final report about the oncological patient" is used for reporting data on the treatment of the oncological patient. This form also consists of three parts /Supplement 14/, and like the notification, each part is sent to different places. The form contains more detailed information than the notification. Apart from the patient's personal data, it contains the number of case history, time of treatment, exact diagnosis, macro- and microscopic features of the tumour, date and type of surgical intervention, description of the tumour at the operation, its localization, blood picture, data on X-ray and radiotherapy, and medical conclusion with regard to the patient. Later the administrative part of the work with the notification was changed as follows: the doctors making final reports on the cancer patient must send them to local oncology centres, from where a certain part of the notification is sent to the National Institute of Oncology.

Thus, all the medical institutions in the country /both outpatient departments and hospitals/ are responsible for filling in the notifications as well as for the examination and treatment of cancer patients. At the same time, it should be pointed out that this registration system has certain insufficiencies. The registration of carcinomas of the breast and female genitalia is more or less acceptable. As regards other localizations, the number of new oncological cases registered annually has always been lower than the mortality index for the same period. On the average, the underestimation is not less than 20 per cent, and for some localizations /systemic diseases/ it is even higher.

The documentation for registration is drawn up on the

This final report is to be filled in by institutions, hospital departments and specialized units for all cancer patients or for suspected cases in duplicate, together with the control form, and sent in a closed envelope to the National Institute of Oncology in Budapest.

....
Stamp of the establish-   Case history No.
ment /hospital/   Department

FINAL REPORT ON THE ONCOLOGICAL PATIENT

Name	
Maiden name	Mother's name:

Year and month of birth:

Permanent place of residence:

Place of work:

Occupation:

Occupation of spouse:

Duration of hospital treatment:		Diagnosis /stage/:	First symptoms of the tumour and the date of its appearance:
From	to		

Has the patient passed through oncologic screening?

Yes   No   Where   When

Characteristic of the tumour:

Date of histologic studies:	Organ examined:	Who prescribed the treatment:	Diagnosis

362

Findings during surgical intervention /localization, origin, distribution, direction of tumour growth, metastases/:

Surgery /date, surgeon's name, radical, non-radical, palliative, experiment, diagnostic operation, excision, puncture, abrasion/:

Type of anaesthesia:

Localization of the remaining tumour:

Postoperative period /apyretic, febrile, recovery, other complications/:

On the basis of permission No 8655/1954
of the head of Central Statistical Office

Case history No: ....

Issue No: ....

....
Stamp of the establishment
sending the conclusion

CONTROL FORM FOR SENDING THE FINAL REPORT ON THE
ONCOLOGIC CASE

Patient's name /Maiden name/: ....

Permanent place of residence: ....

Diagnosis: ....

Organizational-methodological department of the National Institute of Oncology

Blood picture	Urine	ESR	ECG
erythrocytes	amount, ml	Wassermann	
hemoglobin	density	reaction	
leukocytes	phosphorus	blood-group	
strain	protein	blood-sugar	X-ray
bacilli	pus	blood-pressure	
segments	sugar	heart rate	
eosinophils	urobilinogen	weight	
basophils	precipitate		
lymphocytes			
monocytes			

Other analyses: endoscopy

Data on the X-ray treatment

Date, site of irradiation, number and size of fields, factors, dose in the field and total dose:

Irradiation was carried out by:

Date on radiotherapy /date/

The therapy was
prescribed by:

To which establishment the patient
is sent for control and subsequent
treatment:

Course of disease:

Conclusion

Suggestions:

Date of compiling ....

Approved .... Chief physician

Signature of the doctor in charge ....

basis of notifications and final reports delivered to the local centre. /Naturally, after the duplicates have been excluded/. /Supplement 15/

The cardboard envelope used for storing the certificates and descriptions of the analyses and examination of patients is at the same time a form for registration and more detailed information: on one side of the envelope the patient's personal data, localization of the primary tumour and the date of registration are entered. Later the dates of continuous control of patients are noted on the same side. At the oncological outpatient clinics the registration envelopes are kept in chronological order, and in alphabetical order within each year of registration; the envelopes of patients receiving follow-up treatment or deceased are kept separately. To avoid duplication, there are nominal cards for all living and deceased patients, kept in alphabetical order.

Moreover, at oncological outpatient clinics another card is filled in and stored in chronological order for subsequent control examinations; on the basis of these cards home nursing and patient appointments are arranged. The oncological outpatient clinics compile annual reports of all the new cases registered according to the international classification of diseases and causes of deaths /8th revision/, grouping the data according to age and sex. The reports are sent to the Organizational Methodological Department of the National Institute of Oncology where periodic checks are made. After that the collected and checked documentation is sent to the Central Statistical Office where it is put in computer.

Simultaneously with the annual reports the oncologic dispensaries compile reports on carcinomas of the mammary gland and cervix uteri and the stages of these diseases /Supplement 16/. The reports are summarized in the Organizational Methodological Department.

The studies of the incidence of carcinomas of the cervix uteri /Fig. 19/ lead us to important conclusions. The frequency curve of the incidence of cervix uteri carcinoma of stage 0-1 according to Heyman is rising rather abruptly from the age groups of 20-24 to 40-44, then it is stabilized up to the age

Supplement 15

ENVELOPE FOR STORING THE DOCUMENTATION OF THE ONCOLOGIC PATIENT

Mouth, pharyngeal cavity and digestive organs	Lip/s/
	Liver, biliary ducts
	Esophagus
	Stomach
	Salivary glands
	Small, large intestine
	Digestive organs
	Pancreas
	Rectum
	Peritoneum
Respiratory organs	Nose and paranasal sinuses
	Larynx
	Bronchi, lungs
Urogenital organs	Kidneys, adrenal glands
	Urinary bladder
	Other uropoietic organs
	Testicle
	Penis
	Prostate
	Vulva
	Vagina
	Cervix uteri
	Corpus uteri
	Adnexa uteri
	Cardiovascular system
	Lymphatic system
	Hematopoietic organs /leukemia/
	Lymphogranulomatosis
	Thyroid gland
	Soft tissues /sarcoma/
	Bone system
	Nervous system
	Organs of sense
	Skin
	Mammary gland
	Other

Date of first visit to doctor: moth, year

General condition of the patient:

Administrative No:

Name:

Maiden name:

Mother's name:

Place of work:

Occupation:

Occupation of spouse:

Place of birth:

Dates of the treatment prescribed:

Year of birth:

Place of residence:

Dates of control examinations:

Place of registration in the dispensary:

Where does the patient have to apply for control examination:

Screening:

Where   When   Year of primary registration Call for examination to the dispensary:

Personal screening card: Sent   Patient appeared

admitted   enclosed

Died - date

in the medical institution - at home

Post mortem - carried out   yes - no

Distribution of Patients Suffering from Cervix Uteri and Breast Carcinomas in 19...

	0-	1-	5-	10-	15-	20-	25-	30-	35-	40-	45-	50-	55-	60-	65-	70-	75-	80-	85-	Total
Breast																				
Stage I																				
II																				
III																				
IV +registered after death																				
Curable																				
Incurable																				
Unknown																				
Breast total																				
Cervix uteri																				
Stage I																				
II																				
III																				
IV+registered after death																				
Curable																				
Incurable																				
Unknown																				
Cervix uteri total																				
Total																				

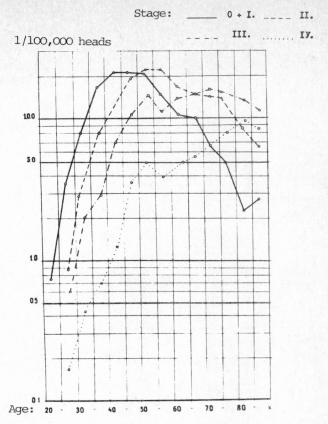

Stage: _____ 0 + I. ____ II.
_ _ _ III. .... IY.

1/100,000 heads

Age: 20 - 30 - 40 - 50 - 60 - 70 - 80 - x

Fig. 19 Incidence of cervix uteri carcinoma by age /1969-1974/

of 50 and drops sharply after that. The frequency curve of
cervix uteri carcinoma of stage 2 has the same shape but
lagging behind it by 6-8 years; it reaches its highest point
between 50 and 60 years and then drops.

The analysis of the incidence of breast carcinoma according to age and stage /stages according to Steinthal /Fig. 20/
gives quite a different picture. The curves of the first and
second stages go up almost parallel, beginning from 20 years
of age and reaching the highest point at the age of 50-54; then
a certain decrease in frequency is observed in both stages; in
some age groups the frequency is almost the same up to 80 years.

The material received from the Central Statistical Office
is compared at the Organizational-Methodological Department

369

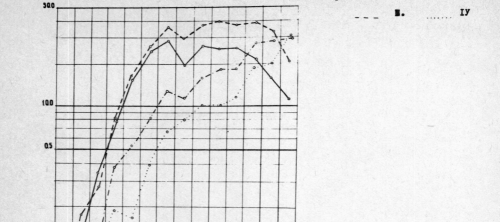

Stage: ——— I.   ____ II.
         _ _ _ Ⅲ.   .... Ⅳ

<u>Fig. 20</u> Incidence of mammary gland carcinoma by age and stages
/1969-1974/

with the data on mortality from cancer of the same localization. Thus, the efficiency of registration can be judged.

ORGANIZATION OF DETECTION AND EXAMINATION OF
ONCOLOGIC PATIENTS

Most often oncologic patients are detected as follows: the patient visits the local medical establishment /usually the panel doctor/ because of certain symptoms. If a malignant tumour is suspected, the patient is sent to the regional out-

patient department of the hospital to be examined by a specialist. According to the results of examination at the outpatient
department /if a more thorough examination is required or the
need for treatment is ascertained/ the patient is sent to one
of the departments of the regional hospital in his place of
residence. If the hospital is not equipped with the necessary
facilities to examine and treat the patient, after being put
on the waiting list, he is assigned to the next medical institution of a higher level, the county hospital, university hospital or the National Institute of Oncology where adequate
facilities are available. The waiting period for patients
varies in different parts of the country and depends of a number of factors, but is usually no more than two to three weeks.

Another way of detecting cancer patients is that of mass
oncologic screenings. At present, in Hungary the oncologic
screenings mainly involve women over 30 years of age /for
carcinomas of the breast and cervix uteri/. In preventive X-ray
examinations for tuberculosis the X-ray pictures are also
checked for possible cancer of the lungs. Furthermore, the
dentists should examine each patient's oral cavity to detect
possible tumours /examination, palpation and, if necessary,
cytologic examination/.

A few centres for the investigation of stomach cancer are
developing methods of mass screening to detect stomach cancer
in small groups of the population. The range of these studies
and the methods used do not allow them to be considered mass
screenings.

The oncologic screenings of women over 30 are envisaged
in the regulations of the oncologic network and those of the
National Institute of Oncology. According to the regulations,
the oncologic network is responsible for the oncologic
screenings of women. It is the task of the heads of oncologic
dispensaries to carry out the screenings and to organize them
in the area of the centre with the participation of oncologic
clinics and specialists in gynecology. The population, however,
is not obliged to undergo the screenings, the participation is
voluntary. The degree of involvement of the population in the

oncological screenings largely depends on the level of health education. On average, 25 per cent of the female population over 30 year of age have been involved in preventive screenings in some areas and at certain periods of time. Attempts are made to encourage women to undergo screenings by arranging them at enterprises where most of the workers are women, by mobile teams of specialists and so on.

Recently, efforts have been made in the capital to introduce compulsory screenings of all women visiting the gynecologist or clinics of family planning.

The history of preventive screenings goes back to the fifties when the screening was still poorly developed. The screenings mostly consisted in palpation of the mammary gland, visual examination of the cervix uteri and an gynecological examination. In the subsequent years /up to the mid-sixties/ the oncological service was able to organize preventive oncological screenings using the colposcope, and to training doctors on colposcopy courses at the National Institute of Oncology. In the mid-sixties the foundations of the oncocytological network were laid down at the Research Institute of Oncopathology, and after a period of development in the seventies it reached the level at which the training of paramedical-cytologists became possible. Every year 20 young paramedical persons are trained for cytologocal analyses on special 10--month courses; at present there are more than 100 paramedical--cytologists working in Hungary. The scientific -methodological guidance of personel is accomplished by pathologists who are also responsible for checking the smears collected.

In the sixties, some facilities were created for mammography mostly by the rearrangement of the available X-ray units. At present, X-ray departments of some hospitals have these facilities.

All in all, the course of preventive oncologic screenings of women for the detection of tumourous and pretumourous diseases may be described as follows: palpation of the breast; women with any symptoms are sent to the department of X-ray diagnosis for mammographic examination. This is followed by the colposcopic examination of the vagina and cervix uteri with the collection of cytological smears in 50 per cent of the cases and then by an ordinary gynecologic examination. Patients with malignant tumours revealed at the screening are sent to the local oncologic committee which decides upon their further treatment. Such committees are organized by the chief oncologist who is usually a gynecologist; the members of the committee are a radiologist, a surgeon, a pathologist and, if necessary, specialists in other fields.

The examination of patients suspected of lung cancer is carried out by a well-organized system of X-ray screening centres covering almost 100 per cent of the adult population in every other year, thus providing the basis for the early diagnosis of lung tumours. Besides, the pulmonological establishments are equipped with endoscopes, and at present the system of bronchocytological diagnosis is being developed. The early diagnosis of tumours of the gastrointestinal tract is a great problem in Hungary. There is a plan to develop a network of gastroenterologic centres equipped with fiberogastroscopes that will be realized in the next five to ten years. It is quite obvious that progress in the early detection of tumours of the gastrointestinal tract can only be achieved by organized gastroenterologic endoscopic centres.

For the women covered by prophylactic screening /Supplement 17/ a special form "Prophylactic screening card" is filled in for the purpose of ensuring repeated screenings in subsequent years, apart from registering personal data of the women covered by screening and the medical conclusion. If the prophylactic screening results in diagnosis of a malignant tumour the registration documentation of the patient is also affixed to the screening card.

The oncologic dispensaries draw up reports about the cancer patients detected at screenings and send them to the National Institute of Oncology. Part of the report contains data on the number of oncologic examinations, as well as the number of pathologic changes revealed.

Such reports are drawn up separately on territorial

PROPHYLACTIC SCREENING CARD

Card of oncologic screening of women	Removed Escaped control Died, diagnosis	Underwent oncologic screening or not. When? Where?	Ensured? Yes. No.	Number

First examination: day   month   19....
Name: Year of birth
Maiden name: Mother's name:
Place of work:
Occupation:
Husband's occupation:
Address:

Stamp of the oncologic dispensary

Establishment

Receives treatment for gyne-cological disease	Yes	No
Gynecological symptoms	Yes	No
Symptoms related to the mammary gland	Yes	No

Father's line /father, father's brother/
Diagnosis:
Mother's line /mother, mother's brothers and sisters/
Diagnosis:
Brothers, sisters, children
Diagnosis:

	During the first examination	At the time of the first examination	At what age died or fell ill
Menstruation	Before menopause After		
Previous illnesses - surgical interventions			
Symptoms:			

Repeated examinations /year, month/

month year   month year   month year   month year
month year

374

A Negative oncologic result

B Disorders of the menstrual cycle /not significant from the point of view of oncology/

C Changed genital position /retroflexion, etc./

D Inflammatory processes in the genitalia /acute, chronic, leukorrhea/

E Benign tumours of genitalia, polyps

F Erosions

G Suspect hemorrhage

H Kraurosis-leukoplakia /of the genitalia/

J Mastopathy, mastodynia, blood discharge from the mammary gland

K Precarcinomas of the skin and visible mucous membranes /except genitals/

L Malignant tumours of the genitalia

M Malignant tumour of the breast

N Malignant tumour of the skin and visible mucous membranes

O Other malignant tumours

Other diseases:

Histology:

Pregnancy:

Notes:

Biopsy:

The patient is sent:

to the oncologic dispensary
to the oncologic outpatient department
for hospitalization

screenings /in villages, places of work, etc./, screenings of hospitalized patients as well as on screenings carried out in oncologic dispensaries /Supplement 18/.

Cases of tumours of the mammary gland and cervix uteri are described in a special report where the data are entered according to stage and five year age groups.

The prophylactic screenings of women started in 1952 covered a large part of the female population then. After the first two years the number of women covered by screenings decreased abruptly, then it stabilized and only later did show a gradual, but slow, growth.

During the first 10-16 years large number of the population had undergone prophylactic screenings in the provinces: the situation has changed lately and at present the mass prophylactic oncologic screenings combined with the ordinary gynecological examination are wide-spread in Budapest.

In 1955-59, on the average about 40 % of all the malignant tumours detected at screenings were carcinomas of the cervix uteri, 25 % carcinoma of the breast, almost 18 % other malignant tumours of the female genital organs, and 16 % skin tumours. The cases of cervix uteri carcinoma detected in 1970-1972 made up 26.8 %, carcinoma of the breast - 37.4 %, and all the other malignant tumours of the female genital organs 5.6 %.

As can be seen from Table 62, 83-92 % of those covered by prophylactic screening do not usually show any pathologic changes. Cervical erosion is revealed in 9.7 - 13.1 % of the cases, mastopathy in 3 - 3.8 per cent and in 1.2 - 1.6 % other pre-malignant diseases. The ratio of malignant tumours detected at prophylactic screenings is 0.21 - 0.31 %.

The ratio between the frequency of cervix uteri carcinoma and carcinoma of the breast has changed over the past decade. While earlier the cervix uteri carcinoma was more common, now carcinoma of the breast is more frequently detected /Table 63/.

The distribution according to the stages of cervix uteri carcinoma and those of the breast detected at prophylactic

Name of the centre of oncologic screenings

Region ....

City ....

Working Form

for annual reports of the oncologic screening centre

.... month 19......

Date of screening	Number of those participating in the oncologic screening			Distribution according to diagnosis								
	Participation in screening for the first time	Participation in oncologic screening for the second time	T o t a l /1+2/	Without oncologic changes A – C	Benign tumour D	Erosion E	Mastopathy F	Other suspect and precancerous diseases G, H, J, K	Malignant tumours of the genitalia L	Malignant tumours of the mammary gland M	Malignant tumours of the skin N	Other malignant tumours O	T o t a l
	1	2	3	4	5	6	7	8	9	10	11	12	

Total

Table 62

Results of Mass Oncologic Screenings of the Female Population in Hungary /Average Annual Data/

	Average number of screenings	Benign tumors	Erythro-plasia	Mastopathy	Other pre-cancerous diseases	Malignant tumours
1957-1959						
absolute number:	402.572	18.068	39.100	13.635		708
percent of the number of screenings		4.5	9.7	3.4		0.18
1960-1964						
absolute number:	428.108	19.953	56.311	13141	6.623	1.201.4
percent of the number of screenings		4.7	13.1	3.1	1.6	0.28
1965-1969						
absolute number:	490.416	21.108	62.517	18.048	6.664	1.511.4
percent of the number of screening		4.3	12.7	3.7	1.4	0.31
1970-1972						
absolute number	492.326	18.785	62.570	18.555	6.271	1.445.2
percent of the number of screenings		3.8	12.7	3.8	1.3	0.29
1973-1975						
absolute number:	395.282	15.452	51.302	13.040	4.826	828.7
percent of the number of screenings		3.9	13.0	3.3	1.2	0.21

Note: the Table does not include results of screenings for Budapest

Table 63

Distribution of Patients According to the Localization of Malignant Tumours
Detected at Oncologic Screenings in Hungary /% of All Detected Cases/

	Cervix uteri	Breast	Other gynaecologic diseases	Skin	Other localiza-tions	Average annual number of all cases detected
1955-59	40.2	25.0	12.7	16.1	6.0	700.4
1960-64	36.8	29.8	13.0	15.5	4.9	1.201.4
1965-69	31.2	32.4	16.6	13.1	6.7	1.511.4
1970-72	26.8	37.4	15.6	14.8	5.4	1.445.2
1973-75	31.1	36.7	16.3	13.0	2.9	828.7

The Table does not include results of screenings for Budapest

Table 64

Stage Distribution of Patients with Carcinomas of the Cervix Uteri and Breast Detected at Mass Oncologic Screenings and by Using Other Methods /%/

Stages	Oncologic screenings		Other methods of detection	
	cervix uteri	breast	cervix uteri	breast
O	11.4		4.3	
I	36.8	40.2	20.8	28.4
II	31.3	40.9	36.6	39.7
III	16.5	13.6	28.5	20.3
IV	4.0	5.3	9.8	11.6

screenings has shown the considerable advantage of active prophylactic screenings as compared to other methods /Table 64/.

The sixties were marked by the intensive development of the oncocytologic service. In 1965-1969 the average annual number of cytologic analyses was 35,390, in 1970-1974 73,610 analyses were performed, due to the prophylactic screenings of the female population. This means that in 1965-1969 there were 7.2 cytologic analyses per 100 preventive screenings, while during the next five years this index has doubled. Naturally, attempts are made to further improve the onco-cytologic network. The oncocytologic service has undoubtedly contributed to the detection of cervix uteri carcinoma in the early stages. While in 1960-1964 the average annual number of 0 and 1 stage carcinomas of cervix uteri detected at screenings was 46.2 %, in 1970-1971 it reached 52.4 %.

ORGANIZATION OF HOSPITALIZATION AND TREATMENT OF CANCER PATIENTS

The leading bodies of the Hungarian health service are of the opinion that it is unnecessary to develop a separate specialized network of establishments for the hospitalization of cancer patients. The only specialized establishment of this type in the country is the National Institute of Oncology with 300 hospital beds. This establishment is also best equipped for all kinds of therapy /together with a few university hospitals/. The task of this establishment is primarily the hospitalization of such patients, for the treatment of which there are no facilities in local hospitals. Thus, cancer patients, like patients suffering from any other disease, first go to a general establishment at their place of residence. If the hospital does not have the equipment required for exact diagnosis or for the treatment of a tumour of a particular localization, the patient may be sent to another general medical establishment equipped with oncoradiological facilities or, if necessary, to the National Institute of Oncology. At present, radiological centres with modern equipment are to be found in one medical establishment in Budapest and four general medical establishments in the provinces. Besides, in the capital and in three other cities in Hungary there are university hospitals with modern equipment for the treatment of malignant tumours.

Thus, if combined or complex treatment is necessary, patients are directed to medical establishments which have appropriate equipment and facilities; other cancer patients are treated in institutions of the general medical network.

DISPENSARIZATION OF CANCER PATIENTS

The main task of oncologic dispensaries is the dispensarization of cancer patients registered at different medical institutions. Some medical establishments /mainly radiotherapeutic centres and departments dealing with the treatment of leukemic patients/ independently organize the follow-up treatment of patients who have been treated there. The patients are placed under observation by the oncologic dispensaries as from the registration and called in for checks every three months during the first year, and every six months during the second and third years; patients who have survived for three years are called in for checks once a year. If the oncologic dispensaries receive information about cancer patients registered in other medical establishments the observation is only a formality. If no information is received from medical establishments about the registered patient, if the patient does not come to the check-ups and there is no notification of death, the general practitioner or the district nurse is charged with the oncologic follow-up treatment. With the help of these measures, either the patient is encouraged to go to the check-ups or information on his condition is obtained through the general practitioner /Table 65/.

A patient registered because of a malignant tumour is examined in the course of the check-up at the oncologic dispensary according to the localization of the primary tumour, to estimate his condition. If metastasis or relapse are suspected the institution where the patient initially received

Table 65

Distribution of Patients with Malignant Tumours According to the Place of Observation for 10 Years After Registration

Years after registration	Cancer patients, including:		
	Patients under control of the		
	Oncologic dispensary /%/	Medical establishment /%/	Panel doctor
1	55.0	16.1	28.9
2	50.7	15.8	33.5
3	49.9	15.6	34.5
4	51.5	13.3	35.2
5	49.9	11.6	38.5
6	50.4	11.8	37.8
7	50.9	8.3	40.8
8	49.1	8.0	42.9
9	50.0	7.7	42.3
10	50.2	6.8	43.0

treatment is consulted. Each patient undergoes usual examinations /roentgenoscopy of the thorax, in the case of tumours
of the female genital organs cytology of vaginal smear, in the
case of breast tumours mammography of the other breast/.

The oncologic dispensaries are obliged to make annual
reports on dispensarization and the results of the observations
of cancer patients registered by them /Supplement 19/. From the
evaluation of these annual reports it is possible to supervise
the work of oncologic dispensaries and their data are used for
studying the survival of cancer patients.

When studying the tendency with regard to the mortality
of cancer patients registered, it may be noticed that during
a 10-year period the logarithm of mortality percentage has
increased in direct ratio to the logarithm of the time passed
/Fig. 21/. The first year is survived by 67 per cent of the
patients /28 % of man and 39 % of women/ /Table 66/.

Table 66

Mortality Rate of Patients with Malignant Tumours
During 10 years After Registration

Years after registration	Deceased, %			% of patients under control
	men	women	total	
1	39.1	27.9	33.3	66.7
2	51.5	37.8	44.4	55.6
3	56.0	42.9	49.2	50.8
4	60.7	47.8	54.0	46.0
5	61.9	51.5	56.5	43.5
6	64.3	53.8	58.9	41.1
7	67.5	55.4	61.1	38.9
8	70.8	58.1	64.1	35.9
9	71.3	60.1	65.3	34.7
10	73.6	61.4	67.1	32.9

Because of the different circumstances the oncologic
dispensaries are not able to exercise a 100 % control over
cancer patients; by the end of the ten-year period after the

Distribution of cancer patients registered by the oncologic
dispensary in 19.... according to sex and tumour localization

/According to International Classification of Diseases, 8th revision/

Code number	Localization	Number of men								Number of women							
		Examined by the chief oncologist	Examined at a medical establishment	Controlled	Not controlled	Control was not possible	Died after registration	Registered after death	T o t a l	Examined by the chief oncologist	Examined at a medical establishment	Controlled	Not controlled	Control was not possible	Died after registration	Registered after death	T o t a l
140	Lip																
141	Tongue																
142	Pancreas																
208	Polycythaemia vera																
209	Myelofibrosis																
	Total																

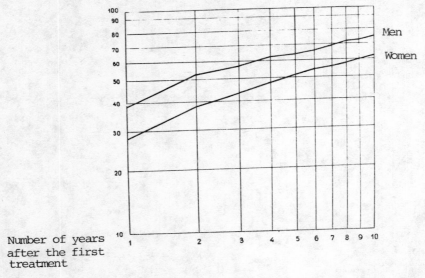

100
90
80   Men
70
60   Women
50

40

30

20

10

Number of years   1   2   3   4   5   6   7   8   9   10
after the first
treatment

Fig. 21 Probability of death in patients with malignant
tumours registered in oncological establishments /all
localizations, 1964/

beginning of treatment 30 to 35 % of the patients have escaped
control /Table 67/.

The survival rate of patients according to certain localizations is studied by similar methods. Thus 58.8 % of women
suffering from breast cancer die within ten years, and 25.6 %
remain under observation. Among patients suffering from cancer
of the cervix uteri 48 % die within ten years and 34.7 %
remain under control. 87.6 % of men with diagnosed cancer of
the stomach die within the 10-year period /55 per cent by the
end of the first year/, and only 5.7 % remain under observation. The survival rate of women suffering from cancer of
stomach is 83 %, while 8.3 % remain under observation.

STUDY OF THE EFFICIENCY OF THE TREATMENT OF PATIENTS

The information received from oncologic dispensaries
about the dispensarization and control of cancer patients /see
above/ form the basis for evaluating the survival rate of cancer patients. Due to the shortcomings of the registration system and notifications the data cannot be extended to evaluate
the efficiency of certain therapy methods. The data are

Table 67

Indices of the Oncologic Dispensary Observations of Patients Suffering from Malignant Tumours for 10 Years After Registration /in % of all patients survived/

Years after re-gistra-tion	M e n			W o m e n			T o t a l		
	Under control of oncologic dispensary	Not con-trolled	Control is not possible	Under control of oncologic dispensary	Not con-trolled	Control is not possible	Under control of oncologic dispensary	Not con-trolled	Control is not possible
1	69.8	25.4	4.8	74.2	24.6	1.2	72.3	24.9	2.8
2	68.1	29.4	2.5	70.2	27.0	2.8	69.3	28.1	2.6
3	65.2	31.8	3.0	69.1	27.7	3.2	67.5	29.4	3.1
4	62.6	33.7	3.7	66.1	29.8	4.1	64.7	31.4	3.9
5	57.4	38.5	4.1	64.8	31.2	4.0	64.4	34.3	4.1
6	57.3	39.4	3.3	63.4	32.4	4.2	60.9	35.3	3.8
7	57.4	37.8	4.8	62.2	33.0	4.8	60.3	34.9	4.8
8	58.9	36.7	4.4	61.5	33.5	5.0	60.5	34.7	4.8
9	58.4	36.4	5.2	61.4	33.2	5.4	60.5	34.4	5.3
10	59.5	34.7	5.8	61.1	32.7	6.2	60.5	33.5	6.1

indirectly characterized by mortality indices of certain localizations of the primary tumour for several years after the
registration of the patient. In view of the fact that the
registration data of oncologic dispensaries are available only
in relation to cervix uteri and breast carcinomas, a special
analysis has been undertaken in areas of the country where the
registration system has appeared to be satisfactory.

For 1955, 1960 and 1965 data from 14 oncologic dispensaries
were studied on patients registered with carcinomas of the
breast and cervix uteri. In 1955, the number of patients registered with breast carcinoma was 284, in 1960 315, and in
1965 394; in 1955, the number of patients registered with
cervix uteri carcinoma was 333, in 1960 370, and in 1965 343.

After 10, 15 and 20 years the number of patients with
breast carcinoma who escaped observation and moved to other
regions of the country was 4.9 % for 1955, 7.6 % for 1960, and
9.4 % for 1965; in patients suffering from carcinoma of the
cervix uteri the indices are 10.4 %, 9.5 %, and 12.3 %,
respectively.

The notifications contained no data on histology in 60.4%
of the cases of breast carcinoma in 1955, in 26.7 % in 1960,
and in 17.5 % in 1965. In cases of cervix uteri carcinoma the
indices were 30.4 %, 24.3 %, and 13.8 %, respectively.

The description of the therapy applied is insufficient
and cannot be evaluated for patients suffering from breast
carcinoma registered in 1955 in 36 % of the cases, in 1960 in
12.1 %, and in 1965 in 9.9 % of the cases; for patients suffering from cervix uteri cancer the indices are 21.5 %, 13.1 %
and 10.2 %, respectively.

In patients suffering from breast carcinoma the stage
distribution according to Steinthal was used; in 1955 the
stages were determined in 64.6 % of the patients, in 1960 in
81 %, and in 1965 89 %; the stage distribution of cervix
uteri carcinoma was calculated according to Heyman: in patients
registered in 1955 the stage was determined in 87.1 % of the
cases, in 1960 in 91.9 % and in 1965 - in 96.5 %.

With regard to the shortcomings mentioned above it should

be concluded that the registration material available is too diverse in content and often lacks extremely important information. Thus the evaluation of the effectivity of treatment for different groups of patients would not produce any significant and acceptable data.

When studying of the data on patients treated for breast carcinoma it may be observed that the mortality rate is rather high in the first 10 years after therapy, whereas after this period it does not differ much from the death rate for the average female population /corrected survival indices/ /Table 68/. This is particularly true in cases treated in stages I and II. All patients with malignant tumours diagnosed in stage IV died within 10 years.

In patients suffering from cervix uteri carcinoma the survival in stage I after therapy greatly differs from the results of stage II therapy. /It would be wrong to evaluate survival indices in the stage "O" because of the very small number of patients registered/. The mortality of patients treated in stage I is higher than the death rate of the ordinary female population only during the first seven years after therapy, whereas later the death indices do not differ to a great extent.

Death rate indices for patients diagnosed and treated in stage II of cervix uteri carcinoma are very high even after 10 years and differ greatly from the indices for the rest of population.

Death rate indices for patients treated in stage III are very high during the first five years after the therapy, whereas the indices for those who have survived this period hardly differ from the indices for the rest of population.

All patients treated in stage IV died within 10 years after therapy.

The fact that the evaluation of the efficiency of different therapeutic methods is impossible on the basis of territorial data points to a shortcoming of data collection and processing in the medical establishments. Some institutions and departments evaluate different treatment methods from

389

Table 68

Indices of 5-, 10-, 15-years Survival of Patients Suffering from Carcinomas of the Breast and Cervix uteri According to stages in %.

Stage according to Steintal	Carcinoma of the Breast			Stage according to Heyman	Carcinoma of cervix uteri		
	5 years	10 years	15 years		5 years	10 years	15 years
I	74.7	51.0	38.8	I	79.9	75.6	66.7
II	53.8	37.8	35.3	II	55.3	43.9	31.6
III	31.9	21.1	5.7	III	26.2	18.3	18.3
IV	2.9	-	-	IV	2.2	-	-

x/ Survival of patients registered in 1955 and 1960

their case histories for reports at congresses or in publications. Usually this is the way for the comparison of results.

ORGANIZATION OF MEDICAL DETERMINATION OF DISABILITY
AND REHABILITATION OF ONCOLOGICAL PATIENTS

In Hungary the medical determination of disability is carried out by a special service organized for this purpose. The leading establishment is the State Bureau of specialists which is supported in its activities by regional specialists. It is their task to collect data on the results of the examinations of the patients as well as on the health state of these patients in time. Thus, with respect to patients treated for malignant tumours the opinion of the chief oncologist is asked for. By comparing the data examination collected from different specialists, a conclusion is drawn about the patient's ability to work. In determining the cancer patient's ability to work, the opinions of all the specialists who have participated in his examination are taken into account.

In Hungary the studies regarding the development of the problem of patients' rehabilitation are still in the initial stage. In inpatient hospitals there are specialists in therapeutic physical training responsible for the physical training of patients, mainly in the postoperational period, aimed at promoting the restoration of the damaged functions of the organism.

After the patient is discharged from hospital the prescribed therapy or the one started is continued in physicotherapy clinics. Since Hungary is rich in medicinal springs, there are extensive opportunities for sending patients to sanatoria where they can receive appropriate balneological treatment.

At the patient's place of work the doctor has to decide whether the patient can continue his job and also to ensure his transfer to a more suitable job within the enterprise through negotiations with his chief. In the course of this work the doctor asks for the opinion of the chief oncologist about patients suffering from malignant tumours. The chief oncologist may suggest that the patient should be transferred to another job, but the possibilities of enterprises are often limited. The problem of transfer to another job can only be solved with the patient's consent. The patient cannot obliged to consent to his transfer, even if he is unable to do his former job.

ORGANIZATION OF TREATMENT OF PATIENTS WITH ADVANCED TUMOURS

The treatment of patients with advanced forms of tumours is the responsibility of the general medical network of the public health service. If a patient with an advanced tumour has not been examined or treated in hospital before, the general practitioner sends him to the general medical establishment in his place of residence. Naturally, patients sometimes refuse hospital treatment or examination and then they are attended and treated in their terminal period by the local doctor on the basis of the diagnosis determined. If the patient agrees to be sent to a medical establishment, where, if possible and indispensable, he is given some palliative treatment. When palliative treatment is not possible, the patient is treated by the local practitioner. In such cases, the local doctor is given recommendations concerning the medical care of a particular patient. Usually it is symptomatic treatment /anaesthesia/; chemotherapy, if any improvement is expected from it, is performed by the medical establishment itself. The local practitioners can organize consultations at the patient's home during the terminal period with the participation of the district's chief oncologist who gives advice to the local practitioner with regard to the patient's further care.

There are no special medical establishments in the country for hospitalizing patients with advanced forms of tumours. The departments for incurable patients in some medical establishments are still scanty and have a small number of hospital beds. Those in charge of the public health service hold the opinion that no special departments should be organized for the hospitalization of patients in terminal condition since the atmosphere of such departments would be painful both for those working in them, and for the patients themselves.

District nurses /on the average one nurse per one general practitioner/ are of great help to district doctors in rendering assistance to incurable patients. These nurses partly take care of patients in terminal condition, partly teach the members of the patient's family the proper professional methods of care.

TEACHING OF ONCOLOGY, TRAINING OF ONCOLOGISTS AND
PARAMEDICAL PERSONNEL FOR ONCOLOGICAL DEPARTMENTS

The teaching of oncology is an integrated part of the teaching at medical institutes in Hungary. Hence the students at medical institutes are given general information on malignant tumours, in studying therapy, surgery, radiology and other branches of medicine. Teaching of oncology as a separate science is not included in the compulsory curriculum of medical institutes in Hungary. At the Semmelweis Medical School in Budapest an optional course of lectures on oncology is given annually for approximately 20 regular students.

Within the system of advanced training of doctors specialized training of oncologists is organized on a much wider scale. Such courses are conducted annually by the Postgraduate Medical School, as the main organizing and guiding body in this system of training, together with the National Institute of Oncology. Other possibilities are also used for teaching oncology. Thus, for example, in the postgraduate courses of other branches of medicine, lectures on some aspects of oncology delivered by the members of the National Institute of Oncology are included.

Over the past five years 22 courses have been organized by the Postgraduate Medical School and the National Institute of Oncology. On these courses the students have been partly practising oncologists, partly clinical surgeons who have been particularly interested in contemporary methods of treatment of malignant tumours.

In Hungary every doctor is obliged to attend postgraduate courses in every four year. It is not necessarily a course of lectures: many doctors take the courses individually, i.e. the doctors are sent to another medical establishment of a higher level for one to two months to become acquainted with its work.

While taking individual postgraduate courses, many doctors visit the National Institute of Oncology. The training of chief oncologists is part of the curriculum. In Hungary, after a basic specialization usually in gynecology or surgery a six-month individual postgraduate course at the National Institute of Oncology is required; only after that can the doctor hold the post of chief oncologist. In the last six years 39 doctors have taken such individual courses at the National Institute of Oncology.

The training of radiologists is based on the resolution about the final examination in the different specialities. According to the resolution, anyone wishing to specialize in radiology must work for three years in an X-ray department. During this period they gain knowledge both in X-ray diagnosis and radiotherapy. The possibility of specialization in the field of radiotherapy is given to oncoradiologists. This requires a three-year practical course, including six months in the X-ray diagnostic department, while the rest of the time is spent in non-radiology department such as surgery, gynecology, internal diseases, etc. so as to make the doctor acquainted with the diagnosis of malignant tumours of these localizations.

The role of the Research Institute of Oncopathology should be mentioned separately with regard to the system of advanced training. The pathologists who are being trained for oncocytological work are taught partly in courses of lectures organized together with the Postgraduate Medical School, partly individually at the Research Institute of Oncopathology. Pathologists wishing to gain a more profound knowledge and practice in the diagnosis of malignant tumours take individual training courses at the Research Institute of Oncopathology for a few weeks or a month.

The paramedical personnel in the field of oncology is trained on courses for nurses who pursued preliminary oncocytologic studies. These ten-month courses are organized and conducted by the Research Institute of Oncopathology. During this period the students receive special training of a high level, and after the final examination they can work independently. The first course was organized in 1972. Over the past four years about 100 students have graduated from these courses. During the training period students receive grants from the medical establishment that has sent them for training, and, after graduating, they are obliged to return to their job. Their work is supervised by the hospital's chief pathologist. Working sessions are held annually at the Research Institute of Oncopathology to provide these paramedical cytologists with advanced training. At these sessions the nurses have to make reports on their work and attend a course of lectures about the latest achievements in this field.

The paramedical staff of radiology departments take courses for assistants on X-ray radiology. The chief oncologists work with general paramedical personnel. At present, a textbook on oncology for courses of nurses is being prepared for publication. For the advanced training of nurses lectures on oncology was organized by the Health Department of the city council of Budapest only once. No postgraduate courses of this type have been organized in any other regions of the country.

HEALTH EDUCATION OF THE POPULATION

In Hungary the leading organization in health education /on a state level/ is the Institute of Health Education of the Ministry of Health. The Institute's local bodies are the health education groups supervised by the chief medical officer and subordinated to the regional councils. The Institute of Health Education is producing health education films and publishing books, leaflets, and posters. From their budget the regional organizations can buy the films issued by the Institute, order the literature published by it, and issue different publications themselves. At present, six films are available on the topic of malignant tumours and primarily on the importance of screening and early diagnosis. /Besides, there are films aimed at control of smoking, improper nutrition partly touching on cancer control/.

The authors of the working regulations of the oncologic network took into account the great importance of health education regarding successful cancer control. Therefore the chief oncologists are responsible for delivering lectures in districts for the health education of the population. From 1970 to 1974 450 lectures were delivered annually by oncologists.

However, health education is not limited by these possibilities. Both the Hungarian Red Cross Society and the Society for Popularization of Scientific Knowledge, the task of which is to raise the cultural level of the population in the field of natural sciences, organize numerous lectures on health education. The lecturers are usually specialists from local hospitals and outpatient departments. Also of great help is the fact that the Hungarian braodcasting system as well as the press /central and local/ systematically report on events related to cancer control /CMEA sessions, international congresses/ and disseminate knowledge on the subject through interviews with specialists.

Table 69

Age-sex Structure of the Hungarian Population as of
January 1, 1970

Age	Total	Men	Women
0-4	703213	362588	340625
5-9	649386	333798	315588
10-14	823908	423016	400892
15-19	917134	469624	447510
20-24	779249	395921	383328
25-29	740865	371769	369096
30-34	671824	326284	345540
35-39	712352	349196	363156
40-44	736856	358101	378755
45-49	731196	345653	385543
50-54	430743	201598	229145
55-59	665574	309219	356355
60-64	575301	264231	311070
65-69	475455	213443	262012
70-74	349451	145160	204291
75-79	205202	78185	127017
80-84	106336	39013	67321
85 and more	48056	16852	31204
Total	10322099	5003651	5318448

Table 70

Absolute Number and Incidence of Malignant Tumours in the
Urban and Rural Population of Hungary in 1970-1973

	1970	1971	1972	1973
Total for Hungary				
Absolute number	20.921	21.075	22.703	21.873
Incidence per 100.000 population	203.0	203.0	219.0	210.0
Budapest				
Absolute number	4.519	4.247	5.011	4.676
Incidence per 100.000 population	232.0	210.0	247.0	229.0
Selected cities				
Absolute number	1.495	1.663	1.491	1.468
Incidence per 100.000 population	208.0	225.0	198.0	185.0
All other regions				
Absolute number	14.907	15.165	16.201	15.729
Incidence per 100.000 population	195.0	200.0	214.0	208.0
Rural areas				
Absolute number	16.402	16.828	17.692	17.197
Incidence per 100.000 population	196.0	202.0	212.0	206.0

Table 71

Absolute Number and Incidence of Malignant Tumours in the
population of Hungary in 1970-73

Years	Lips /140/	Skin /172/	Breast /174/	Cervix uteri /180/
Total population				
1970				
Absolute number	519	2.871	2.036	1.212
Incidence per 100.000 population	5.0	27.8	19.7	11.8
1971				
Absolute number	587	3.050	2.066	1.285
Incidence	5.7	29.4	19.9	12.4
1972				
Absolute number	583	3.160	2.234	1.291
Incidence	5.6	30.5	21.6	12.5
1973				
Absolute number	584	3.242	2.323	1.341
Incidence	5.6	31.0	22.3	12.9
Budapest				
1970				
Absolute number	36	496	614	357
Incidence	1.8	24.7	30.5	17.8
1971				
Absolute number	56	556	628	343
Incidence	2.8	27.5	31.0	17.0
1972				
Absolute number	53	620	703	404
Incidence	2.6	30.5	34.6	19.9
1973				
Absolute number	70	620	772	383
Incidence	3.4	30.3	37.8	18.7
Regions				
1970				
Absolute number	483	2.375	1.422	855
Incidence	5.8	28.5	17.1	10.3
1971				
Absolute number	531	2.494	1.438	942
Incidence	6.4	30.3	17.3	11.3
1972				
Absolute number	530	2.540	1.531	887
Incidence	6.4	30.4	18.3	10.6
1973				
Absolute number	514	2.622	1.551	958
Incidence	6.1	31.3	18.5	11.4

399

Table 72

Prevalence of Patients with Malignant Neoplasms of Certain Localizations According to the Data of the Hungarian Oncological Registration 1971-1974

Local-izations	Absolute numbers			Prevalence per 100.000 population		
	1971	1973	1974	1971	1973	1974
All malignant tumours	128.607	107.757	121.445	1.242.13	1.034.57	1.162.32
Skin /172/	31.610	29.551	32.513	305.30	283.72	311.17
Breast /174/	14.519	14.081	14.007	272.18[x]	262,44[x]	260.27[x]
Cervix uteri /180/	14.501	14.123	13.226	271.85[x]	263.23[x]	245.77[x]

[x]/ in terms of female population

Table 73

Distribution of Patients with Malignant Neoplasms by Survival Time Following Diagnosis 1971-74

Localization	Total Abso-lute number	Number of living patients registered by the end of the years							
		Abso-lute number	% of total number of patients	Abso-lute number	% of total number of patients	Abso-lute number	% of total number of patients	Abso-lute number	% of total number of patients
1971 Total	128.607	25.584	19.89	2.030	15.57	34.963	27.19	32.269	25.09
Skin /172/	31.610	5.259	20.56	4.934	24.63	9.838	28.14	8.710	27.00
Breast /174/	14.519	3.009	11.76	2.249	11.23	3.770	10.78	3.762	11.66
Cervix uteri /180/	14.501	2.057	8.04	1.725	8.61	3.940	11.27	5.639	17.48
In the percentage of female population									
Breast /174/			20.67		19.26		17.67		11.66
cervix uteri /180/			14.13		14.76		18.47		25.68
1973 Total	107.757	24.306	22.56	17.569	16.30	31.364	29.11	34.518	32.03
Skin /172/	29.551	5.860	22.05	4.534	25.81	9.387	29.33	10.270	29.75
Breast /174/	14.081	3.247	13.36	2.368	13.48	4.007	12.76	4.459	12.92
Cervix uteri /180/	14.123	2.064	8.49	1.678	9.55	3.710	11.83	6.671	19.33
In the percentage of human population									
Breast /174/			23.63		23.13		21.17		19.18
Cervix uteri /180/			15.02		16.39		19.60		28.70

Table 73 /cont'd/

Localization	Total Absolute number	Number of living patients registered by the end of the years							
		Absolute number	% of total number of patient	Absolute number	% of total number of patients	Absolute number	% of total number of patients	Absolute number	% of total number of patients
1974 Total	121.445	26.016	21.42	19.309	15.90	36.124	29.74	39.996	32.93
Skin /172/	32.513	5.809	22.33	4.940	25.58	10.155	28.11	11.609	29.03
Breast /174/	14.007	3.345	12.86	2.493	12.91	4.068	11.26	4.101	10.25
Cervix uteri /180/	13.226	1.992	7.66	1.632	8.45	3.622	10.03	5.980	14.95
In the percentage of human population									
Breast /174/			22.38		22.02		18.89		15.36
Cervix uteri /180/			13.33		11.42		16.82		22.40

Table 74

Number of Deaths and Mortality from malignant tumours in the Hungarian Population in 1970-74

	1970	1971	1972	1973	1974
Total population					
Number of deaths	22.263	23.231	23.383	23.888	25.112
Mortality per 100.000 population	216	224	225	230	240
Budapest					
Number of deaths	5.311	5.856	5.843	5.965	6.204
Mortality per 100.000 population	264	289	287	293	302
Selected cities					
Number of deaths	x	1.518	1.585	1.693	1.758
Mortality per 100.000 population	x	205	209	213	216
Regions /except the selected larger cities/					
Number of deaths	16.931	15.857	15.955	16.230	17.150
Mortality per 100.000 population	203	209	210	214	225

The selected cities are cities with over 100.000 population according to the data of the Demographical Annual for 1970, -71, -72, -73, -74.   x = no data

Table 75

Number of Deaths and Mortality from Malignant Tumours of
Certain Localizations in the Hungarian Population in 1970 - 1974

1 9 7 0

ICD /8th revision/ Code Number	Localization	Total population		Budapest		All other regions	
		Number of deaths	Mortality	Number of deaths	Mortality	Number of deaths	Mortality
140-209	All malignant tumours	22.263	216	5.311	264	16.952	204
140-149	Lips, oral cavity	373	3,6	66	3,3	307	3.7
150-159	Digestive organs	10.188	98,9	2.230,	110,7	7.958	95,9
150	Esophagus	207	2,0	47	2,3	160	1,9
151	Stomach	4.725	45,8	742	36,8	3.983	48,0
152-153	Large and small intestines	1.434	13,9	472	23,4	962	11,6
154	Rectum	999	9,7	247	12,3	752	9,1
160-163	Respiratory organs	3.859	37,4	984	48,9	2.875	34,7
162	Lungs	3.390	32,9	881	43,7	2.510	30,3
170-171	Bones,connective tissues	386	3,7	82	4,1	304	3,7
172-173	Skin	337	3,3	69	3,4	268	3,2
174	Breast	1.314	12,7	397	19,7	917	11,05

Code	Localization						
180–184	Female genital organ	1.903	18.45	492	24.4	1.411	17.0
180	Cervix uteri	498	4.8	93	4.6	405	4.9
185–187	Male genital organs	1.046	10.1	270	13.4	776	9.4
185	Prostate	970	9.4	252	12.5	718	8.7
188–189	Uropoietic organs	880	8.5	266	13,2	614	7.4
200–209	Lymphatic and haemopoietic organs	1.234	12.0	315	15.6	919	11.1
204–207	Leukaemia, aleukaemia	641	6,2	144	7,15	497	6.0

1 9 7 1

Code	Localization						
140–209	All localizations	23.231	224.	5.856	289	17.375	209
140–149	Lips, oral cavity	387	3.7	78	3,8	309	3.7
150–519	Digestive organs	10.372	99.9	2.406	118,9	7.966	95.7
150	Esophagus	205	2,0	54	2.7	151	1,8
151	Stomach	4.659	44.9	776	38.2	3.883	46.7
152–153	Large and small intestines	1.608	15.5	527	26.0	1.081	13.0
154	Rectum	1.019	9.8	262	12.9	752	9.1
160–163	Respiratory organs	4.229	40.7	1.155	57.1	3.074	36.9
162	Lungs	3.653	35.2	1.008	49.8	2.645	31.8

/cont'd/

Table 75/cont'd/

ICD /8th revision/ Code Number	Localization	Total population		Budapest		All other regions	
		Number of deaths	Mortality	Number of deaths	Mortality	Number of deaths	Mortality
170-171	Bones, connective tissues	404	3.9	92	4.5	312	3.7
172-173	Skin	329	3,2	67	3.3	262	3.2
174	Breast	1.459	14,0	445	22.0	1.014	12.2
180-184	Female genital organs	1.952	18.8	577	28.	1.375	16.5
180	Cervix uteri	484	4.7	89	4,4	395	4.7
185-187	Male genital organs	1.104	10.6	270	13.3	834	10.0
185	Prostate	1.024	9.9	243	12.0	781	9.4
188-189	Uropoietic organs	913	8.8	273	13.5	640	7.7
200-209	Lymphatic and haemopoietic organs	1.282	12.4	348	17.2	934	11.2
204-207	Leukaemia, aleukaemia	667	6.45	179	8.8	488	5.9
				1 9 7 2			
140-209	All localizations	23.383	225	5.843	287	17.540	210

140–149	Lips, oral cavity	399	3.85	88	4,3	311	3.7
150–159	Digestive organs	10.374	100.0	2.415	118.8	7.959	95.4
150	Esophagus	231	2.2	53	2.6	178	2.1
151	Stomach	4.479	43.2	776	38.2	3.703	44.4
152–153	Large and small intestines	1.650	16.7	530	26.1	1.120	13.4
154	Rectum	1.078	10.4	273	13.4	805	9.6
160–163	Respiratory organs	4.198	40.45	1.122	55.2	3.076	36.9
162	Lungs	3.656	35.2	986	48.5	2.670	32.0
170–171	Bones, connective tissues	359	3.8	101	5.0	294	3.5
172–173	Skin	315	3.0	49	2.4	266	3.2
174	Breast	1.484	14.3	478	23.5	1.006	12.1
180–184	Female genital organs	1.962	18.9	561	27.6	1.401	16.8
180	Cervix uteri	528	5.1	100	4.9	428	5.1
185–187	Male genital organs	1.106	10.7	252	12.4	854	10.2
185	Prostate	1.026	9.9	232	11.4	794	9.5
188–189	Uropoietic organs	928	8.9	291	14.3	637	7.6

Table 75 /cont'd/

1 9 7 3

ICD /8 th revision Code Number	Localization	Total population		Budapest		All other regions	
		Number of deaths	Mortality	Number of deaths	Mortality	Number of deaths	Mortality
200–209	Lymphatic and haemopoietic organs	1.394	13.4	339	16.7	1.055	12.6
204–207	Leukaemia, aleukaemia	708	6.8	183	9.0	525	6.3
140–209	All localizations	23.888	230	5.965	292	17.923	214
140–149	Lips, oral cavity	405	3.9	98	4,8	307	3.7
150–159	Digestive organs	10.508	101.1	2.452	120.0	8.056	96.3
150	Esophagus	201	1.9	62	3.0	139	1.7
151	Stomach	4.384	42.2	740	36.2	3.644	43.5
152–153	Large and small intestine	1.630	15.7	509	24.9	1.121	13.4
154	Rectum	1.178	11.3	323	15.8	855	10.2
160–163	Respiratory organs	4.358	41.9	1.196	58.5	3.162	37.8
162	Lungs	3.862	37.15	1.059	51.8	2.803	33.5

Code	Site						
170—171	Bones,connect. tissues	365	3.5	73	3.6	292	3.5
172—173	Skin	377	3.6	55	2.7	322	3.8
174	Breast	1.496	14.4	462	22.6	1.034	12.4
180—184	Female genital organs	2.072	19.9	606	29.7	1.466	17.5
180	Cervix uteri	515	4,95	107	5.2	408	4.9
185—187	Male genital organs	1.117	10.75	239	11.7	878	10.5
185	Prostate	1.033	9.9	217	10.6	816	9.75
188—189	Uropoietic organs	1.000	9.6	284	13.9	716	8.6
200—209	Lymphatic and haemopoietic organs	1.364	13.1	329	16.1	1.035	12.4
204—207	Leukaemia, aleukaemia	684	6.6	166	8.1	518	6.2
				1 9 7 4			
140—209	All malignant tumours	25.112	239.6	6.204	320.2	18.908	221.4
140—149	Lips, oral cavity	450	4.3	89	4.6	361	4.2
150—159	Digestive organs	10.790	103.0	2.530	130.6	8.260	96.7

Table 75 /cont'd/

ICD /8th revision Code Number	Localization	Total population		Budapest		All other regions	
		Number of deaths	Mortality	Number of deaths	Mortality	Number of deaths	Mortality
150	Esophagus	242	2.3	51	2.6	191	2.2
151	Stomach	4.341	41.4	721	37.2	3.620	42.4
152–153	Large and small intestines	1.817	17.3	585	30.2	1.232	14.4
154	Rectum	1.183	11.3	308	15.9	875	10.2
160–163	Respiratory organs	4.712	45.0	1.264	65.2	3.448	40.4
162	Lungs	4.191	40.0	1.137	58.7	3.054	35.75
170–171	Bones, connective tissues	443	4.2	109	5.6	334	3.9
172–173	Skin	391	3.7	66	3.4	325	3.8
174	Breast	1.558	14.9	446	23.0	1.112	13.0
180–184	Female genital organs	2.065	19.7	534	27.6	1.531	17.9
180	Cervix uteri	521	5.0	107	5.5	414	4.85

185–187	Male genital organs	1.288	12.3	288	14.9	1.000	11.7
185	Prostate	1.196	11.4	266	13.7	930	10.9
188–189	Uropoietic organs	1.032	9.8	276	14.2	756	8.85
200–209	Lymphatic and haemopoietic organs	1.458	13.9	394	20.3	1.064	12.5
204–207	Leukaemia, aleukaemia	752	7.2	213	11.0	539	6.3

Table 76

Number of Deaths and Mortality from Malignant Neoplasms in the Hungarian Population by Administrative Regions / 1970 - 1974 /

Administrative regions of the country	Number of deaths					Mortality per 100.000 population				
	1970	1971	1972	1973	1974	1970	1971	1972	1973	1974
Budapest	5.311	5.856	5.843	5.965	6.204	264	289	287	292	302
Regions :										
Baranya	514	481	528	563	600	188	176	194	207	221
Bács-Kiskun	1.222	1.269	1.301	1.267	1.307	216	225	231	225	231
Békés	974	983	996	1.024	1.063	223	226	230	237	246
Borsod-Abauj-Zemplén	1.062	1.093	1.068	1.191	1.243	179	185	181	202	210
Csongrád	755	790	784	769	788	235	247	246	267	274
Fejér	687	755	819	753	861	175	191	206	188	213
Győr-Sopron	863	649	653	662	707	213	215	216	220	234
Hajdu-Bihar	727	773	723	725	708	201	216	203	204	221
Heves	795	821	808	793	820	234	241	237	233	240
Komárom	546	576	575	570	604	179	188	186	184	194
Nógrád	465	483	466	460	520	199	206	199	197	222
Pest	1.775	1.826	1.863	1.947	2.076	201	205	206	213	224
Somogy	761	804	773	826	896	212	224	215	229	248

Szabolcs-Szatmár	1.002	952	852	976	980	177	170	152	174	172
Szolnok	971	943	1.000	999	1.128	223	215	229	229	256
Tolna	526	564	617	551	573	207	223	245	219	227
Vas	636	681	682	662	675	229	245	245	238	242
Veszprém	855	822	879	880	891	211	199	212	211	212
Zala	542	585	557	598	619	208	224	213	229	237
Selected cities:										
Debrecen	327	342	366	343	391	199	203	213	196	217
Győr		246	223	251	259	169	229	204	224	226
Miskolc	310	356	370	395	424	199	191	195	206	218
Pécs	300	300	316	346	300	199	194	202	218	187
Szeged	316	274	310	358	384	256	211	235	219	231
Total:	22.263	23.231	23.383	23.888	23.112	216	224	225	229	237

Mortality /per 100.000 Population/ from Malignant Neoplasms
by Age and Sex

	Males					Total	
	-30	30-39	40-49	50-59	60 and older	per 100.000 popu-lation	Stand-ardized indices /Segi/
All malignant tumours /140-149/							
1970	9.80	27.23	89.95	311.85	1.214.45	236.11	174.66
1971	10.52	31.25	101.40	327.55	1.236.79	246.58	181.97
1972	9.79	26.06	102.71	318.68	1.231.71	246.45	180.67
1973	9.79	31.54	102.36	317.21	1.225.99	249.28	181.28
1974	10.72	30.94	111.24	324.33	1.301.94	265.55	191.48
Esophagus /150/							
1970	-	0.15	1.99	4.11	15.85	3.11	2.28
1971	-	-	1.55	5.68	16.46	3.32	2.39
1972	-	0.30	2.42	4.28	18.61	3.71	2.68
1973	-	-	2.42	6.02	13.49	3.08	2.25
1974	-	0.29	1.73	7.89	18.58	4.05	2.94
Stomach /151/							
1970	0.59	4.00	21.46	75.57	293.18	55.81	40.76
1971	0.17	4.02	18.64	69.94	289.27	54.75	39.70
1972	0.34	4.77	18.47	67.50	276.87	53.32	38.49
1973	0.34	4.59	18.70	63.09	263.06	51.42	36.87
1974	0.30	3.98	19.43	60.40	163.00	51.55	36.46

of Selected Localizations in the Hungarian Population
/1970 - 1974/

		F e m a l e s			T o t a l	
- 30	30-39	40-49	50-59	60 and older	per 100.000 popu-lation	Stand-ardized indices /Segi/
7.53	32.88	115.40	257.56	761.48	195.82	120.83
7.94	38.48	118.82	263.29	773.55	202.94	124.25
8.08	39.48	110.35	264.17	774.65	204.56	123.91
7.82	34.43	110.57	264.68	789.71	209.88	125.12
8.67	40.09	118.86	256.80	798.86	215.15	127.56
-	0.14	0.13	1.37	4.09	0.96	0.56
-	-	0.26	0.51	3.22	0.71	0.39
-	0.14	0.27	1.01	3.85	0.82	0.47
0.04	-	0.27	1.51	3.08	0.84	0.52
0.04	-	0.54	0.33	2.66	0.67	0.38
0.35	2.40	10.73	28.69	164.82	36.20	20.72
0.27	3.55	10.77	30.58	157.34	35.70	20.24
0.40	3.99	9.96	27.22	145.15	33.43	18.67
0.27	2.56	7.93	24.75	144.98	33.18	18.02
0.44	3.55	9.91	22.80	135.30	31.89	17.33

Table 77 /cont'd/

	Males					Total	
	-30	30-39	40-49	50-59	60 and older	per 100.000 popu- lation	Stand- ardized indices /Segi/
Trachea, bronchi, lungs /162/							
1970	0.13	2.66	18.33	82.81	286.83	54.75	39.26
1971	0.42	3.42	23.59	91.10	297.56	58.91	42.37
1972	0.30	2.98	22.87	77.62	302.77	58.73	41.84
1973	0.21	3.11	25.41	82.70	304.66	60.67	43.10
1974	0.47	5.75	29.07	88.50	330.07	66.78	47.38
Breast /174/							
1970	0.04	0.15	0.28	0.39	3.04	0.58	0.44
1971	0.04	0.15	0.42	0.59	2.07	0.48	0.36
1972	-	0.15	0.57	0.78	2.30	0.54	0.40
1973	-	0.15	0.57	0.58	2.75	0.59	0.43
1974	0.04	0.29	-	0.77	2.46	0.53	0.40
Uterus /180/							
1970							
1971							
1972							
1973							
1974							
Organs of lymphatic and haemo- poietic sys- tems /200- 209/							
1970	2.25	2.96	4.55	7.44	27.22	13.61	10.81
1971	2.88	2.68	4.66	7.84	29.29	14.64	12.11
1972	2.16	2.53	5.97	10.12	28.06	14.94	12.21
1973	2.50	4.44	5.00	9.32	26.48	15.16	12.17
1974	2.37	1.47	3.89	8.85	32.49	15.84	12.48

		F e m a l e s				
- 30	30-39	40-49	50-59	60 and older	T o t a l	
					per 100.000 popu- lation	Stand- ardized indices /Segi/
0.13	1.98	6.41	17.93	47.46	12.15	7.48
018	1.99	5.51	20.38	49.90	12.96	7.75
0.22	1.71	3.85	18.32	51.67	12.97	7.61
0.36	1.42	6.31	17.22	58.13	14.76	8.93
0.31	2.13	6.78	17.81	56.65	14.77	8.61
0.22	6.21	23.30	48.33	77.47	24.13	15.66
0.22	8.09	27.44	46.20	86.96	26.87	17.27
0.13	8.27	25.76	52.43	85.16	27.20	17.50
0.31	6.54	24.86	50.83	86.31	27.28	17.30
0.22	6.68	25.78	51.43	89.83	28.37	17.81
0.27	6.63	28.39	49.70	76.48	24.93	16.48
0.44	5.82	26.26	43.66	80.72	25.01	16.12
0.31	7.13	24.70	43.36	81.91	25.33	16.18
0.27	7.54	24.59	46.65	85.75	26.78	17.00
0.40	7.54	24.56	42.27	80.57	25.50	16.06
1.99	1.88	4.19	8.03	15.36	10.36	7.63
1.82	3.27	4.20	5.95	14.72	10.22	7.36
1.82	2.99	2.92	9.41	17.80	11.97	8.43
1.56	2.42	4.97	6.69	15.97	11.11	7.72
2.18	1.85	5.56	8.32	17.97	12.10	8.53

REFERENCES

1. Évkönyv 1974 /Az Egészségügyi Minisztérium statisztikai év-
   könyve/ Eü. Min. Bp. 1975
   Annual for 1974 /Statistical Annual of the Ministry of
   Health/. Ministry of Health, Budapest, 1975
2. Magyarország népessége /a Központi Statisztikai Hivatal de-
   mográfiai évkönyvei/ KSH Budapest, az 1957-1964. években
   The population of Hungary /Demographic Annuals of the
   Hungarian Central Statistical Office/. Central Statistical
   Office Budapest, issues of 1957-1964 years.
3. Demográfiai Évkönyv Központi Statisztikai Hivatal
   Budapest, 1965-1974
   Demographic Annuals, Central Statistical Office Budapest
   issues of 1965-1974 years.
4. Hospitalizált morbiditás 1972-73. II. kötet Eü. Minisztérium,
   Budapest, 1974
   Data on Hospitalization for 1972-1973, Volume II, Ministry
   of Health, Budapest, 1974

CANCER CONTROL IN THE
MONGOLIAN PEOPLE'S REPUBLIC

B. Dorzhgotov, M. Ochirbay and N. Nyamdavaa

GEOGRAPHICAL, ECONOMIC AND DEMOGRAPHIC CHARACTERIZATION OF THE COUNTRY. HISTORICAL SURVEY OF CANCER CONTROL

The Mongolian People's Republic occupies a vast territory in Central Asia - 1,565,000 square kilometres.

The Mongolian People's Republic is a mountainous country; its lowest point is the Eastern plain in the area of the drying up Chöch-Nuur lake, at an altitude of 532 metres, while the highest peak in the Mongolian Altai Range rises up to 4,653 metres above sea level.

The average elevation of the territory of the Mongolian People's Republic above sea level is 1,580 metres. The high level of the northern half of the Central Asian plateau and remoteness from the ocean explain the sharply continental climate of the country with its long winter, harsh spring, a relatively dry and warm summer and clement autumn. The high hypsometric position of the country can be seen from the following figures: 15.3 per cent of the territory rise from 500 to 1,000 metres above sea level, 40 per cent from 1,000 to 1,500 metres, 22.4 per cent from 2,000 to 3,000 metres, 2.4 per cent from 3,000 to 4,000 metres and 0.02 per cent over 4,000 metres.

In the Table 78 the different altitudes above sea level of aimak /regional/ centres of the Mongolian People's Republic are revealed.

The ploughland in the Republic lies between 600-800 and 1,200-1,400 metres above sea level.

The explicit altitudinal relations determine the duration of the vegetation period, it varies from 76 to 166 days.

The Mongolian People's Republic has four major natural

419

Table 78

Altitudes of Regional Centres of the Mongolian People's Republic

A i m a k s	Aimak Centres	Altitude above sea level /metres/
Capital of the Mongolian People's Republic	Ulan-Bator	1,351
Arkhangai	Tsotserlig	1,695
Bayan-Ulgei	Ulgei	1,710
Bayan-Khongor	Bayan-Khongor	1,845
Bulgan	Bulgan	1,210
Gov-Altai	Altai	2,160
East Gobi	Sainshand	952
Eastern	Choibalsan	752
Central Gobi	Mandalgov	1,435
Zavkhan	Uliastai	1,754
Ubur-Khangai	Arvai-Kher	1,844
South Gobi	Dalanzadgad	1,470
Sukhe-Bator	Barun-Urt	850
Selenga	Sukhe-Bator	650
Central	Zunmod	1,510
Ubsanur	Ulan-gom	935
Kobdo	Kobdo	1,395
Khubsugul	Muren	1,281
Khentei	Undurkhan	1,027

and climatic regions each with its distinctive physical-geo-graphical features:

1. Region of the Khangai-Khentei Mountain;

2. Region of the Altai Mountain;

3. Region of the East steppe;

4. Region of the Gobi desert-steppe.

1. <u>Region of the Khangai-Khentei mountain</u> The region spreads over a vast area /527,500 sq km/ comprising 30 per cent of the total area of the country. It plays a very important role in the economy, for it has the best pastures, many rivers, good hay meadows, rich forests, industrial, agricultural and livestock complexes.

Dark-chestnut and chestnut soils prevail in the region. Light-chestnut soils occur in the southern part. The average annual precipitation is 200-300 mm.

2. <u>Region of the Altai mountain</u> It covers an area of 248,900 square kilometres. In the area of the Mongolian Altai Range the annual precipitation is about 200-300 mm, while in the area of large lakes it is less than 100 mm. According to its positive temperatures the depression of the big lakes belongs to a moderately warm zone. Frequent gales and snow storms are specific features of the region.

3. <u>Region of the East Steppe</u> It covers 247,600 square kilo-metres. The plains of Eastern Mongolia reveal a diversified relief. In the east, especially in the area of Lake Buyr-nur and the Khalhin-Gol River, ideal plains lie. One of the

specific features of the region is the penetration of summer monsoons from the eastern coast of Asia.

In cold seasons northern and north-eastern winds, while in warm periods western and north-western winds are dominant. As regards the temperatures of the vegetation period this territory belongs to a moderately warm zone. Prevalent soils are chestnut and in the east of the region dark-chestnut soils. It is a region of agricultural and livestock-breeding state farms.

4. Region of the Gobi Desert-Steppe It occupies an area of 545,800 square kilometres. The climate is pronouncedly continental. This is the most arid zone of the country with the annual precipitation not more than 200 mm, in the south less than 100 mm. The summer is hot and dry. Prevalent soils are brown, while in the valleys of brooks meadow and light-chestnut soils occur. There are no rivers in the Gobi zone.

The climatic conditions of the Mongolian People's Republic are typical of the northern half of Central Asia and constitute a transitional zone between the taiga mountains of Southern Siberia and Gobi desert of Central Asia. The climate is markedly continental, with insufficient precipitation, large temperature variations during the day and the year, and sharp alternation of the seasons. The absolute variations of extreme temperatures reach 90° and those within one day $20-30^{\circ}$. The small number of cloudy days characteristic of the Mongolian winter is an additional factor contributing to the amazing cooling down. The consequence of these factors is a cold winter without thaws.

As mentioned above, the specific features of the Mongolian climate are due to the great altitude, remoteness from the ocean, and to the high mountains surrounding the whole of Central Asia.

Prevailing winds in the whole country are northerly, western and north-western. During summer southern winds prevail.

The average precipitation in the country is 200-220 mm. 80-95 per cent, in some years even more, of the annual precipitation between May and September. The main season of precipitation is July-August /66-78 per cent/. During winter the amount of precipitation is very low /5-10 per cent/.

In a brief historical period the Mongolian people have eliminated the extreme economic and cultural backwardness. the legacy of feudalism, and achieved great successes in building and developing socialist industry, an entirely new branch of material production in the country, and in transforming the Mongolian People's Republic into an agrarian-industrial state.

The completion of socialist cooperation of individual arat /peasant/ farms put an end to all pre-socialist economic structures and ensured the creation of a uniform socialist economy.

In the early 1960's the Mongolian People's Republic entered the period of completing the building of socialist society. The main content of this period is the all-round development and completion of the material and technical basis of socialism.

Between 1960 and 1975 the Mongolian People's Republic made definite progress in the accelerated expansion of coal mining, power generation, mining, metal-working and metallurgical, leather, footwear, textile, meat and dairy, flour, woodworking and other industries.

In the past fifteen years the basic funds in industry have increased 4.7 times, the volume of per capita industrial output 2.4 times. In 1971-1975 the total national production increased by 44 per cent, the increase in the national income due to industrial growth was 38 per cent /against 23 per cent in 1966--1971/. The structure of the Mongolian economy is steadily improving, acquiring a distinct industrial orientation. In the last five years alone labour productivity has increased by 25 per cent, thus amounting to three quarters of the increase in the national income.

The deep agricultural changes of the past 15 years had a favourable effect on the intellectual and labour image of the traditional arats and cattle-breeders. A new generation of people has grown up on the virgin-soil state farms and cooperatives. They have mastered the latest agricultural machinery and modern technology of production of grain, vegetables, meat, milk and wool.

In the rate of provision of farming machinery, tractors, combines and trucks the state farms and cooperatives occupy one of the leading places in the world. In the past five years alone agriculture has received 4,500 tractors, 1,500 combines, more than 3,000 trucks and many other vehicles.

In 1971-1976 the cultivated area has grown by 12 per cent and the yields of basic cereals and vegetables have risen. Fodder production has doubled.

At present the country annually produces on an average 410,000 tons of grain, 400,000 tons of meat, 320,000 tons of milk and 28.3 thousand tons of wool. In the number of livestock per head the Mongolian People's Republic is among the first seven countries of the world. 58.3 per cent of the total livestock are sheep, 20 per cent goats, 10 per cent horses, horned cattle 9 per cent and camels 2.7 per cent.

Growing vegetables and grain are the main branches of socialist agriculture in the Mongolian People's Republic today.

At present, the total ploughland of state farms and co-operatives amounts more than 700,000 hectares. Till the end of the Sixth Five-Year Plan 230 thousand hectares of virgin--soil will be broken.

The dynamics of the birth and death rates of the population have always been closely connected with the socio-economic structure of the Mongolian society.

As it is known, earlier no precise registration of the population and the volume of births and deaths had been kept in Central Asia. Various investigators of the pre-revolutionary Mongolian People's Republic had differed in their estimates of the population, putting it between 400,000 and 1,400,000. Academician I.M. Maisky was the first to obtain comparatively precise data from the 1918 census which show that before the revolution the population of the Mongolian People's Republic was 647,504 /"Modern Mongolia", Irkutsk, 1921/.

According to the 1956 census the population of the Mongolian People's Republic was 845,500, in 1963 it increased to

1,017,000, in 1975 to 1,500,000 and in 1976 to 1,377,900. The population density varies from 0.5 to 0.9-1.5 per square kilometre.

While in 1956 the inhabitants of towns and town-type settlements comprised 32.8 per cent of the total population, in 1973 this ratio rose to 46.3 per cent. The rest of the population is engaged in agricultural production and livestock-breeding and lives in the countryside.

Etnographically, the Mongolian People's Republic is inhabited by peoples of two linguistic groups /Table 79/. 90 per cent of the population are represented by Mongol-speaking groups which comprise several nationalities. The backbone of the population consists of Khalkha-Mongols /75.3 per cent/ inhabiting vast territories from the Altai mountains and depressions of big lakes to Mandzhuria. Smaller nationalities of Mongol tribes inhabit the western regions of the country, the territory of the Uvsanur and Kobdo aimaks. They are Dyurbets, Bayads, Mingats, Torguts, Olets, Zakhchins, etc. From among them Dyurbets comprise 3 per cent and inhabit the Uvsanur aimak. Torguts inhabiting the Kobdo aimak comprise 0.6 per cent of the population and the same proportion /0.6 per cent/ is accounted for by other groups. Among Khalkha-Mongols Sartuls, Khotgoits and Darigangans or Khalkhasians have historically evolved. Darigangans comprise 1.7 per cent of the population. The north of the country in the area of Lake Khuvsgul is inhabited by a small tribal group of Darkhat hunters, deer and cattle breeders. Buryats comprise 2.5 per cent of the population.

The Turkic linguistic group, includes Kazakhs, Uryankhaitses /Tuvins/, Chotons /Turkmen/. Kazakhs from the most numerous Turkic tribe inhabiting the Bayan-Ulgei aimak and comprising 5.2 per cent of the total population. In a very small number there are also Chinese.

The ethnic traits of the peoples and nationalities inhabiting the Mongolian People's Republic are certainly different. But concerning their way of life as it has evolved during the years of people's power and socialist construction, the peoples of the country are basically alike, with the exception of

Table 79

Ethnic Composition of the Population of the Mongolian
People's Republic /According to the 1969 Census/

Ethnic groups	Population in thousands	Percentage of the total
Khalkha-Mongols	901.2	75.3
Kazakhs	62.8	5.2
Dyurbets	34.7	2.9
Buryats	29.8	2.5
Bayads	25.5	2.1
Daringangans	20.6	1.7
Tuvins	15.7	1.3
Zakhchins	15.0	1.3
Torgouts	7.1	0.6
Olets	6.9	0.6
Others	78.3	6.5
Total	1,197.6	100.0

certain national traditions and customs.

After the victory of the People's Revolution and the establishment of the popular democratic system the dynamics of
population growth changed decisively. Mass training of doctors
and para-medical personnel and the organization of a broad network of medical institutions have brought about amazing changes
in the demographic picture. In the last 20 years the population
of the country has more than doubled as compared to the pre-
-revolutionary times. The rate of growth is steadily rising due
to the steep increase of birth rate and the reduction of mortality.

While in 1940 the rate of birth was 26.1 and mortality was
21.8 per 1,000 inhabitants /natural growth 5.7/, in 1969 the
respective figures were 38.6, 10.0 and 28.6 per 1,000 inhabitants.

In the past 20 years the demographic processes in Mongolia
have undergone substantial changes. On one hand, the population
became younger /0-14 years old children comprise 44.5 per cent

of the total population/ and, on the other hand, life expectancy
is longer now /60 years old and older people comprise 9.2 per
cent/. In the past fifty years the average life expectancy in
the Mongolian People's Republic has increased by 43 years, of
which 10 years have been added just in the period from 1956 to
1969 /Table 80/.

Table 80

Dynamics of Average Life Expectancy in the Mongolian People's
Republic

Years	1915	1925	1940	1956	1963	1969
Number of years	22	30	40	55	63	65

According to the latest census /1969/ average life expectancy in 1968-69 was 62.42 for men, 66.18 for women and 64.54
for both sexes.

Apart from the important indicator of average life expectancy, the level of longevity in the country is characterized
by the indicators of the proportion of aged and old people in
the age structure /Table 81/. This circumstance must be taken
into consideration when oncological aid for the population is
organized.

Table 81

The Size of Population of Elderly Age Groups /According
to the Census Data/

Age	Size of population		
	1956	1963	1969
55-59	38,046	42,111	43,575
60-69	54,050	63,307	63,562
70-79	20,239	30,605	31,529
80-89	3,621	3,573	6,426
90 years and older	213	337	414

The number of people reaching the age of 60 and more is rising from year to year. In 1963 their number was 14.7 per cent higher than in 1956 and in 1969 it increased by 25.5 per cent. According to this indicator, the Mongolian People's Republic may be referred to Group II under Rosset's classification and is on the "threshold of ageing". The number of 70 years old and older persons increased by 37.3 per cent from 1956 to 1969. Thus, the Mongolian People's Republic holds one of the first places in Asia with respect to longevity.

One of the conspicuous achievements of the Mongolian People's Republic is the development of the health service - a completely new feature in the social and cultural life of the country. Prior to 1921 the population had been actually deprived of medical care. The country had neither doctors nor hospitals. At present the Mongolian People's Republic occupies one of the leading places in the world in the number of doctors per 10,000 population. According to the latest data of the Mongolian Central Statistical Office, there are 20.8 doctors per 10,000 inhabitants. Formerly sick people had to turn to ignorant lama quack doctors who practised "curing" by incantation and various magic formulas.

One of the outstanding achievements of the Mongolian people is the creation of an integral socialist system of public health the basis of which was laid with the aid of the Soviet Union and with the direct participation of Soviet doctors and specialists. As a result of this in the 1960's a special oncological service was introduced in the public health system.

Previously the patients with malignant tumours were treated in the general therapeutic and prophylactic institutions of the country. Thus, the Mongolian oncological service was shaped together with the development of the public health system.

One the initiative of home specialists, the foundations of a specialized oncological service were laid in the middle of the 1950's in a former republican surgical hospital. A thoracic surgery ward was opened where surgical aid was given to patients with the cancer of esophagus, stomach and lungs.

In 1959 a radiotherapeutic section was opened at the Republican Central Hospital. Thus the development of radiotherapy of malignant tumours has begun.

All these preparatory measures led to the opening of a Republican Oncological Hospital on December 25, 1961, which marked the foundations of a special oncological service in the country.

Since then the number of hospital beds has increased 2.4 times, the number of oncologists four times and also the equipment and technical facilities of the hospital have been considerably expanded.

At present, the hospital has surgical and gynecological departments, a radiotherapeutic department and chemical therapy beds. It gives oncological aid to the population on a country-wide scale.

In the first years of its existence the hospital treated mainly patients admitted to the hospital. In recent years the range of its activity has considerably expanded. Now it conducts prophylactic observation of patients with precancerous conditions and malignant tumours and annual examinations of the population.

Though there is now an independent oncological service in the country, which constantly expands its activity, it still falls short of modern requirements. Therefore effective measures are taken to improve oncological aid for the population, including the building of a new oncological centre.

Apart from practical oncological aid to the population, on the initiative of young specialists and doctors the publication of research works in the field of oncology was started. A considerable number of these works written by Mongolian authors are devoted to regional features of the spread of malignant neoplasms. This is not accidental. In the Mongolian People's Republic, owing to the specific climatic and geographical conditions, as well as to the specific way of life, customs and habits of people, the spread of malignant tumours differs in many ways compared with the majority of other countries.

From the very beginning, the study of the spread of

malignant tumours in the Mongolian People's Republic, as in other countries, was based on the materials of hospital statistics and autopsies.

Data on the high incidence of the cancer of the esophagus and cardiac part of the stomach in the Mongolian People's Republic were first published in 1961 by T. Shagdarsuren. Having studied the archives of the Central Surgical Hospital for 1955--1958, B. Dorzhgotov /1961/ showed the high incidence of the cancer of the esophagus and the cardiac part of the stomach which accounted for 37.7 per cent among other malignant tumours.

In 1965 a monograph by B. Dorzhgotov on "The Cancer of the Esophagus and the Cardiac Part of the Stomach" was published. This was the first book on oncology in the Mongolian People's Republic. The author pointed to the relatively high incidence of the cancer of esophagus and the cardiac part of the stomach and described some regional features of the spread of these cancer localizations.

According to the data of the statistical office of the Ministry of Health of the Mongolian People's Republic for 1975, among the causes of deaths the third place is taken by malignant tumours. Among people aged 40 and over, malignant neoplasms occupy the first place among the causes of death.

The materials of postmortem examinations carried out at major clinical hospitals of the country /the First and Third Oncological Hospitals in Ulan-Bator/ revealed that in the structure of mortality caused by malignant tumours a high proportion is accounted for by the cancer of the esophagus and stomach and primary carcinoma of the liver /G.Boshigt and G.P. Zlatin 1969, E. Bodkhu 1970, D. Dashdorzh 1971/.

REGISTRATION OF PATIENTS WITH PRIMARILY DIAGNOSED MALIGNANT NEOPLASMS

In 1971 a uniform system was introduced throughout the country for the registration of patients with a malignant neoplasm diagnosed for the first time in their lives, using the Registration Form 26 /Supplement 20/.

Notifications on Form 26 are filled in by doctors of all

Mongolian People's Republic
    Ministry of Health

Endorsed by the Ministry of
Health of the Mongolian
People's Republic in 1970

Report about a patient with malignant neoplasm, trachoma,
fungus disease and venereal disease diagnosed for the first
time in his life

1. Name, surname _____ 2. Age _____

3. Male, female /underline/ ___ 4. Address _____

5. Place of work _____ 6. Job _____

7. Education -- higher, secondary, primary, no education
   /underline/

8. Profession _____

9. Local citizen--1, from other area--2 _____

10. Date of application _____

11. Diagnosis _____

12. Confirmation of the diagnosis 1. by X-rays, 2. by biopsy,
    3. by endoscopy, 4. by other investigations, 5. no confir-
    mation

13. Measures taken by doctor to identify disease _____

14. Entries about the report by the recipient institution ____

    a/ Diagnosis confirmed, not confirmed /underline/ _____

    b/ Date of receipt _____

    c/ Clinical diagnosis _____

       a. Date _____

          Report written by _____

       b. Medical institution _____

       c. Doctor _____

          Report received by _____

       a. Date _____

       b. Medical institution _____

       c. Doctor _____

prophylactic and therapeutic institutions for every patient
with newly diagnosed malignant neoplasm /cancer,
sarcoma, leukosis/. This form is used also of the malignant
neoplasm is identified only at autopsy.

The doctor who fills in the Registration Form 26 must
forward it to an aimak or town oncological centre within a week.
The latter, following the registration of the collected forms,
forward them to the organizational-methodological department of
the Republican Oncological Hospital in every three month.

The Republican Oncological Hospital receives compiled notifications from 18 aimaks, two towns, three republican clinics
and three interdepartmental sanitary services.

The organizational-methodological department of the Republican Oncological Hospital checks the names of patients in
the alphabetical order, removes duplicates and on this basis
determines the malignant neoplasm incidence on the republican
scale.

This method of registering patients with malignant neoplasms diagnosed for the first time has definite shortcomings
which leads to under-registration of patients. Taking this into
consideration, at present reports based on Form 26 are compared
with death certificate from malignant neoplasms.

At present the Mongolian People's Republic is not provided
with complete information about the incidence of malignant tumours among the population. The structure of mortality for 1966-
-1970 is presented on Table 82.

Table 82

Structure of Mortality by Main Cancer Localizations

Localizations	Total	Men	Women
Stomach	35.97	37.73	33.31
Esophagus	17.59	19.41	15.29
Liver	15.52	17.98	12.88
Lungs	7.66	3.14	5.81
Uterus	7.60	-	17.07
Other sites	15.66	15.74	15.64
Total	100	100	100

Mortality from malignant neoplasms in 1966-1970 is
revealed on Table 83.

Table 83

Mortality from Malignant Neoplasms among the Population
of the Mongolian People's Republic in 1966-1970 /per 100,000/

A i m a k s	Indices	
	Crude	Standardized
Ulan-Bator	132.0	164.0
Khentei	137.0	179.0
Eastern	121.0	134.0
Bulgan	93.0	132.0
Khuvsgul	121.0	125.0
Sukhe-Bator	102.0	125.0
Selenga	86.0	105.0
Gov-Altai	94.0	106.0
South Gobi	94.0	102.0
Central Gobi	72.0	99.0
Central	95.0	96.0
East Gobi	81.0	93.0
Khobdo	72.0	72.0
Arkhangai	58.0	63.0
Uburkhangai	62.0	63.0
Bayan-Ulgei	58.0	61.0
Zavkhan	53.0	59.0
Bayan-Khongor	53.0	54.0
Darkhan town	47.0	51.0
Uvs-Nur	34.0	4.0
T o t a l	89.0	96.0

The mortality structure testifies the high susceptibility
of the population to the cancer of the esophagus and primary
carcinoma of the liver, which indicates the specific regional
features of their spread. The lower mortality from malignant
tumours can apparently be explained by the shortcomings of the
recently organized tumour registration.

ORGANIZATION OF DETECTION AND EXAMINATION OF ONCOLOGICAL PATIENTS

Prior to 1961 the early identification of patients with malignant neoplasms was carried out by doctors of medical institutions as part of the general prophylactic examinations of the population. After the creation of the Republican Oncological Hospital and the organization of independent oncological aid for the population in 1961, prophylactic oncological examinations began to be carried out aimed at the identification of tumourous and precancerous cases.

In 1969, in conformity with the decision of the Council of Ministers of the Mongolian People's Republic passed in 1968 and the order of the Ministry of Health, a permanent mobile oncological team was set for identifying precancerous and tumourous cases. Following the formation of this oncological team the prophylactic examinations have become more effective, wide-scale and permanent.

The team includes a surgical oncologist, a gynecological oncologist, cytologist, roentgenologist and sanitary statistician. In carrying out prophylactic oncological examinations in districts the team relies on local roentgenologic centres, laboratories of aimak /regional/ and inter-somon /inter-district/ hospitals and takes into consideration the services of local doctors of some specialities.

On account of the vastness of territory and small density of the population two- or three-stage prophylactic examinations are preferred. Aimak and somon doctors conduct primary oncological examinations of the rural population. These examinations cover rural dwellers working on livestock farms and teams, in field-camps or engaged in household work. In towns and populated centres examinations have a mass character.

At the second stage the mobile oncological team examines and investigates persons selected by the doctors of general medical service at the first stage.

During oncological examinations various health educational activities are undertaken. Medical workers explain the aims and tasks of oncological examinations over the radio, at meetings and in the press. Besides, they instruct local doctors in the peculiarities and specificities of diagnosis of malignant tumours and some methods of their treatment and perform surgical operations in local medical institutions whenever circumstances permit. They carry out roentgenologic, cytological and histological investigations of persons with suspected cancerous and precancerous conditions. Such prophylactic examinations are conducted every year in three or four aimaks embracing 25-30 per cent of the adult population.

By now examinations have been carried out by the mobile oncological team among the population of 12 aimaks /out of the 18/ and the town of Nelaikh, this concerns altogether about 120,000 inhabitants.

As a result of these examinations malignant tumours have been identified in 0.32 per cent of examined persons, benign tumours in 0.38 per cent and precancerous conditions in 4.56 per cent. Special gynecological examinations of women are organized with the aim of revealing tumourous and precancerous conditions of the female genitals. The results of these examinations are presented in Tables 84 and 85.

It can be seen from the above data that the percentage of malignant and benign tumours revealed at oncological surgical examinations increases in the senior age groups /1.02 per cent in the age group of 50-59 and 6.25 per cent in the age group of 70 and more years/. As regards precancerous conditions, indicators begin to rise in the age group of 30-39 years /0.38 per cent/ and reach their maximum in the age group of 60-69 years /0.83 per cent/. The general number of identified cases begins to increase in the age group of 40-49 /1.77 per cent/ and reaches its maximum in the age group of 70 and more years /7.91 per cent/. The general number of sick people revealed during oncological surgical examinations comprises 1.10 per cent of the total number of examined persons. Onco-gynecological examinations have revealed that the rise in the number of malignant tumours begins in the age group of 40-49 /0.40 per cent/ and reaches its maximum in the age group of 70 years and more /1.44 per cent/.

Table 84

Mass Prophylactic Examinations of the Population

		Age					Total
		Below 29	30-39	40-49	50-59	60-69	70 and more	
Number of persons examined		21,975	16,857	13,811	7,920	3,369	847	64,779
Malignant tumours	Cancer of esophagus	-	1	9	15	32	25	82
	Cancer of stomach	-	-	7	18	19	16	60
	Cancer of liver	2	1	7	17	9	3	39
	Cancer of lungs	-	1	7	14	16	4	42
	Malignant tumours of other localizations x	5	8	4	17	17	5	56
	Absolute number	7	11	34	81	93	53	279
	Per cent	0.03	0.06	0.24	1.02	2.76	6.25	0.43
Benign tumours	Absolute number	22	25	40	47	19	12	165
	Per cent	0.10	0.14	0.28	0.59	0.56	1.41	0.25
Precancerous conditions	Absolute number	35	65	88	53	28	2	271
	Per cent	0.15	0.38	0.63	0.66	0.83	0.23	0.41
Total of identified cases	Absolute number	64	101	162	181	140	67	715
	Per cent	0.29	0.59	1.17	2.28	4.15	7.91	1.10

x With the exception of the female genitalia

Table 85

Results of Oncogynecologic Examinations

		Age					Total
		Below 29	30-39	40-49	50-59	60-69	70 and more	
Number of persons examined		17,346	15,730	12,208	5,492	2,350	484	53,610
Malignant tumours	Cancer of the cervix uteri	1	11	37	14	8	3	74
Malignant tumours of ovaries		1	5	7	3	3	–	19
Malignant tumours of other localizations of female genitals		1	3	5	2	1	4	16
Total	Absolute number	3	19	49	19	12	7	109
	Per cent	0.01	0.12	0.40	0.34	0.51	1.44	0.20
Benign tumours	Absolute number	11	73	115	59	24	3	285
	Per cent	0.06	0.46	0.94	1.07	1.02	0.61	0.53
Precancerous condition	Erosion of the cervix uteri	1,763	1,677	1,014	328	137	1	4,920
	Polyp	9	24	46	56	11	–	146
	Leukoplakia	7	18	23	11	5	–	64
Total	Absolute number	1,779	1,719	1,083	395	153	1	5,130
	Per cent	10.25	10.92	8.87	7.19	6.51	0.20	9.56
Total of identified cases	Absolute number	1,793	1,811	1,247	473	189	11	5,524
	Per cent	10.33	11.51	10.21	8.61	8.04	2.25	10.30

437

The degree of identification of benign tumours begins to increase in the age group of 30-39 /0.46 per cent/ and reaches its maximum in the age group of 50-59 /1.07 per cent/, showing a tendency to fall in the subsequent age groups. An increase in the extent of identified precancerous conditions is observed in the age group of 20-29 /10.25 per cent/ and from the age of 30 to 39 years /10.92 per cent/. Then the appropriate indicators begin to decline, reaching a minimum in the age group of 70 and more years. The proportion of identified cases to the general number of examined persons comprises 10.3 per cent.

The above data show that the percentage of cases identified during prophylactic examinations is rather high. This is due to the fact that the calculations have been carried out in relation to persons identified at the second stage of examinations /identified cases include patients revealed at the first stage, but indicators of the degree of identification are calculated only for the second stage of examinations/.

It is generally known that the immediate and remote results of treatment depend on the timely and comprehensive examination of oncological cases and on the early diagnosis of a malignant neoplasm. Despite successes achieved in the early diagnosis and investigation of patients, the solution of the problem still falls short of modern requirements.

The primary examination of patients with malignant neoplasms and persons with suspected malignant tumours identified in rural localities is carried out chiefly at aimak hospitals, where clinical and roentgenologic examinations are performed and materials are taken for cytologic and histologic investigations conducted at the Republican Oncological Hospital.

Patients who have undergone appropriate examinations at aimak or town hospitals and clinics and received special anti-tumour treatment, are sent to the central oncological hospital where they are subjected to repeated examinations and their further treatment is decided upon. In complicated cases when the question cannot be settled at an aimak hospital, a specialist is called in from the centre. This gradual approach to the investigation of oncological cases is accounted for by the low density of the population.

At the outpatient and inpatient departments of the Republican Oncological Hospital the oncological patients are subjected to the necessary examinations, which include laboratory, cytologic, histologic and roentgenologic investigations. In the recent years various endoscopic investigations have been carried out on a wide scale using modern instruments, such as gastro-fiberoscope, bronchofiberoscope, etc.

Ordinary roentgenologic investigations are extensively combined with contrast radiography, including double contrasting.

The diagnosis of a malignant neoplasm is confirmed by cytologic and histologic investigations. Throughout the republic about 50 per cent of patients with a malignant neoplasm diagnosed for the first time are subjected to cytologic and histologic investigations.

For the purposes of early identification of primary carcinoma of the liver the application of the alphafetoprotein test has begun. To evaluate the results of such tests, we have 631 patients with different liver complaints were investigated. In 62 cases out of the 99 patients with primary carcinoma of the liver alphafetoprotein was found. Besides, in four cases in which the diagnosis of the carcinoma of the liver was rejected, alphafetoprotein was found during the investigation. Later on, the primary carcinoma of the liver of those patients was confirmed by cytologic and histologic investigations. This shows good prospects for the early identification of primary liver cancer by means of the alphafetoprotein test.

ORGANIZATION OF THE HOSPITALIZATION AND TREATMENT OF PATIENTS WITH MALIGNANT NEOPLASMS

Every person residing in the Mongolian People's Republic has the right to free medical aid in case of illness, and this fully applies to patients with malignant tumours. The basic factors for improving remote therapeutic results are timely hospitalization and correct choice of treatment methods.

After a preliminary outpatient examination oncological

patients, if necessary, are hospitalized and subjected to additional examinations for the confirmation of the diagnosis. Then appropriate treatment begins.

In most cases persons admitted to a hospital receive combined and complex treatment /surgical, radiotherapeutic and cytostatic/. On the average surgical treatment is applied in 20 % of the cases, radiotherapy in 30 % while cytostatic treatment in 50 % of the cases.

In the course of radiotherapy long-distance gammatherapy and roentgenotherapy as well as treatment with radioactive isotopes /^{226}Ra, ^{60}Co/ are performed.

In the course of cytostatic treatment mostly anti-tumour preparations produced in the socialist countries are given.

Almost in all cases combined methods of treatment are applied on a wide scale. In some long-neglected cases, however, radiotherapy and drug therepy are used separately for palliative treatment.

At present there is a certain number of clinically healthy persons who in the first years of the existence of the Republican Oncological Hospital /1962, 1963/ underwent radical treatment of the cancer of the stomach, esophagus, cervix uteri and are now under observation.

FOLLOW-UP EXAMINATIONS OF PATIENTS WITH MALIGNANT NEOPLASMS

As already mentioned, in the early period of its activity the Republican Oncological Hospital mainly provided medical treatment and only in the last few years started to reveal precancerous and tumourous conditions and to accomplish the regular follow-up of oncological patients.

The prophylactic examination of oncological patients is carried out on the basis of experience accumulated in the Soviet Union and other socialist countries. It should be pointed out that in the Mongolian People's Republic, with its vast territory and low density of the population, where oncological aid is centralized, the hospitalization of oncological patients involves considerable difficulties, first of all because patients who are to be kept under the observation of an oncological dispensary often live at a distance of up to 2,000 km from it. In these conditions patients from aimaks who have been treated at the Republican Oncological Hospital are placed under the observation of doctors of the aimak hospitals, mainly surgeons and gynecologists, who regularly examine the patients and, if necessary, call in an oncologist from the centre to examine patients on the spot.

Patients with tumourous and precancerous conditions revealed by the mobile oncological team are placed under the control of doctors of hospitals /in aimaks and somons/ in the place of their residence.

The Republican Oncological Hospital is responsible for the observation of oncological patients living in Ulan-Bator.

Observation of oncological patients is based on the classification of clinical groups Ia, Ib, II, III and IV applied in the Soviet Union.

ORGANIZATION OF MEDICAL DETERMINATION OF DISABILITY AND REHABILITATION OF ONCOLOGICAL PATIENTS

Malignant neoplasms affect literally all organs and systems and the results of treatment and related functional disturbances are different in the various localizations, all the more so since the concept of complete curing of a patient with a malignant neoplasm is still unclear.

Patients with malignant neoplasms are regarded as cured if in the course of five years do not develop metastases and relapses. In some cases, however, metastases and relapses occur after the five-year observation. At the same time, the five-year period is taken as the basis for establishing the grade of disability for patients with malignant neoplasms. The post-treatment period is undoubtedly of great importance for determining the working capacity of an oncological patient. But this capacity considerably depends on the severity of the illness and the localization of the malignant tumour, the character of its growth, the data of histologic investigation, the type of medical measures taken, complications, immediate and remote results of treatment, the age of the patient, his general condition, the character of local changes, profession, conditions of work and also on the patient's desire to accomplish a certain job.

In the Mongolian People's Republic the working capacity of oncological patients is determined on the basis of the instruction on disability groups and of the list of diseases leading to disability, both were endorsed in 1975. According to the instruction, three groups of disability have been established in the Mongolian People's Republic.

1. The first group of disability is established for persons who, as a result of a chronic disease and grave damage of the organism and its functions, have lost their ability to work, cannot take care of themselves and require supervision and care of other people, being confined to bed.

2. The second disability comprises those persons who, despite their chronic disease, grave damage to the organism and its functions and loss of ability to work completely or for a long period of time, do not require constant supervision and care on the part of other people and under medical control can perform certain types of work not contraindicated for the damaged organ.

3. The third group is established for persons who, due to their chronic disease damaging the organism and its functions and prolonged loss of ability to work, cannot accomplish their usual job in the former volume either quantitatively or qualitatively, but are mentally healthy and able to take full care of themselves and perform an appropriate work.

Apart from these three disability groups, the Medical and Labour Examination Commission issues a certificate for reduced working hours for persons whose health and ability to work are reduced or tend to deteriorate and who cannot perform their usual work, in terms of quantity and quality, within the time schedules fixed for them.

In accordance with the above principles of determining the working capacity, patients in the third or fourth stage of the malignant tumour who cannot be completely cured, are included in the first disability group without time limits set, while patients in the first or second stage of the malignant tumour are included in the second and third disability groups, depending on the extent of damage and localization of the malignant tumour, on the type of medical treatment, complications, and on the patient's general condition, age and type of work. Likewise, patients who have undergone gastrectomy and pulmonectomy and other major operations are included in disability groups without time limits set. Patients suffering from acute and often aggravating leukosis, especially in the case of the generalization of the process, are included in the first and second disability groups, while patients with leukosis and persistent remissions are included in second and third disability groups.

Despite the fact that the determination of the working capacity of oncological patients is based on the above principles, the question of disability of patients with malignant tumours of superficial localizations /cancer of the lip, skin and the mammary gland/ cured in the first and second stages of the disease is settled on the bases of other principles. There is no disability group established for these patients and, on completing appropriate treatment, they resume working and are kept under dispensary observation. Moreover, there are quite a few cases in which no disability group is established either, namely for patients who underwent treatment in the first and second stages of the disease, including resection of the distal section of the stomach and extirpation of the uterus. These patients are reinstalled in their former jobs.

It follows from the above that in the Mongolian People's Republic the work of oncological patients is regulated on the basis of an individual approach in conformity with a number of conditions which take into account the character of disease and the general state of the patient. Under this type of regulation an important role is played by the doctor, the medical control commissions and medical and labour examination commissions.

443

ORGANIZATION OF THE MEDICAL ASSISTANCE TO PATIENTS WITH ADVANCED FORMS OF TUMOURS

The organization of medical service for patients with advanced forms of tumours is one of the complex and still unsolved problems.

Most patients with this form get symptomatic treatment at home.

Patients with an advanced form of tumour who cannot be subjected to radical treatment in hospital conditions, must receive medical aid, if necessary, at the place of their residence. This procedure of taking medical care of patients with advanced forms of tumours operated until 1973. Quite often, however, there were cases when patients with advanced tumour had undergone treatment at the oncological hospital occupying thus a hospital bed.

In 1972 home treatment medical beds were made available beside the oncological hospitals. All types of medical service for patients on home treatment beds are provided free of charge just as for patients admitted to a hospital. Thirty medical home treatment beds are serviced by a doctor and a nurse who have a special vehicle at their disposal. The doctor examines these patients three times a week and a laboratory assistant carries out routine clinical laboratory investigations, such as blood count, etc.

Emaciated patients are given general analeptical drugs, injections and blood substitution. If necessary, the doctor in charge invites a highly qualified specialist for consultation at the home of the patient. This form of medical service for patients with advanced tumours has a great psychological and moral effect on critically·ill patients and also serves as a moral and material support for their family.

When patients with advanced tumours need special care on the part of other people in home conditions /whether they occupy a home treatment bed or not/, persons taking care of them are issued sickness benefits.

In the remote districts patients with advanced forms of tumours are given medical aid in hospital and home conditions by regional and inter-district hospitals and district medical centres.

TEACHING OF ONCOLOGY, TRAINING OF ONCOLOGISTS AND PARA- MEDICAL PERSONNEL FOR ONCOLOGICAL INSTITUTIONS

In the Mongolian People's Republic teaching of oncology and the training of oncologists are carried out as follows.

At the Ulan-Bator Medical University oncology is taught from the third year at several chairs. Since the 1974-1975 academic year sixth-year students of the surgical department of the Institute are taught clinical oncology at an oncological hospital /12 hours of lectures and 39 hours of practical training/.

The training of oncologists and improvement of their qualifications are carried out in the following this pattern:

Specialization in oncology is obtained through individual education by highly skilled native and foreign oncologists and also through training directly at the workplace. Besides, 3-month courses are being introduced according to a special programme.

Teaching at the place of work and postgraduate courses are carried out by sending doctors, successfully working in oncological hospitals for three years, to the Soviet Union and other socialist countries. The paramedical personnel for oncological institutions is trained by individual instruction and short-term courses.

HEALTH EDUCATIONAL WORK AMONG THE POPULATION

The programme of the Mongolian People's Republic Revolutionary Party envisages wide-ranging measures which express concern for the protection and improvement of the health of the population, for the further improvement of the conditions of life and work for working people and extension of the prophylaxis of diseases and health education.

As regards the health educational work, the medical prophylactic institutions conduct extensive health educational propaganda among the population. Each week lectures and talks are given using posters and other visual aids and question-and--answer sessions are organized which promote the establishing of hygienic habits among the people.

Weekly "Wednesdays" are part of the general health educational work conducted all over the country. Health education is also affected in central and local newspapers and journals, over radio and television. The oncological hospitals take an active part in this work. Oncologists publish articles in central and local newspapers and deliver lectures and talks over radio and television on questions of prophylaxis of malignant tumours, the importance of their early diagnosis, the curability of tumours and negative consequences of people's bad habits.

Besides, persons are interviewed who have lived many years ago since the complete cure of malignant tumours. This method has a number of advantages, bringing it home to people that malignant tumours are curable after all.

Using the above methods and forms of work, doctors of the permanent mobile oncological teams conduct wide propaganda among the population of aimaks for the regular prophylactic examinations. Wherever this work is well organized, people readily attend prophylactic oncological examinations. This testifies to the need to conduct health educational work on a broader scale and scope. Oncologists from oncological hospitals deliver lectures and talks to local doctors and medical workers on the latest achievements of oncology, cancer control in the country and questions of tumour treatment and prophylaxis.

PROSPECTS FOR THE IMPROVEMENT OF THE ORGANIZATION OF
THE ONCOLOGICAL SERVICE IN THE MONGOLIAN PEOPLE'S REPUBLIC

After the beginning of the 1960's a special oncological service has been established in the country and since then definite development has been made in concerning the material facilities of the oncological service and the training of specialists.

At present a series of measures are planned to bring

oncological service closer to the people, to reveal precancerous conditions and improve early diagnosis of tumours.

Since a considerable role in tumour control is played by early diagnosis and treatment of malignant tumours and precancerous conditions, it is planned to improve the work of mobile oncological teams and to increase their number and capacity.

An oncological sector is now being formed at the Research Institute of Medicine of the Ministry of Health of the Mongolian People's Republic.

In order to improve oncological service for the rural population, measures will be taken to build oncological departments in towns and regional centres and to improve their work.

In improving the diagnosis and treatment of malignant tumours great attention will be given in future to the training of oncological personnel within the country and abroad, at postgraduate and other courses and also through training in member countries of the Council for Mutual Economic Assistance. As a result, in 1976–1980 the number of oncologists will be almost trebled.

In 1976–1980 the material facilities of the oncological service will be further expanded. An oncological hospital of 200 beds provided with the modernest equipment will be built in Ulan-Bator with the help of the Soviet Union.

In connection with the growing international cooperation in the field of oncology and the implementation of the comprehensive programme "Malignant neoplasms" in the CMEA countries, it is planned to augment the volume of research in oncology. In 1976–1980 this research will be centred on the epidemiology of malignant neoplasms.

REFERENCES

1. B. Dorzhgotov — Развитие онкологической службы в МНР /Вопросы онкологии, 1977, У. 23, № 10, стр. 27-29./

   Development of Oncological Service in the Mongolian People's Republic - /an article from Mongolia/-/Voprosy Onkoligii, 1977, v. 23, No. 10, pp. 27-29./

2. G. Zhamba, Zg. Kupul and Ye. Avilov — The Ways and Main Stages of the Development of the Sanitary-and-epidemiologic Service in the Mongolian People's Republic - /an article from Mongolia/ - Hygiene and Sanitation, 1977, No 7, pp. 87-90

3. B. Dorzhgotov, R. Gur and Doris — Смертность от злокачественных опухолей в МНР /Вопросы онкологии, 1973, У. 19, № 1, стр. 63-65./

   Mortality Rate from Malignant Tumours in the Mongolian People's Republic - Voprosy Onkologii, 1973, v. 19, No. 1, pp. 63-65.

CANCER CONTROL IN POLAND

I. R. Sosinski

GEOGRAPHICAL, ECONOMIC AND DEMOGRAPHIC CHARACTERIZATION
OF THE COUNTRY

Poland occupies the eastern part of Central Europe. Its
territory is bounded by the following points:

on the North - 54°50' Northern latitude,

on the South - 49°00' Northern latitude,

on the West - 14°07' Eastern longitude,

on the East - 24°08' Eastern longitude.

The territory of the country is 312,677 sq km, average
height above the sea level is 173 metres, the highest point is
Mount Rysy /2,499 m/, the lowest point lies 1.8 m below the
sea level.

As of December 31, 1970, Poland's population was 32,700
thousand: 52.3 % living in towns and 47.7 % in the countryside.
In 1975 the population exceeded 34,000 thousand and the proportion of urban inhabitants rose to 54.6 %. In 1970, 18,300
thousand people were employed in production - 70.2 % of them
in various industries, while 29.8 % in the agriculture.

In 1970 the natural population growth was 8.5 per 1,000
population. In the same year the proportion of women to men
was 106 to 100.

Poland is an industrial-agrarian country with a constantly growing industrial potential. From 1950 to 1970 the national
income increased by 374 %.

Poland is rich in mineral resources, first of all in coal,
sulphur, copper ores, common salt, iron ores, natural gas, etc.

The climate is moderate, the average annual temperature
ranges from 6 to 8.8°C.

Epidemiological Information

In 1970 56,278 new cases of malignant tumours were registered in Poland. When analyzing the data on malignant tumour incidence, lethality and mortality, registered since 1952, it is apparent that there is a constant rise in the incidence of this disease group. This rise is undoubtedly affected by the improvement of diagnosis and perfection of the organization of the health service, but there is also an absolute growth caused by the actual rise in the number of cases.

Epidemiological Characterization of the Incidence of Malignant Tumours in Poland in 1963-1972

On the basis of the data of malignant tumour registration carried out on a country-wide scale it is possible, with a certain measure of probability, to assess the dynamics of the incidence of malignant neoplasms. These data can be used for comparative evaluation with regard to selected areas /the city of Warsaw and five districts of the Warsaw region - Gostynin, Minsk, Mazowecki, Plock, Siedlce, Serpc/ where registration is particularly well organized. The indicator of disease incidence among men rose from 106.6 in 1963 to 178.4 in 1972. Among women the incidence was 123.7 in 1963 and 173.8 in 1972. In 1963-1972 the average incidence was 148.5 among women and 141.0 among men. The sex ratio equals 0.9 /Table 86, Fig.22/.

Indicators of the average annual rate of disease among men and women by age groups are given in Table 87 and Fig. 23. The 10-19 age group is characterized by the low incidence indicators while in the other age groups there is a considerable rise. A more rapid rise is particularly characteristic of men. Indicators for men older than 20 years at least double every ten-year age span. Among women the indicators grow more rapidly in the 30-39 and in the older age groups.

When analyzing the data according to localization, it is shown that among men the cases of stomach and lung cancer occur most frequently, comprising more than 40 % of all cancer cases. They are followed by skin neoplasms /6.4 %/. Other malignant tumours did not exceed 5 % of the total number of neoplasms /Table 88, Fig. 24/.

450

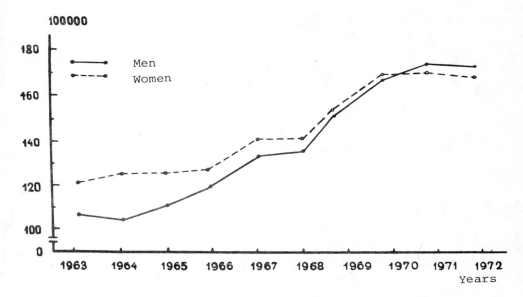

Fig. 22 Incidence of malignant tumours among the Polish
population by sex /per 100,000 population, 1963-1972/

Table 86

Incidence of Malignant Tumours Among the Polish Population
by Sex /per 100,000 population in 1963-1972/

Year	Men	Women
1963	106.6	123.7
1964	105.1	128.1
1965	111.4	128.1
1966	120.7	129.4
1967	136.6	144.1
1968	138.0	145.2
1969	155.1	158.9
1970	172.1	173.7
1971	179.8	176.5
1972	178.4	173.8
1963-1972	141.0	148.5

Among women carcinomas of the cervix uteri and of the
mammary gland occupy first and second places /33.9 % of all

451

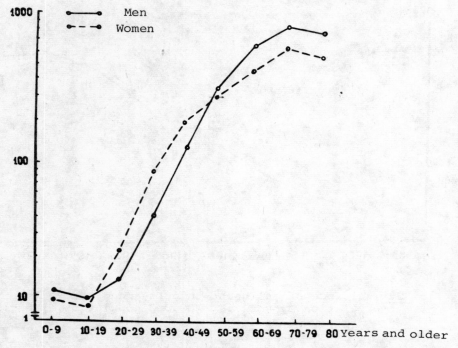

<u>Fig. 23</u> Incidence of malignant tumours among the Polish
Population by age and sex /per 100,000 population,
1963-1972/

Table 87

Malignant Tumour Incidence in Poland, by Age and

Sex /per 100,000 population in 1963-1972/

Age groups	Men	Women
0-9	10.7	9.0
10-19	9.6	8.3
20-29	14.8	22.3
30-39	41.8	85.1
40-49	130.6	204.6
50-59	350.6	335.2
60-69	739.4	487.1
70-79	1,020.5	601.2
80 years and older	874,4	549.1

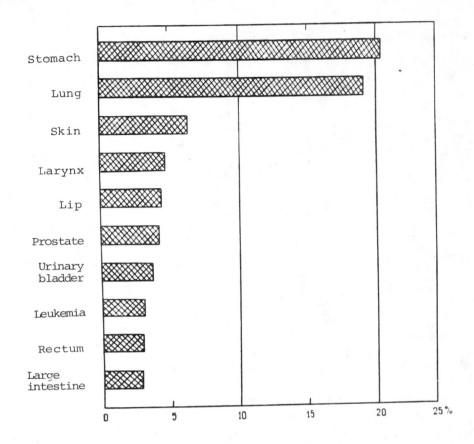

Fig. 24   Structure of the incidence of malignant neoplasms of
          different localizations in men /1963-1972/

neoplasms/. Together with other neoplasms of the female
genitals /ovary 5.2 %, body of the womb 4.8 %/, this indicator
reaches 43.9 per cent. Noteworthy is a rather high percentage
of neoplasms of the stomach /10.9 %/, the gallbladder and
liver /7.3 %/ and also of the lungs /3.3 %/ /Table 89, Fig.25/.

The history of cancer control in Poland

        In 1906 a Commettee for Cancer Research and Control was
formed at the Warsaw Society of Hygiene. The first City Polyclinic for Patients with Tumours was set up in 1917 in Łódz
and some years later similar polyclinics were opened in other
Polish towns.

Table 88

Incidence of Malignant Neoplasms of Different Localizations among Men in Poland /per 100 patients with malignant neoplasms of all localizations, 1963-1972/.

ICD /8th Rev. Code No.	Localization	Number of cases	Per cent
140-209	Total	219,257	100.0
151	Stomach	45,481	20.7
162, 163	Lung	43,716	19,9
173	Skin	14,126	6.4
161	Larynx	10,162	4.6
140	Lip	9,748	4.4
185	Prostate	9,003	4.1
188	Urinary bladder	7,953	3.6
204-207	Leukemia	6,443	2.9
154	Rectum	6,218	2.8
153	Large intestine	6,108	2.8

Table 89

Incidence of Malignant Neoplasms of Different Localizations among Women in Poland /per 100 patients with malignant neoplasms of all localizations, 1963-1972/.

ICD Code No	Localization	Number of cases	Per cent
140-209	Total	244,710	100.0
180	Cervix uteri	51,587	21.1
174	Mammary gland	31.233	12.8
151	Stomach	26.635	10.9
155, 156 197.7, 197.8	Liver and gallbladder	17,971	7.3
173	Skin	16,155	6.6
183	Ovary	12.815	5.2
182	Body of the womb	11,801	4.8
162, 163	Lung	8,058	3.3
153	Rectum	6,516	2.7

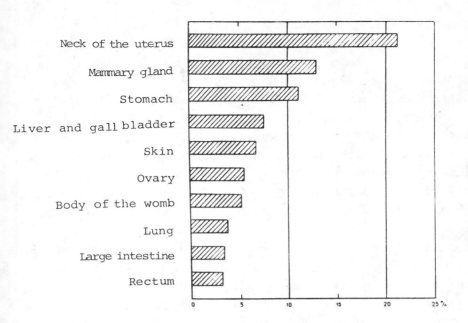

Neck of the uterus					
Mammary gland					
Stomach					
Liver and gall bladder					
Skin					
Ovary					
Body of the womb					
Lung					
Large intestine					
Rectum					

Fig. 25   Structure of the incidence of malignant neoplasm
           incidence of different localizations in women
           /1963-1972/

Around 1920, on the initiative of the great Polish scientist, Marie Sklodowska-Curie, a Committee for the Building
of an Institute of Radiotherapy was formed in Warsaw.

In 1923, "Neoplasms", one of the world's first journals,
fully devoted to the questions of oncology, began to be
published in Warsaw. Except the years of the war /1939-1945/,
this journal has been published up to now as a special organ
of the Marie Sklodowska-Curie Institute of Oncology and the
Polish Oncological Society.

In 1925, in the presence of Marie Sklodowska-Curie, a
ceremony was held for laying the foundation stone of the
Institute of Radiotherapy in Warsaw. The building of the Institute financed by contributions of the Polish public continued
till 1932. From that time on till the Warsaw uprising of 1944
the Institute treated patients using about one gram of radium
which it received from Marie Sklodowska-Curie. In 1944, during
the uprising, the nazis killed all patients at the Institute

and then ransacked and burnt the building.

In 1945, immediately after the liberation of Warsaw, the restoration of the Institute was started. The rebuilt Institute of Radiotherapy in Warsaw began to function in 1947. Cancer institutes were opened in Gliwice /1946/ and Krakow /1951/. In 1952, on the basis of the three oncological institutes, a scientific research institute was formed under the auspices of the Ministry of Health and Social Insurance which was called Institute of Oncology named after Marie Sklodowska-Curie with its headquarters in Warsaw and branches in Gliwice and Krakow. This organizational structure of the Institute of Oncology has remained unchanged up to this day.

The socialist model of organization of the medical service introduced in People's Poland which guarantees free medical services for some 98 % of the population has made it possible to launch an offensive against the increase of the tumour cases according to a uniform plan.

In 1952 the staff of the Institute of Oncology worked out a social plan of the struggle against tumour diseases two principal aims:

1. Achievement of an organizational and professional level of oncological aid to the population that would ensure malignant tumour patients treatment corresponding to the present state of science in this field. Patients whose radical treatment is impossible should be provided with medical care and symptomatic treatment.

2. Creation of proper working conditions for Polish scientists who work on the problem "Malignant Neoplasms" thereby promoting Poland's contribution to world achievements in the knowledge of the essence, therapy and diagnosis of neoplasms.

The first aim of this plan can be fulfilled only on the condition of active involvement of the entire health service. Experience shows that about 50 % of newly identified malignant neoplasm cases in the course of a year require surgical treatment and may be treated in special hospital departments depending on the localization of the tumour.

However, not less than 50%of the newly identified cases

of malignant neoplasms require a combination of treatment methods which may be applied exclusively at specially equipped
oncological hospitals. The planning of the network of oncological hospitals is carried out on the basis of the above estimation that about 50 % of newly identified malignant tumour
cases require specialized treatment. For an early diagnosis of
malignant tumours the establishment of a network of specialized
oncological dispensaries is planned which would be able to examine
all patients treated with suspected malignant neoplasms by other
medical institutions /specialized but not oncological/.

The implementation of the second aim of the social anti-
-tumour plan is the task of the Institute of Oncology.

All the above elements of the social anti-tumour plan are
contained in the three theses formulated by Professor Tadeusz
Koszarowski on the basis of a broad discussion among Polish
oncologists.

Oncology is a science dealing with the etiology, pathology,
epidemiology, prophylaxis, identification and complex treatment
of malignant neoplasm cases and their further observation, with
the care for incurable cases and organization of social struggle
against this disease.

Oncologist is a specialist /pathologist, surgeon, radiotherapist, gynecologist, etc./ who has received special training
in the field of oncology according to an established programme
and passed an examination. Such a physician is prepared for
coordinating and guiding the work of a collective connected
with prophylaxis, identification, treatment and with the organization of social endeavours against neoplasms.

Cancer control is a complex of measures /investigation and
study, prophylaxis, identification, treatment and further
permanent care and also restoration of the ability to work/
aimed at reducing the incidence of the disease, increasing the
number permanently cured cases with the lowest rate of invalid-
ization, and lowering the mortality from malignant neoplasms
among the population.

Since 1952 the gradual implementation of the social plan
of tumour control has been under way in Poland. At the first
stage, with the help of specialists from the Institute of
Oncology who carried out the tasks of wojewodztwo /county/
specialists, in some wojewodztwos Wojewodztwo Oncological
Dispensaries were set up the work of which was regulated by
the instruction of the Minister of Health and Social Insurance.

The gradual increase in the number of oncologists made

possible to set up the first integrated oncological institutions of open and closed types on the territory of certain 'wojevodztows'.

The scope of the work of 'wojewodztwo' institutions was defined in 1966.

1. Comprehensive diagnosis and treatment of tumours.

2. Consultation of patients at institutions engaged in the treatment of tumour cases and also consultation of patients treated by other medical institutions.

3. Organization and conduct of dispensary examinations of patients with a suspected malignant tumour registered at the 'wojewodztwo' oncological complex.

4. Registration of oncological patients, analysis of the results of treatment depending on the methods applied and the reasons of advanced forms among oncological cases.

5. Organization of mass prophylactic examinations, participation in them, and control over the quality of examinations carried out by other health service institutions.

6. Organizational and methodological activity in the oncological help to the population.

7. Improvement of the qualifications of oncologists and also of other specialists in the field of oncology.

8. Participation in the pre-graduation training of students of medical institutes in general oncology and in the training of students of medical institutes in clinical oncology.

9. Participation in organizing aid for patients with advanced forms of oncological diseases not subject to radical treatment.

10. Implementation of measures connected with the prophylaxis, identification and treatment of neoplasms in the extent established by the national specialists in oncology /the Marie Sklodowska-Curie Institute of Oncology/.

By 1975 Poland had full-scale oncological institutions in 10 wojewodztwo towns, oncological radiotherapy or surgery departments in five wojewodztwos and only wojewodztwo oncological dispensaries in two wojewodztwos. In 1975 the oncological institutions had altogether 2,134 beds /Fig. 26/.

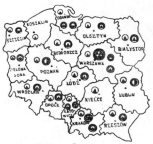

⊛   The Centre of the Institute of Oncology

⊜   The Branch of the Institute

◔   The Clinic of Pediatric Oncology of the Institute of mother and child

⊙   The Oncological Department of the Medical Academy

◑   Wojewodztwo oncological hospital

◕   Oncological department /or departments/ of wojewodztwo hospital

◌   Wojewodztwo oncological dispensary

<u>Fig. 26</u>   The network of oncological institutions in Poland
/as of May, 31, 1975/

Organization of tumour control in Poland today

On June 1, 1975, Poland enacted a law on the reorganization of the administrative division of the country under which
49 smaller wojewodztwos appeared instead of the 17 wojewodztwos
of the previous period. As a result of this, the organization
of specialized oncological institutions distributed in 17 wojewodztwo towns, had to be restructured. /Fig. 27/

Besides, the experience gained in the organization of the
network of oncological institutions in Poland over 22 years
made it possible to draw the following conclusions:

1. It is expedient to organize oncological institutions
capable of providing oncological service in a district, conducting comprehensive treatment of patients and periodic control
examinations of patients who have undergone radical treatment,
and reducing the number of cases with advanced forms of tumour
in those districts of the country where oncological institutions of a full-scale type operate.

2. Organization of full-scale oncological institutions is
expedient only in towns having Medical Academies. This combination provides the cooperation of the oncological institution
in question with different specialists from the Academy.

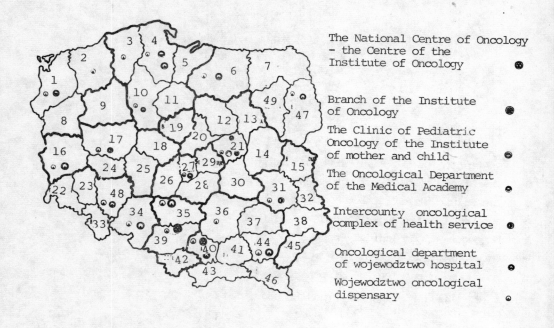

The National Centre of Oncology
- the Centre of the
Institute of Oncology

Branch of the Institute
of Oncology

The Clinic of Pediatric
Oncology of the Institute
of mother and child

The Oncological Department
of the Medical Academy

Intercounty oncological
complex of health service

Oncological department
of wojewodztwo hospital

Wojewodztwo oncological
dispensary

Fig. 27   The network of oncological institutions in Poland
/as of December 31, 1975/

1 - Szczecin, 2 - Koszalin, 3 - Slupsk, 4 - Gdansk,
5 - Elbąg, 6 - Olsztyn, 7 - Suwałki, 8 - Gorzów, 9 -
Piła, 10 - Bydgoszcz, 11 - Torun, 12 - Ciechanóv, 13-
Ostrołęka, 14 - Siedlce, 15 - Biała Podlaska, 16 -
Zielona Gora, 17 - Poznan, 18 - Konin, 19 - Wloclawsk,
20 - Płock, 21 - Warsaw, 22 - Jelenia Góra, 23 - Leg-
nica, 24 - Leszno, 25 - Kalisz, 26 - Sieradz, 27 -
Lodz, 28 - Piotrków, 29 - Skierniewice, 30 - Radom,
31 - Lublin, 32 - Chełm, 33 - Walbrzych, 34 - Opole,
35 - Częstochowa, 36 - Kielce, 37 - Tarnobrzeg, 38 -
Zamość, 39 - Katowice, 40 - Krakow, 41 - Tarnow, 42 -
Bielsko-Biała, 43 - Nowy Sącz, 44 - Rzeszow, 45 -
Przemysl, 46 - Krosno, 47 - Bialystok, 48 - Wroclaw,
49 - Zomia

3. To ensure effective operation of a full-scale oncological institution, it is necessary to unite organizationally
the staffs of open- and closed-type institutions and to have
an efficient organizational-methodological department as well
as a highly skilled head oncologist.

The experience gained so far and the new administrative
division of the country introduced on June 1, 1975, necessitated the elaboration of a new concept about the organization

460

of the specialized oncological service.

This concept takes into account the possibilities of Polish oncology with regard to skilled personnel, provision of hospital beds and equipment, the new administrative division as well as to the forecast of relative population growth in the different regions of the country and to the anticipated number of onco-logical cases by the year 2000.

The head institution of cancer control is the Marie Sklodowska-Curie Institute of Oncology in Warsaw with its two branches in Kraków and Gliwice. The Institute of Oncology con-ducts its work according to the Statute issued on the instruc-tion of the Minister of Health and Social Insurance which sets the following tasks:

1. Planning, organization and conduct of investigations in the experimental and clinical oncology as well as organiza-tion of cancer control.

2. Coordination of work in experimental and clinical on-cology conducted by other institutions subordinated to the Minister of Health and Social Insurance.

3. Elaboration of comprehensive plans of work in cancer control for the health service and control and evaluation of the fulfilment of the plans.

4. Direct specialized supervision over oncological insti-tutions /departments/ and participation in supervision over other social health service institutions, conducted by other specialists, especially in connection with the methods of can-cer control.

5. Keeping level with the development of research in the country and abroad, review and evaluation of works connected with the achievements of science and technology in the given field.

6. Participation and help in introducing scientific achievements in the practice of the health service.

7. Specialization and improvement of scientific and professional knowledge of the staff of the Institute and other establishments.

8. Cooperation with the Polish Academy of Sciences, higher

461

educational establishments, research institutes and other
research bodies, professional and scientific societies of the
country as well as cooperation and contacts with appropriate
scientific organizations and institutions abroad.

9. Drafting and provision of documentation and scientific
and technical information and publishing activity connected
with the work of the Institute.

10. Fulfilment of other assignments of the Minister of
Health and Social Insurance.

At the instance of the Institute of Oncology, the Minister
of Health and Social Insurance issued a decision on July 31,
1975, providing for the regionalization of oncological establishments.

In accordance with this decision, Poland was divided into
ten districts with head institutions in Warsaw, Gliwice,
Kraków, Szczecin, Gdansk, Poznan, Łódz, Wrocław, Białystok and
Lublin. In the first three districts the oncological service
is headed by the Institute of Oncology and its two branches
/Warsaw, Gliwice, Kraków/, while in the other districts
by interwojewodztwo oncological complexes of the health service.
It is planned to establish the eleventh oncological district
in Bydgoszcz by reducing the size of the Gdansk, Poznan and
Łódz districts. The territories of the corresponding districts
are shown in Fig. 28. In the provinces which have not inter-
-wojewodztwo oncological complexes, wojewodztwo oncological
dispensaries and, if possible, hospitals are formed. Administrative schemes and the structure of the oncological network
and institutions are represented on Figs 29, 30, 31 and
Table 90.

SYSTEM OF REGISTRATION OF PATIENTS WITH
PRIMARILY DIAGNOSED MALIGNANT NEOPLASMS

In Poland the registration of patients with primarily
diagnosed malignant neoplasms and patients suspected of having
malignant neoplasms has been compulsory since 1952. A circular
of the Minister of Health and Social Insurance had pledged all
institutions of the health service to report newly diagnosed

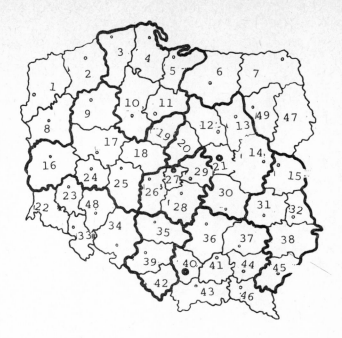

Fig. 28   Oncological service centres in Poland

cases and mortalities from malignant neoplasms.

In order to ensure the registration of tumour cases by medical institutions not subordinated to the Ministry of Health and Social Insurance, in 1962 an instruction was published by the Ministers of Health and Social Insurance, Defence, Internal Affairs, Communications and Justice concerning the compulsory registration of malignant neoplasms and suspects of malignant tumours. This instruction is still valid now.

According to the instruction, all open- and closed-type medical establishments are obliged to report diagnosed and suspected cases of malignant neoplasms and also deaths from malignant neoplasms by filling in a special "Report on a Malig-nant Neoplasm" /Supplement 21/.

All medical institutions submit reports about tumour cases to a corresponding wojewodztwo oncological dispensary within time-limits indicated in the instruction. The wojewodztwo on-cological dispensaries submit the cards to the Cancer Control

Stamp of the institution reporting the case	The card is filled in for patients with diagnosed or a suspected malignant neoplasm in the first and subsequent communications and also in the event of death /see Polish Monitor No.30 dated April 7, 1962/	Not to be filled in No. /1/ Hospital /2/ Check-out /3/

Registration Card of a Malignant Neoplasm

1. a/ Date of admission   For patients treated
   b/ Date of discharge   in medical institu-
                         tions of closed type

2. Name /in block letters/
   .... | Resident /3/

3. Permanent address /exact/
   Town .... Str............ No....
   Village .... Str........... No....
   Powiat .... Wojewodztwo ....

4. Date of birth .... Age ..... | Born /3/

5. Sex: Male Female /underline/ | Sex /1/

6. Occupation ....|Profession /1/

Back side   Not to be filled in

7. Clinical diagnosis and primary localization of the neoplasm
   .... | Disp. /4/

8. Result of histopathological investigation[x]
   .... | Hist. /1/

9. Another confirmation of the diagnosis indicated in Point 7 /underline/: cytological, endoscopic investigation, diagnostic operation, biopsy of the metas-
   tatic focus | Disp. /1/

10. Treatment conducted so far
    .... | Treatment /1/
    /indicate where the patient is sent
    without treatment/

11. When was the neoplasm indicated in Point 7
    first diagnosed /year/ ....

....
Date

Stamp and signature of the person making
the report

[x] Note: All points must be answered | Death /3/

                                    | Name and surname

If the patient did not undergo histopathological investigation,Point 8 should read:"Did
not undergo". If the result of the investigation,for example,of a section, has not yet been
received or if the result is negative,one should
indicate"under investigation" or give the negative result

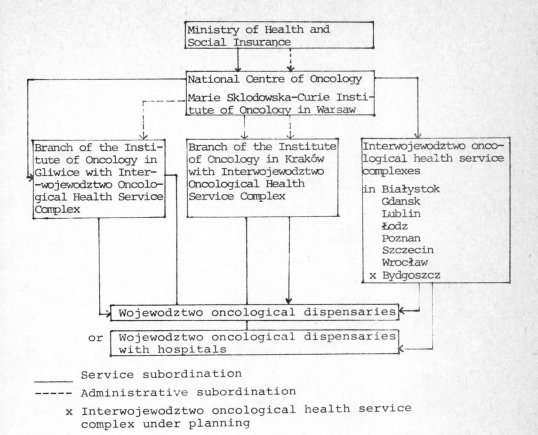

Ministry of Health and Social Insurance

National Centre of Oncology
Marie Sklodowska-Curie Institute of Oncology in Warsaw

Branch of the Institute of Oncology in Gliwice with Inter-wojewodztwo Oncological Health Service Complex

Branch of the Institute of Oncology in Kraków with Interwojewodztwo Oncological Health Service Complex

Interwojewodztwo onco-logical health service complexes

in Białystok
  Gdansk
  Lublin
  Łodz
  Poznan
  Szczecin
  Wrocław
x Bydgoszcz

Wojewodztwo oncological dispensaries

or Wojewodztwo oncological dispensaries with hospitals

_____ Service subordination

----- Administrative subordination

x Interwojewodztwo oncological health service complex under planning

Fig. 29   Organizational scheme of the oncological service in Poland

Department of the Marie Sklodowska-Curie Institute where the central register of tumour cases is kept.

Information about prophylactic medical examinations is reported once a year which makes possible to calculate the rate of incidence of malignant tumours in the register of neoplasms. Every member of the oncological service has the right and duty to demand proper filling-in of "Declaration Cards of Malignant Neoplasms" in his district and to see to the registration of all malignant tumour cases.

The Ministry of Health and Social Insurance issues annual

465

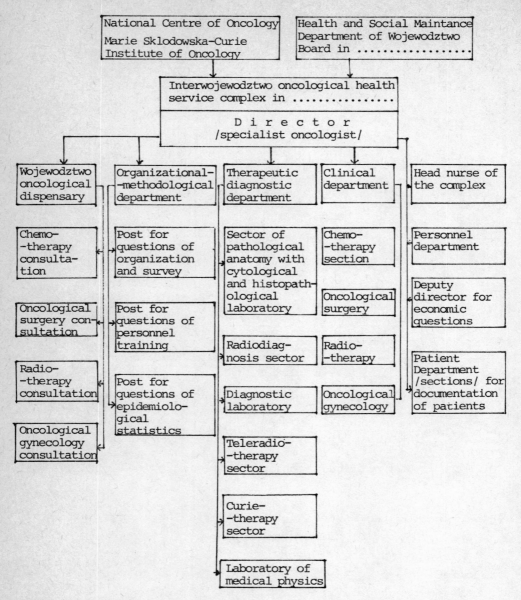

Fig. 30 Scheme of organization of an interwojewodztwo onco-
         logical health service complex

statistical bulletins which contain data on the incidence,
lethality and mortality of malignant tumours.

466

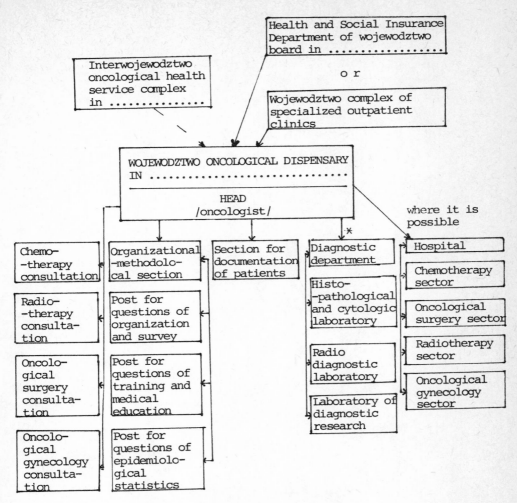

X Diagnostic department may be common for the
wojewodztwo complex of specialized outpatient
clinics

Fig. 31 Organizational structure of wojewodztwo oncological
dispensary

Once in two or three years the Institute of Oncology
issues extensive and detailed studies concerning the epidemiology of neoplasms which take into account the age structure,
sex, profession, place of residence, the degree of neglect of
different tumour localizations.

Table 90

Poland's Oncological Service as of December 31, 1975, and its Planned Development up to 1990

Town	Organizational unit	County /wojewodztwo/	Population		Number of beds		Megavolt therapy instruments		Specialist in oncology	
			1975	1990	1975[x]	1990	1975	1990	1975[xx]	1990
Warsaw	National centre Centre Institute	Warsaw Plock	4,633,000	5,513,000	314 0.06	820 0.15	1	7	56 +/10/	85
	Oncological clinic of the Child Health Centre	Ciechanow Ostroleka Siedlce Radom								
Gliwice	Branch of the Institute Interwojewodztwo Oncological Health Service Complex	Katowice Bielsko Czestochowa	4,939,000	5,877,000	375 0.07	820 0.15	1	7	32 +/7/	85
Kraków	Branch of the Institute Interwojewodztwo Oncological Health Service Complex	Krakow Kielce Tarnow Tarnobrzeg Rzeszow Nowy Sacz Krosno	4,854,000	5,776,000	246 0.04	820 0.15	1	7	22 +/3/	85

Region	Complex	Cities								
Poznan	Interwojewodztwo Oncological Health Service Complex	Poznan, Pila, Zielona Gora, Konin, Kalisz, Leszno	3,450,000	4,106,000	200 0.05	620 0.15	2	5	22 +/8/	65
Łódz	Interwojewodztwo Oncological Health Service Complex	Łódz, Sieradz, Skiemiewice, Pjotrkow, Włocławek	2,824,000	3,360,000	201 0.07	505 0.15	2	4	12 +/3/	55
Biały-stok	Interwojewodztwo Oncological Health Service Complex	Białystok, Olsztyn, Suwalki, Lomza	2,000,000	2,380,000	12 0.06	360 0.15	1	3	14 +/4/	35
Wrocław	Interwojewodztwo Oncological Health Service Complex	Wrocław, Jelenia Gora, Legnica, Walbrzych, Opole	3,575,000	4,255,000	300 0.05	640 0.15	1	5	14 +/7/	65

Table 90 /cont'd/

Town	Organizational	County /wojewodztwo/	Population		Number of beds		Megavolt therapy instruments		Specialist in oncology	
			1975	1990	1975x	1990	1975	1990	1975xx	1990
Lublin	Interwojewodztwo Oncological Health Service Complex	Lublin Biała Podlaska Chelm Zamosc Przemysl	2,224,000	2,646,000	80 0.03	400 0.15	1	3	15 +/5/	40
Gdansk	Interwojewodztwo Oncological Health Service Complex	Gdansk Slupsk Eldlag Torun Bydgoszcz	3,556,000	4,232,000	178 0.05	635 0.15	1	5	10 +/1/	65
Szczecin	Interwojewodztwo Oncological Health Service Complex	Szczecin Koszalin Gorzow	1,698,000	2,020,000	45 0.02	300 0.15	–	3	2 +/1/	30
Poland /total/			33,753,000	40,165,000	2,061	6,040	11	50	199	610

xAbsolute numbers and index per 1,000 population.
xxThe figure + /in brackets/ means the number of doctors who started specializing in oncology.

470

ORGANIZATION OF THE IDENTIFICATION AND EXAMINATION
OF ONCOLOGICAL CASES

The Wojewodztwo Oncological Dispensary is responsible for the early identification of tumours and for sending the patients for appropriate treatment.

The Wojewodztwo Oncological Dispensary receives patients sent by general medical institutions /district doctors, doctors of rural health centres/, all specialized outpatient clinics and all other medical institutions. In other words, any doctor in Poland, wherever he works, has the right and duty to send a patient suspected of having tumour to the Wojewodztwo Oncological Dispensary. Besides, the Wojewodztwo Oncological Dispensary receives patients without a doctor's direction, if these patients have suspicions of a neoplasm. Patients who come without doctor's direction make up about 20 per cent of the total number examined in the Wojewodztwo Oncological Dispensary. In principle, the Wojewodztwo Oncological Dispensary has every facility necessary for making a diagnosis. In cases when the diagnosis is particularly difficult or when hospitalization is needed to identify the disease, the Wojewodztwo Oncological Dispensary sends the patient to the hospital of the Interwojewodztwo Health Service Oncological Complex.

This procedure of identifying tumours is characteristic of 60-80 % of oncological patients with different localizations of neoplasms; for 20-40 % per cent of oncological patients the diagnosis of malignant neoplasms is made at non-oncological outpatient clinics or clinics of the Medical Academies, with the exeption of neoplasms of female genital organs, since the majority of women's clinics in Poland have the facilities and ability to carry out cytological investigation. Thus the identification of neoplasms of the uterus is made chiefly by women's clinics.

Mass prophylactic examinations in Poland cover first of all working women above 25 years of age. Periodic /once a year/ cytological investigations are carried out among them to identify cancer of the cervix uteri. In different areas of the country these examinations include 20 to 80 % of women above 25 years of age. Owing to the good organization and training in the gynecological service and the prophylactic examinations mentioned above, the number of cases with the stage III cancer of the cervix uteri is steadily declining in Poland from year to year. Cases in which patients apply to medical institutions with the stage IV of this type of cancer are already exceptionally rare.

The prophylactic examinations conducted over many years by the industrial health service among the workers of chemical plants producing anilin dyes or applying gas tar products in production technology have made it possible to work out appropriate norms of the duration of working day for workers who have a prolonged and direct contact with carcinogenic agents. As a result of the introduction of these norms no new cases of the urinary bladder cancer have been observed for several years among workers of large chemical plants, while previously several cases were registered every year. In the near future such prophylactic examinations will be carried out at petrochemical plants and in coal industry.

ORGANIZATION OF HOSPITALIZATION AND MEDICAL AID FOR PATIENTS WITH MALIGNANT NEOPLASMS

The network of specialized oncological institutions in Poland is designed to meet the therapeutic requirements of about 50 % of new malignant neoplasm cases in a year. The provision of appropriate therapeutic equipment and highly skilled specialists at oncological hospitals make possible to treat cases which require the application of combined therapeutic methods, e.g. X-ray therapy and megavolt radiotherapy, surgery, hormonotherapy and chemotherapy. According to expert data, about half of all malignant tumour cases require the use of combined therapeutic methods.

The other half of malignant neoplasm cases are treated with a positive result by using one method, most often surgical intervention. These patients must be and are treated according to the localization principle at specialized hospitals or departments of the Medical Academies. If, in the course of observation after treatment, some patients of this group need additional treatment, e.g. radiotherapy, they are sent to oncological hospitals.

In principle all radiotherapy instruments are concentrated at specialized oncological hospitals. Presently the insufficient number of beds at oncological hospitals is responsible for the fact that after a tumour is diagnosed, patients have to wait from three to six weeks /depending on the district of the country/ for a vacancy at a hospital.

At present oncological hospitals have 0.05 beds per 1,000 population; by 1990 it is planned to raise this indicator up to 0.15, which will fully meet the needs of the country.

The director of each oncological hospital compiles annual reports containing information about the number of treated patients, the average duration of the treatment of one patient, the number of patients treated during a year per one hospital bed, the length of the patient's stay at the hospital prior to the beginning of treatment, the degree of the gravity of the disease at the beginning of treatment, etc. These reports are subjected to the thorough analysis by the local health service organs and the National Team of Specialists at the Marie Sklodowska-Curie Institute of Oncology in Warsaw. Based on this analysis, appropriate decisions are taken to perfect the organization and raise the level of medical service for the population.

FOLLOW-UP OF PATIENTS WITH MALIGNANT NEOPLASMS

The functions of the wojewodztwo oncological dispensary in identifying malignant neoplasm cases and directing them for treatment have been enumerated above.

Following the treatment of their tumour patients are subjected to periodic control examinations at a corresponding wojewodztwo oncological dispensary at the place of residence.

Every patient discharged of a hospital is appointed for the first checkup at a wojewodztwo oncological dispensary.The dispensary in question is also notified of the date of the checkup.

The number of post-treatment checkups depends on the character of the tumour case and the state of the patient. As a rule, control checkups are carried out first once a month or every three months and later once or twice a year.

Each patient who received anti-tumour therapy, is kept under observation by a wojewodztwo oncological dispensary to the end of his life.

Once a year the wojewodztwo oncological dispensary transmits information about every patient under observation to the Central Registry of Malignant Neoplasms kept at the Marie Sklodowska-Curie Institute of Oncology in Warsaw according to the "Report on a Malignant Neoplasm" /see Supplement 20/.

Irrespective of these data, the Central Registry of Malignant Neoplasms receives information from population registration offices about deaths from malignant tumours.

This organization of post-treatment control examinations of patients makes possible the follow-up of about 70 % of the patients with treated malignant neoplasms in the country. Approximately 30 % of the treated patients do not report for checkups, despite the fact that the wojewodztwo oncological dispensary repeatedly summons patients who failed to appear on the appointed date.

An example of the form of summons for control checkups:

Wojewodztwo oncological
    dispensary

Poznan, Barbara Str. 4,   Poznan ....
Doctor

You are urgently required to report for a checkup at the wojewodztwo oncological dispensary.

If you cannot come for some reason, please inform us in a letter about the state of your health.

Checkups are daily, except ....
Saturdays and Sundays, in mornings.

Please present this letter at the dispensary at the checkup.

                                    Head of the Medical
                                      Secretariat

Control examinations of patients after treatment serve as basis for deciding further therapeutic methods rending on the given disease and also for determining the efficiency of the treatment.

ORGANIZATION OF MEDICAL AID FOR PATIENTS WITH ADVANCED FORMS OF TUMOURS

Specialized oncological hospitals cannot take care of patients with malignant tumours, who, due to the neglect of the tumour process, are not subject to radical treatment and are only hospitalized for medical care and palliative /symptomatic/ treatment.

The reasons are the following:

1. The expensive therapeutic equipment of oncological hospitals must be used to the maximum extent for the radical treatment of patients, thus every patient admitted to an oncological hospital for medical care only decreases the utilization of therapeutic equipment.

2. It is of great importance for getting the consent of a patient with malignant tumour to treatment in an early stage of the disease to convince him that a large percentage of cases leave the oncological hospital cured. Hospitalization of patients in an advanced stage whose stay at an oncological hospital may have a lethal end has a negative effect on patients in early stages of the disease, often making them refuse the proposed treatment.

There is no consensus among Polish oncologists as to the organization of medical aid for patients with malignant tumour that are not amenable to special treatment. A group of oncologists believes that for solving the problem properly it is necessary to create special departments or homes for incurable cases where they may be taken care of in a qualified way. Another group regards this solution incorrect both organizationally and from the humane point of view and suggests: their hospitalization at general town or district hospitals where the available beds are not always fully used.

At present both versions of the hospitalization of such

patients are applied in Poland. The experience accumulated has revealed a number of positive and negative aspects of both solutions. On the whole it may concluded that either solution may be correct depending on the involvement of people directly responsible for these patients. In the ambulatory observation of patients with malignant neoplasms in an advanced stage there is a rule that a patient requiring specialized treatment stays under the observation of the wojewodztwo oncological dispensary or of a district doctor who is guided by the instructions of the dispensary. If only analgetic treatment is possible, the patient is placed under the observation of a district doctor in his residential area who is obliged to visit the patient at home.

Patients needing the care of a nurse in domestic conditions are looked after by nurses of the Polish Red Cross through social insurance departments of the local councils.

TEACHING OF ONCOLOGY; TRAINING OF ONCOLOGISTS AND PARAMEDICAL PERSONNEL FOR ONCOLOGICAL INSTITUTIONS

The paramedical personnel /nurses, laboratory assistants/ is trained at oncological institutions /Institute of Oncology in interwojewodztwo oncological health complexes/. Students of medical nurse schools and medical technical schools are trained according to a programme taking into acount the requirement of each particular institution.

The oncological training of medical students is carried out in the following ways:

1. Pregraduate training of students of therapeutic and stomatologic faculties of Medical Academies.

2. Postgraduate training:

a/ basic courses for doctors having the first contact with the patient;

b/ courses for increasing the knowledge in oncology of doctors of different specialties;

c/ courses for improving the qualification of oncologists.

3. Specialization in oncology

In January, 1974 the Minister of Health and Social

Insurance standardized the pregraduate training of oncology students. The local oncological institutions and their staffs were recommended to be the bases of training. The programme of training in oncology was worked out by the Marie Sklodowska--Curie Institute of Oncology.

The training of fifth /or sixth/ year students of therapeutic and stomatologic faculties of medical colleges includes the following topics:

General oncology - the training is carried out by the Institute of Oncology or Interwojewodztwo Oncological Health Service Complex.

1. Organization of the oncological service /historical survey, organization of the oncological service in the world and in Poland, participation of general medical institutions in the treatment of neoplasms/.

2. Epidemiology of neoplasms in the world and in Poland, the system of registration of tumour case, disease incidence, mortality, legislation in oncology.

3. Classification of neoplasms /clinical, histological, etc./.

4. Diagnostic methods in oncology:

a/ Histopathology /biopsy, puncture, trephine-biopsy, examination in the course of a surgical intervention/;

b/ cytology significance of the method, mass prophylactic examinations of female population;

c/ X-ray diagnosis;

d/ isotope diagnosis;

e/ thermography, etc.

5. Modern principles of treating neoplasms:

a/ Surgical methods /principles of oncological radicalism, electrosurgery, cryosurgery and so on, radical and palliative cure/;

b/ ionizing irradiation treatment /teleradium therapy, cobalt-60, cesium, radium, isotopes; radical and palliative cure/;

c/ chemotherapy and hormonotherapy;

d/ complex and combined methods of treating neoplasms.

6. Evaluation of the effect of the treatment of malignant neoplasms.

Special oncology the training is carried out at hospitals of Medical Academies in the following specialities: surgery, dermatology, neurosurgery, ophthalmology, laryngology, urology, gynecology, internal disease, etc. according to programmes compiled by an oncologist-coordinator at every Medical Academy.

Postgraduate training of doctors having the first contact with patients /panel doctors/ is carried out in the form of one-to-three-day conferences organized jointly by the postgraduate training centres of the wojewodztwo health and social insurance departments and by Medical Academies and by the organizational-methodological departments of the interwojewodztwo oncological health service complexes. The programme includes problems of the organization of oncological aid in a given district and also fundamental questions of the diagnosis and therapy of neoplasms. The aim of training is to acquaint district doctors with the symptoms which may indicate the presence of a tumour and thus lead to the immediate direction of the patient to a wojewodztwo oncological dispensary.

Courses improving the knowledge in oncology for doctors of different specialties are organized by the Postgraduate Medical Training Centre at the departments of the Institute of Oncology or of the Medical Academies. The programmes of these courses lasting 2-6 weeks or three months are worked out separately for each specialty and are compiled with due regard to the modern achievements of oncology in the given specialty.

Training courses for oncologists are organized at the Institute of Oncology and last one or two weeks. These courses give an insight into the achievements of modern oncology. Every oncologist working far from scientific oncological centres participate in training courses at least once in every other year.

The decision of the Minister of Health and Social Insurance of March 10, 1973, created conditions for specializing in three oncological specialties: oncological surgery, oncological

478

radiotherapy and oncological pathology.

In oncological surgery one can specialize after first--degree specialization in general or pediatric surgery. Second--degree specialization in oncological surgery requires a 24--month training, at an oncological surgery department or hospital, and taking an examination before a commission in the Institute of Oncology in Warsaw according to the following programme:

1. General pathology of neoplasms /identification of a neoplasm, the principles of classification of neoplasms, biological properties of neoplasms, types and stages of the tumour process, sensitivity of normal and tumour tissue to irradiation and chemical preparations/.

2. Principles of   special pathology of neoplasms.

3. Principles of the surgery of neoplasms; technical and biological operability of neoplasms, indications and contra--indications of surgical treatment of neoplasms, surgical treatment of primary localizations, metastases and relapses, rules of special techniques and their application in treating neoplasms.

4. The clinical picture and surgical treatment of neoplasms.

5. Endoscopic investigation of the esophagus and stomach larynx and bronchi, rectum and sigmoid colon.

6. Radiotherapy: biological and physical fundamentals of radiotherapy, sensitivity of various tissues and neoplasms to irradiation, indications and contra-indications of radiotherapy as the only method of treatment or as a pre- or post-operation component of combined treatment. Substantiation of indications for chemotherapy: indications, principles and results of combined and complex treatment /surgical, radiotherapeutic and chemotherapeutic/, the course of radio- and chemotherapy and possible complications.

7. Principles of joint work of the oncological collective /cooperation with the pathologist, radiodiagnostician, radiotherapist and chemotherapist/.

8. Epidemiology and organization of cancer control.

Specialization in radiotherapy has two degrees. The first--degree specialization requires a 24-month training at a radiotherapeutic institution and an examination before a commission of the wojewodztwo health and social insurance department according to the following programme:

1. Physical and technical questions

Structure of material. Natural and artificial sources of ionizing irradiation used in radiotherapy. Principles of the construction and operation of radiotherapeutic equipment. Physical properties of irradiation. Absorption phenomena of irradiation. Measurements of irradiation: units, principles of the construction and operation of measuring instruments, principles and methods of measuring irradiation, practice in a given field. Distribution of irradiation in tissues.

2. Fundamentals of radiobiology

Biological effects of irradiation. Sensitivity of normal and pathological tissues to irradiation. Postradiation damage: somatic /early and late/ and genetic.

3. Radiological protection

Professional and general risks of being exposed to ionizing irradiation. Safety rules and labour hygiene in radiotherapy. Principles of radiological protection. Practical knowledge of safety rules and labour hygiene. Rules and technology of radiotherapeutic work.

4. Documentation

Clinical radiotherapeutic documentation and general documentation of a radiotherapeutic institution. Knowledge of the methods of observation and evaluation of the results of treatment.

5. Organization of a medical institution

Principles of the organization of radiotherapeutic institutions and principles of organization of cancer control in Poland. Basic information on the epidemiology of neoplasms.

6. Pathology

Classification of neoplasms: practical knowledge of nomenclature. Precancerous conditions. Basic information on the pathology of non-tumours diseases treated by radiotherapy.

7. Clinical picture

The clinical picture, development and course of patholo-gical conditions, chiefly neoplasms subjected to radiotherapy. Methods of diagnosis of neoplasms and critical evaluation of their effect. Practice in the examination of patients. Perform-ance of diagnostic procedures /punctures, biopsies/. Classifica-tion of clinical stages of neoplasms. Main indications for tumour treatment. Principles of treating neoplasms: radical, palliative, symptomatic, and care of incurable cases.

8. Radiotherapy

Theoretical foundations of radiotherapy of neoplasms and non-tumourous diseases. Methods of irradiation. The aim of radiotherapy /radical or palliative treatment/. Indications for radiotherapy. Planning and conduct of treatment by surface beams, interstitial and intracavitary applicators. Post-radia-tion changes and complications.

Second-degree specialization in oncological radiotherapy may be undertaken by a specialist, who has had first-degree training in radiotherapy or internal diseases, pediatrics or in gynecology, after a 36-month training at an institution of oncological radiotherapy and examination before a commission of the Institute of Oncology in the following topics:

1. Radiobiology

Theoretical knowledge on the biological action of ionizing irradiation. Detailed information on questions of the sensitiv-ity of cells, tissues and human organism to irradiation and ability of applying it in the practice of radiotherapy.

2. Radiological protection

Ability of independently organizing and guiding radio-therapeutic work in a way ensuring proper conditions of radio-logical protection. Ability of using technological information in the practice of radiological protection.

3. Organization of a therapeutic institution

The basic elements of the organization of an oncological hospital. Practice of the organization of prophylaxis of neo-plasms and that of occupational tumour diseases and other related problems. Advancing of the early identification of neoplasms.

4. Epidemiology of neoplasms

Detailed information about the incidence and mortality from malignant neoplasms in Poland and other countries, the role and importance of endogenic and exogenic factors in the incidence of malignant neoplasms.

5. Pathology

Modern data about the etiology and pathogenesis of neoplasms. Morphological properties of neoplasms and their connection with clinical course.

6. Clinics

Independent application of diagnostic methods of neoplasms. Basic information for the independent guidance of a clinical department /oncological dispensary/ and knowledge of the principles of cooperation with other specialists. Skill in chemo- and hormonotherapeutics of neoplasms.

7. Radiotherapy

Independent practical knowledge of the methods of radiotherapy: planning of treatment, irradiation techniques, care of irradiated patients, methods of irradiation in the case of post-irradiation complications and damage, theoretical knowledge of the results of radiotherapy and other methods, including combined treatment, and skill in assessing the results of treatment.

Medical-judicial questions:

1. Medical-judicial practice: knowledge of general rules and special medical conclusions

2. Rules of drug control

3. Responsibility of the doctor /civil and criminal/

Note: For doctors having their first-degree special examination in internal diseases, pediatrics, gynecology and obstetrics, the specialization programme includes also the following elements covered by the first-degree specialization:
1. Physical and technical questions:
The structure of material. Natural and artificial sources of ionizing irradiation used for radiotherapy. Principles of the construction and operation of radiotherapeutic equipment. Physical properties of irradiation. Absorption phenomena of irradiation. Measurement of irradiation: units, principles of the construction and operation of measuring instruments, principles and methods of irradiation measurement, practice in the given field. Distribution of irradiation in tissues.

2. Radiological protection

Occupational and general risks of exposition to ionizing irradiation. Safety rules and labour hygiene in radiotherapy.

Specialization in oncological pathology may be undertaken by a specialist with the second degree in pathomorphology after a 12-month training at the pathology department of the Institute of Oncology and an examination before a commission of the Postgraduate Medical Training Centre in Warsaw according to the following programme:

1. General pathology of neoplasms /the notion of a neoplasm, pathogenesis of malignant neoplasms, principles of classification and terminology of neoplasms, biological properties of tumours and stages of malignancy, sensitivity of normal and tumour tissues to irradiation/.

2. Detailed pathology of neoplasms /macroscopy, microscpy and dynamics of the development of the tumour/.

3. General clinical questions /foundations of clinical diagnosis and treatment of neoplasms, principles of selecting the most adequate therapeutic methods, connection between tumour pathology and clinical localization, methods of taking biopsy material/.

4. Macroscopic and microscopic diagnosis of neoplasms /microscopy techniques, description techniques, extent and principles of histopathological conclusions, use of clinical data, formulation of answers/.

5. Ability of conducting urgent investigation.

6. Investigation of the material of punctures and cytological smears.

7. Knowledge of the foundations of medical statistics to an extent essential for interpreting characteristic indicators of malignant neoplasms /incidence of the disease, mortality, lethality, effect of treatment, etc./.

Independently from the above forms of postgraduate training, local organs of the Polish Oncological Society jointly with other scientific societies organize scientific conferences on topics selected to widening the oncological knowledge of doctors of various specialtics.

HEALTH EDUCATIONAL WORK AMONG POPULATION

General questions of health education in Poland are dealt with by the Polish Red Cross and the Institute of Hygiene in Warsaw. The publishing activity of the National Institute of Hygiene also deals with problems of oncology. The Institute of Oncology supplies the necessary material or recommends authors for compiling popular scientific pamphlets intended for broad circulation among the population.

Apart from this, the Department of Organization of Cancer Control at the Institute of Oncology releases several scientific educational popular scientific films devoted to health education in oncology. The research workers of the institute regularly deliver lectures, also in the radio and television, popularizing oncological problems.

The organizational-methodological departments of the inter-wojewodztwo oncological health service complexes conduct broad activity in their territory using all available means for the health education in oncology. As an example, a publication of the Białystok Interwojewodztwo health service complex is shown. /see also Fig. 32/

Białystok oncological complex

EARLY TREATMENT OF CANCER SAVES LIFE

EVERY WOMEN PARTICIPATES IN THE PREVENTION AND EARLY IDENTIFICATION OF CANCER OF THE MAMMARY GLAND

The cancer of the mammary gland is one of the most widespread malignant neoplasms among women. The incidence of the disease must be reduced and the number of cured cases increased.

Every women must consciously participate in this campaign by periodically checking mammary glands. Checks must be made regularly, at least once a month; optimally immediately after the menstruation.

DURING CHECKS ATTENTION MUST BE DRAWN TO:
- symmetry, outlines and form of mammary glands;
- indurations and clear definable tumour in the mammary glands;
- changes in the nipples in the form of upward or downward shifts, recraction of the nipple, ulcer or excretion;
- palpable enlargement or sensitivity of armpit lymph nodes.

EVEN IF THE SLIGHTEST CHANGE IS FOUND WITHIN THE MAMMARY GLAND OR IN THE ARMPIT, VISIT IMMEDIATELY A DOCTOR.

HOW MAMMARY GLANDS MUST BE CHECKED

The mammary gland may be divided into four sections:

The mammary gland may be
devided into four sections:

    I - upper medical
   II - lower medical
 III - lower lateral
  IV - upper lateral

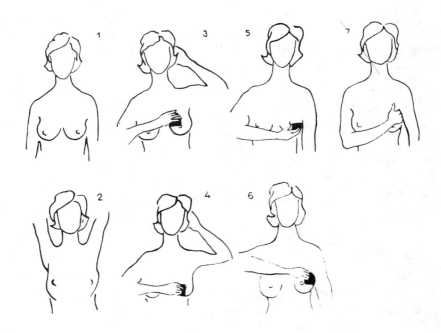

Fig. 32 How mammary glands should be checked

    I   - upper medial
   II - lower medial
  III - lower lateral
   IV - upper lateral
STAND IN FRONT OF A MIRROR UNDRESSED TO THE WAIST
1/ let your hands down along the body and then
2/ raise your hands and cross palms at the back of the
head.
    Movements 1 and 2 enable you to evaluate the symmetry,
outlines and form of mammary glands.
    3. Checking by palpation begins with the upper medical
section of the mammary gland. The hand on the side of the
gland checked should be raised and rest on the back of the

485

head. Fingers of the palpating hand move slowly from ribs and
the breast bone to the nipple of the mammary gland.

4/ Without changing position similar checking is done of
the lower medical section of the gland.

5/ Letting your hand freely down along the body, feel the
lower lateral section of the gland, shifting fingers from the
outer edge of the gland in the direction of the nipple.

6/ The upper lateral section is checked in the same way.

7/ At the end feel carefully the armpit cavity.

The same procedure is followed in checking the
mammary gland and the armpit on the other side.

In its 1976-1980 scientific plan the Marie Sklowska-Curie
Institute of Oncology envisages the elaboration of the most
adequate and effective forms of health education of the population.

COORDINATION OF RESEARCH ON THE PROBLEM "SCIENTIFIC
FOUNDATIONS OF THE ORGANIZATION OF CANCER CONTROL"

The first two clauses of the Statute of the Marie Sklodowska-Curie Institute of Oncology read:

"1. Planning, organization and conduct of research in
experimental and clinical oncology and organization of fight
against tumourous diseases.

2. Coordination of work specified in Clause I and conducted
by other institutions subordinated to the Minister of Health
and Social Insurance to an extent regulated by the Minister."

The organizational unit responsible for the conduct and
coordination of research connected to organization of cancer
control is the Department of Organization of Cancer Control
and Neoplasm Epidemiology at the Institute of Oncology in
Warsaw and its two laboratories at the branches institutes
in Gliwice and Kraków.

In connection with the scientific foundations of the
organization of cancer control the Department carries out
research to estimate the applicability of different organizational models of oncological service under Polish conditions,
works out standards of equipment supply for oncological institutions, scientific principles of cooperation between onколo-
gical institutions and other bodies of the health service,
studies the extent of oncological knowledge of doctors and
paramedical personnel as well as the spread of knowledge

486

concerning neoplasms in the population, moreover it works out
methods for propagating health education and training programmes
in oncology for various groups of medical personnel.

The Institute of Oncology entrusts the elaboration of
certain scientific topics in the organization to other, cancer
control both medical and non-medical scientific institutions
in Poland.

PERSPECTIVES OF THE IMPROVEMENT OF ORGANIZATION OF ONCOLOGICAL AID IN POLAND

After the end of the Second World War, in 1945, Poland
was a country with a ruined industry, towns destroyed to a
different extent, some of them up to 80 % /e.g. Warsaw, Gdansk,
Wrocław, Szczecin/ and gutted railway system. About one quarter
of the population died in the war /as compared to the population in 1939/. After the war Poland had only 8,000 doctors /in
1974 about 57,000/. The entire population made   great efforts
to restore the country, including health service. Naturally,
oncology, a new branch of medicine in the country after the
war, was to be developed proportionally to the other branches.
At present oncology in terms of number of hospital beds, equipment, instruments and training of oncologists meets about 50 %
of the requirements as regards the treatment of oncological
patients at specialized oncological institutions and will meet
about 33 % in 1990, taking into account the increase in the
incidence of the disease and the size of the population.

A team of eminent specialists has been formed to work out
a long-term plan for the development of the oncological service
in Poland. The plan submitted by the team in 1974 was adopted
by the Political Bureau of our Party and was recognized by the
decision of the Presidium of the Government of June 27, 1975
called "Tumour Control" to be one of the seven Government
programmes of research and long-term development /Fig. 33/.

The basic guidelines of the Government programme of
research and long-term development "Tumour Control" worked out
by the Marie Sklodowska-Curie Institute of Oncology and approved
by the Presidium of the Government of the Polish People's

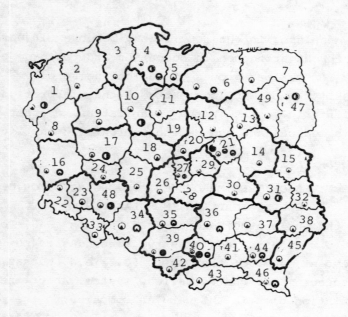

Fig. 33 Plan of the organization of the oncological service
in Poland

◉ - Centre of the Institute of Oncology, ◕ - Branch
of the Institute of Oncology, ⦿ - Department of
Pediatric Oncology of the Institute of Mother and
Child, ◔ - Oncological Department of a Medical Academy,
◕ - Interwojewodztwo oncological health service
complex, ◕ - Oncological department of a wojewodztwo
hospital, ◔ - Wojewodztwo oncological dispensary /or
consultation/
/For explanation of numbers see Fig. 27/

Republic, envisage that, along with basic oncological research,
the number of beds and equipment and also qualified personnel
should be trebled by 1990.

Statistical data on the incidence of and mortality from
malignant neoplasms are presented on Tables 91-93.

COOPERATION WITHIN THE FRAMEWORK OF THE CMEA

Poland's main partners in the scientific cooperation in
oncology are the member countries of the Council for Mutual
Economic Assistance.

Poland participates in the elaboration of all the nine problems included by the Agreement on Scientific and Technical Cooperation of the CMEA countries on the overall problem "Malignant Neoplasms".

The extent of Poland's participation in the elaboration of particular problems depends on the possibilities and, first of all, on the personnel available. It is envisaged that along with the development of Polish oncology our participation in the scientific cooperation with the CMEA countries will be more significant.

Table 91

Absolute Number and Incidence of New Cases of Malignant Neoplasms of the Polish Population by Age and Sex 1974

Age groups	Total				Male				Female			
	Male		Female		Urban		Rural		Urban		Rural	
	Absolute number	per 100.000 population	Absolute number	per 100.000 population	Absolute number	per 100.000 population	Absolute number	per 100.000 population	Absolute number	per 100.000 population	Absolute number	per 100.000 population
Total	31.042	189.5	30.879	178.4	17.554	199.6	13.438	177.7	19.302	202.7	11.577	148.7
0-4	186	13.1	147	10.9	102	14.6	84	11.6	83	12.5	64	9.3
5-9	117	9.0	103	8.3	49	7.9	68	10.0	52	8.8	51	7.8
10-14	136	9.2	98	6.9	57	8.2	79	10.1	44	6.6	54	7.2
15-19	238	13.4	194	11.3	125	13.4	113	13.3	98	10.8	96	11.9
20-24	260	15.3	288	17.5	149	14.6	111	16.3	153	14.5	135	22.8
25-29	296	23.0	410	32.5	184	22.7	112	23.4	274	33.6	136	30.4
30-34	281	29.0	573	59.4	167	27.9	114	30.9	387	64.0	186	51.6
35-39	666	61.6	1.060	97.2	397	61.9	269	61.3	681	103.5	379	87.6
40-44	1.366	120.7	1.848	160.9	856	130.6	510	107.1	1.189	179.3	659	135.8
45-49	2.209	217.7	2.777	245.6	1.273	224.4	936	209.2	1.803	287.9	974	193.1
50-54	2.862	350.2	3.202	330.9	1.662	383.6	1.200	312.5	1.892	266.7	1.310	290.9
55-59	2.535	495.6	2.551	400.7	1.412	561.7	1.123	431.8	1.523	462.6	1.028	334.3

60–64	4.948	747.5	4.168	499.5	2.706	855.8	2.242	648.5	2.481	575.6	1.687	418.1
65–69	5.849	1.056	4.435	607.9	3.168	1244.8	2.681	895.5	2.729	722.1	1.706	485.1
70.74	4.912	1.322.9	4.082	723.1	2.751	1.663.2	2.161	1.049.5	2.540	878.9	1.542	559.7
75–79	2.668	1.419.1	2.832	814.0	1.546	1.853.7	1.122	1.072.7	1.889	1.020.5	943	579.2
80–84	1.041	1.316.1	1.355	791.5	654	1.863.2	387	879.5	937	1.028.5	418	521.8
85 years	369	1.048.3	668	719.8	245	1.570.5	124	632.7	496	1.004.0	172	396.3
older	103	88			51	52		51				37

Table 92

Distribution of Malignant Neoplasms by Sex and Age in Poland, 1974

Age groups	Total				Male				Female			
	Male		Female		Urban		Rural		Urban		Rural	
	Absolute number	per 100.000 population	Absolute number	per 100.000 population	Absolute number	per 100.000 population	Absolute number	per 100.000 population	Absolute number	per 100.000 population	Absolute number	per 100.000 population
Total	52.595	321.0	76.823	443.9	29.329	333.5	23.266	306.5	49.450	519.4	27.373	351.5
0-4	246	17.3	203	15.1	135	19.4	111	15.4	115	17.4	88	12.8
5-9	267	20.5	210	16.9	132	21.3	135	19.9	103	17.4	107	16.4
10-14	273	18.5	210	14.9	121	17.4	152	19.4	115	17.3	95	12.7
15-19	427	24.0	356	20.8	206	22.1	221	25.9	170	18.8	186	23.1
20-24	508	29.8	592	35.9	287	28.1	221	32.4	348	32.9	244	41.3
25-29	603	46.8	901	71.3	393	48.6	210	43.8	611	74.9	290	64.7
30-34	586	60.6	1.406	145.7	352	58.8	234	63.4	953	157.6	453	125.6
35-39	1.268	117.4	3.000	275.0	757	118.0	511	116.5	2.000	303.9	1.000	231.1
40-44	2.559	226.1	5.426	472.4	1.502	229.2	1.057	221.9	3.619	545.7	1.807	372.3
45-49	4.033	397.5	8.845	782.3	2.271	400.4	1.762	393.8	5.828	930.5	3.017	598.3
50-54	5.097	623.6	10.292	1.063.6	2.946	679.9	2.151	560.2	6.434	1.247.1	3.858	853.9
55-59	4.496	879.0	7.555	1.186.6	2.457	977.3	2.039	783.9	4.653	1.413.4	2.902	943.7

Age												
60-64	8.424	1.272.7	11.016	1.320.1	4.586	1.450.3	3.838	1.110.2	6.793	1.576.1	4.223	1.046.6
65-69	9.555	1.725.0	10.473	1.435.4	5.134	2.017.3	4.421	1.476.6	6.749	1.785.9	3.724	1.058.9
70-74	7.764	2.091.0	8.177	1.448.5	4.260	2.575.6	3.504	1.701.8	5.317	1.839.8	2.860	1.038.1
75-79	4.118	2.190.4	4.908	1.410.8	2.342	2.808.2	1.776	1.697.9	3.364	1.817.4	1.544	948.4
80-84	1.632	2.063.2	2.079	1.214.4	981	2.794.9	651	1.479.5	1.440	1.580.7	639	797.8
85 years and older	572	1.625.0	970.	1.045.3	374	2.397.4	198	1.010.2	707	1.431.2	263	606.0
Age un- known	167	204		93		74		131		73		

Table 93

Number of Deaths and Mortality per 100.000 Population from Malignant Neoplasms of the Polish Population, by Age and Sex, 1974

Age groups	Absolute number	Mortality per 100.000 population	Absolute number	Mortality per 100.000 population	Absolute number	Mortality per 100.000 population	Absolute number	Mortality per 100.000 population	Absolute number	Mortality per 100.000 population	Absolute number	Mortality per 100.000 population
Total	27.092	165.4	23.317	134.7	14.700	167.2	12.392	163.8	13.757	144.5	9.560	122.8
0-4	117	8.2	88	6.5	53	7.6	64	8.9	46	7.0	42	6.1
5-9	86	6.6	69	5.5	39	6.3	47	6.9	34	5.7	35	5.4
10-14	102	6.9	50	3.5	45	6.5	57	7.3	23	3.5	27	3.6
15-19	139	7.8	85	5.0	62	6.7	77	9.0	37	4.1	48	6.0
20-24	175	10.3	116	7.0	90	8.8	85	12.5	58	5.5	58	9.8
25-29	168	13.0	169	13.4	109	13.5	59	12.3	97	11.9	72.	16.1
30-34	183	18.9	232	24.0	104	17.4	79	21.4	153	25.3	79	21.9
35-39	396	36.7	517	47.4	244	38.0	152	34.6	332	50.4	185	42.7
40-44	890	78.7	954	83.1	544	83.0	346	72.6	586	88.4	368	75.8
45-49	1.557	153.5	1.480	130.9	916	161.5	641	143.3	900	143.7	580	115.0
50-54	2.231	273.0	1.923	198.7	1.285	296.6	946	246.4	1.119	216.9	804	178.0
55-59	2.180	426.2	1.691	265.6	1.206	479.7	974	374.5	955	290.1	736	239.4

60–64	4.519	682.7	3.204	383.9	2.379	752.4	2.140	619.0	1.778	412.5	1.426	353.4
65–69	5.411	976.9	3.805	521.5	2.825	1.110.0	2.586	363.7	2.218	586.9	1.587	451.2
70–74	4.706	1.267.4	3.765	667.0	2.475	1.496.4	2.231	1.083.5	2.216	766.8	1.549	562.3
75–79	2.701	1.436.7	2.889	830.4	1.473	1.766.2	1.228	1.174.0	1.736	937.9	1.153	708.2
80–84	1.117	1.412.1	1.470	858.6	617	1.757.8	500	1.136.4	943	1.035.1	527	657.9
85 years and older	414	1.176.1	810	872.8	234	1.500.0	180	918.4	526	1.064.8	284	654.4

REFERENCES

1. Hanna Kolodziejska:
   Neoplasm Pathology and Clinics.
   State Medical Literature Publishers, 1965.

2. Tadeusz Koszarowski:
   Practical Oncology in the Surgical Department.
   State Medical Literature Publishers, 1972.

3. Tadeusz Koszarowski:
   Organization of the Care of Malignant Tumour Cases.
   Published by the Department of Prophylaxis and Treatment
   of the Ministry of Health and Social Insurance.
   State Medical Literature Publishers, 1970.

4. Tadeusz Koszarowski, Helena Gadomska, Zbigniew Wronkowski
   and B. Romejko: Epidemiology of Malignant Neoplasms in
   Warsaw and Selected Rural Areas in 1963-1972. Malignant
   Tumour Incidence in Poland - a Forecast.
   Institute of Oncology, 1975.

5. Richard Sosinski:
   Organization of Cancer Control in Poland.
   Institute of Oncology, 1974.

6. Richard Sosinski and Zbigniew Wronkowski:
   Organization of Cancer Control.
   Institute of Oncology, 1975.

7. Richard Sosinski and Tadeusz Naganski:
   The use of Cancer Register for Reducing the Number of
   Long-neglected Cases. Vol. 3,
   State Medical Literature Publishers, Bialystok, 1974.

CANCER CONTROL IN THE USSR

GEOGRAPHIC, ECONOMIC AND DEMOGRAPHIC DESCRIPTION
OF THE COUNTRY AND THE HISTORY OF CANCER CONTROL

V. P. Demidov, N. P. Napalkov and A. V. Chaklin

The Union of Soviet Socialist Republics stretches over
9 thousand kilometres from west to east and more than 4.5
thousand kilometres from north to south. The difference between the northernmost and southernmost points is $46°42'$. The
territory of the Soviet Union is divided into the European and
Asian parts. The overall area of the country is 22.4 million
square kilometres.

The geological structure and relief of the country's
territory is extremely diverse, comprising the Russian and
East-European plain, the West Siberian lowland, the Central
Siberian highland, the mountains of the Far East, the Turansk
plain, the mountain systems of the Caucasus, the Pamirs, the
Tien-Shan, the Altai and the Sayans.

All this determines the climate of the country from cold
arctic in the north to subtropical and desert in the south;
from an oceanic climate to sharply continental-monsoon from
west to east. On the whole, whatever its variety is, the climate of the USSR can be described as temperate and also continental. The following climatic and natural zones can be
singled out: arctic deserts, tundra, forest-tundra, steppe,
the deserts and semi-deserts of the temperate zone, subtropical and elevation zones. The highest point of the country
is the Communism Peak /7,495 m above sea level/, the lowest
point is on the Mangyshlak Peninsula /132 m below sea level/.

The seas of the USSR belong to three oceans: the Arctic,
the Pacific and the Atlantic. The coast in the north is washed

497

by the Barents, White, Kara, Laptev, East-Siberian and the Chukotka Seas; in the east by the Bering Sea, the Sea of Okhotsk and the Sea of Japan; in the west by the Baltic Sea, while in the south by the Black and the Azov Seas.

Large rivers create and determine the water regimen in the central areas of the country. More than half of the rivers drain into the seas of the Arctic Ocean /the Northern Dvina, Pechora, Ob, Yenisei, Angara, Lena and others/. The Amur belongs to the basin of the Pacific Ocean while the Danube, the Dniester, the Don, the Dnieper, the Neva, the Western Dvina, the Neman and others to that of the Atlantic Ocean. The Volga, the Ural, the Amu-Dariya, the Syr-Dariya and some others are draining into the land-locked seas.

There are more than 250,000 lakes in the country, the four biggest ones /the Aral, the Baikal, the Balkhash and the Ladoga/ have an area of more than 10,000 sq km each.

The soils of the Soviet Union are also rather diverse: in the flat part of the country seven soil zones are distinguished: the arctic and tundra podsolic and marshy soils, the grey wood soil, the chernozyom, the brown earth, the brown semidesert soil and the desert soils.

The USSR is rich in all kinds of minerals which fully meet the country's needs. As regards its stocks of reserves of coal, oil, natural gas, shale, iron ore the USSR holds one of the first places in the world; there are large reserves of titanium, manganese, chromium and also non-ferrous and noble metals - copper, lead and zinc, aluminum /bauxites/, tin, nickel and cobalt, tungsten, molybdenum, mercury, antimony, gold, silver and platinum. The extraction of non-metallic minerals - potassium salts, phosphorites and appatites, flour spar, mica, asbestos, magnesites, diamonds, salt, gypsum and anhydrite, building materials and many others account for a considerable part of the country's national economy.

The population of the USSR

In 1970 /according to the census of that year/ the total population of the Soviet Union was 241,700,000, from which 111,400,000 men and 130,300,000 women. In 1976 the population reached 255,500,000, from which 118,700,000 were men and 136,800,000 women.

In 1970 the urban population was 136,000,000 while the rural population 105,700,000. In 1976 156,600,000 people lived in the cities and 98,900,000 in the countryside.

Comparing the figures for 1913, 1970 and 1976, we note, besides the general growth of the population, a considerable increase in the urban population and a corresponding drop in the proportion of the rural population. In the period from 1959 to 1969 alone urban population increased by 36 million; this included 14,600,000 due to natural growth, 5 million on account of transforming villages and settlements into towns, and more than 16 million due to the migration of the rural population to the cities.

In 1970 men made up 46.1 % and women 53.9 % of the population /in 1976 these figures were 46.4 % and 53.6 %, respectively/. In the cities men and women made up 46.3 and 53.7, and in the countryside 45.8 % and 54.2 %, respectively. /For age and sex distribution of the population in 1970 see Table 94/.

The birth rate in 1974 was 18.0 per 1,000 population.

Assuming that the mortality rate of different age groups remains at the present level, the average life expectancy of the generation now born will be 64 years for men and 74 years for women /1971-1972/. In the USSR the average population density is 11.2 per sq km; this indicator varies in the different Union Republics /110.4 for the Moldavian SSR, whereas it is 4.8 for the Turkmenian SSR/. In 1975 the Soviet Union had 13 cities with a population exceeding 1 million.

The USSR is a multinational state. In 1970 the basic ethnic groups were the following: Russians - 129 millions, Ukrainians - 40.8 millions, Uzbeks - 9.2 millions, Byelorussians - 9.1 millions, Tatars - 5.9 millions, Kazaks - 5.3 millions, Azerbaijanians - 4.4 millions, Armenians - 3.6 millions, Georgians - 3.2 millions, Lithuanians - 3.1 millions, Moldavians - 2.7 millions, Jews - 2.2 millions, Tadzhiks - 2.1 millions, Germans - 1.8 millions, Chuvash - 1.7 millions, Turkmens - 1.5 millions, Kirghiz - 1.4 millions, Latvians - 1.4 millions,

Table 94

Distribution of the Population of the USSR by Age and Sex in 1970

Age	Total	Males	Females
Total	241.720.134	111.399.377	130.320.757
0-4	20.509.889	10.434.611	10.075.278
5-9	24.475.707	12.474.611	12.000.986
10-14	24.988.366	12.730.029	12.258.337
15-19	21.999.236	11.225.249	10.773.987
20-24	17.105.210	8.626.904	8.478.306
25-29	13.770.411	6.813.420	6.956.991
30-34	21.144.685	10.408.341	10.736.344
35-39	16.593.854	8.139.761	8.454.093
40-44	19.003.071	8.758.628	10.244.443
45-49	12.255.572	4.743.540	7.512.032
50-54	9.077.740	3.429.835	5.647.905
55-59	12.013.176	4.273.019	7.740.157
60-69	17.595.299	5.922.428	11.672.871
70-79	8.024.761	2.505.750	5.519.011
80 and more	3.163.157	913.141	2.250.016

the peoples of Daghestan - 1.4 millions, Moldavians - 1.3 millions, Bashkirs - 1.2 millions, Poles - 1.2 millions, Estonians - 1 million.

According to the census the number of persons employed in the national economy was 115 million or 47.8 % of the population /75.6 million men and 57.4 million women/.

Of the 130,500,000 persons capable of work those employed in the national economy and students made up 120,600,000 or 92.4 % of the population capable of work /in 1959 - 82 %/.

In 1976 the social composition of the country's population was characterized by the following figures: factory and office workers accounted for 83.6 % from which, factory workers 61.2 %, while collective farm peasantry and cooperated craftsmen account for 16.4 %.

Epidemiology of malignant tumours

Epidemiological studies so widely developed in the last 15-20 years have shown that only a few types of malignant tumours had the same incidence in all countries. Moreover, epidemiological studies have made it possible to establish that the development of malignant tumours in men depends on living conditions to a much greater extent than it had been earlier presumed. Differences in the morbidity pattern of malignant tumours in different countries are a rule rather than on exception. Thus, we can say that in their investigations epidemiologists encounter an experiment presented by nature herself.

The data obtained as a result of epidemiological studies are of special interest, since they permit to reveal and study the interrelationships between the factors affecting man and the morbidity pattern. Thus, it has been proved that in areas of increased ionizing radiation the incidence of leukemia rises notably both in children and adults.

The differences in the incidence of cancer among certain groups of the population and their correlation with the specific features in the dissemination of a possible etiological factor may serve as the basis for discovering of new factors causing the disease.

Hypotheses regarding the causes of cancer may be verified

by comparing individual features pertaining to the patient and the degree to which he was exposed to agents of the environment. Finally, the reality of the causal relationship can be checked by clarifying such questions as whether the disease can be prevented by reducing the dissemination of the suspected agent.

Practical measures based on the above-mentioned information can be used to prevent and remove the risk of malignant tumours. In some branches of industry these methods can be highly successful. In fact, a number of investigations resulted in revealing a provoking role of a number of chemicals and preventive measures were outlined and implemented at major industrial enterprises.

In the study of tumour epidemiology the data of the morbidity pattern and mortality of malignant tumours in different parts of the world are of great importance; moreover, clinical and pathomorphological information can be used for epidemiological studies in cases when the data on morbidity and mortality of a certain zone qualitatively differ from those of other parts of the world. An instance of such a zone are areas with a rather high incidence of cancer of the esophagus on the northern coast of the Caspian Sea /city of Guryev/, in Iran and on the African continent /the Cape Province and the city of Bulawayo/.

Similar places with a high incidence of cancer of the stomach, lung, cervix uteri are found in certain areas of the world and should be carefully studied and investigated. Since the causes of a higher or lower dissemination of individual forms of malignant tumours are by no means the same and ought to be subjected to comprehensive investigation, the tasks of epidemiological studies may be formulated as follows:

1. To reveal the effect of a complex of different climato-geographic, working, housing and other conditions, as well as a number of endogenic factors /genetical, hormonal, etc./ on malignant tumour morbidity.

2. To determine the significance of assumed causal factors in the etiology and pathogenesis of individual forms of

malignant tumours in man.

3. On the basis of the obtained data, to elaborate rational measures for preventing cancer.

Questions pertaining to the epidemiology of malignant tumours began to be elaborated in the USSR in the 1950s. Since then a large amount of material has been accumulated, epidemiological studies have been launched at the republican oncological and roentgenological institutes, and methodological aspects for studying the problem have been worked out. New facts have been revealed with regard to the pecularities in the dissemination of malignant tumours in various climato-geographic zones of the country, among different ethnic and occupational groups of the population, the effect of environmental factors on malignant tumour morbidity and mortality; epidemiological approaches to and the assessment of the role of carcinogenic agents /physical, chemical, biological/ in the development of tumours in man, are elaborated tests are being carried out for the epidemiological study of certain tumours, studies are going on into the epidemiology of malignant tumours of proven and suspected viral origin. Immunological, cytological and serological methods for of tumour identification have begun to be used when studying the epidemiology of certain forms of malignant neoplasms.

In organizing cancer control very important were the experiments exploring and analyzing morbidity and mortality which indicated territorial peculiarities in the dissemination of malignant neoplasms in the USSR. Medico-geographic mapping, the grouping and analyzing of morbidity and mortality patterns according to the individual territories of the Soviet Union made it possible to assess the basic tendencies and formulate specific features in the spread of malignant tumours on territories with common characteristics.

Multi-purpose experiments organized for studying the epidemiology of malignant tumours have permitted to develop methods for examining certain groups of the population /ethnic, occupational, etc./ under individual programs in different territories of the country. This is the only way of studying this problem under real conditions, which permits to compare not only statistical indices but factors affecting morbidity and mortality due to malignant tumours. The possibility of carrying out a retrospective study in a single program by special analytical methods, and using computers makes it possible to study parallel the morbidity of malignant tumours and that of pretumourous diseases.

Descriptive and analytical studies which established the specific features in the dissemination of malignant tumours have made it possible for the health workers to make a differentiated approach to these problems in planning to organize concrete cancer control measures in the individual Union Republics.

In the recent years in the epidemiology of malignant tumours great attention has been paid to the elaboration and study of the factors of risk, which play a certain role in tumour morbidity of a number of sites and, to a certain extent, can explain the non-uniformity of their dissemination in individual areas of the country.

In the USSR there are characteristic differences in the distribution of cancers of the skin, stomach, mammary gland, cervix uteri, esophagus, those of the oral cavity, and of the primary cancer of the liver.

Differences in the distribution of c a n c e r o f t h e   s k i n   are expressed by the high morbidity indices characteristic of several areas of the country. The morbidity index for the whole of the USSR is 21.7; the highest indices are recorded for the Estonian SSR - 30.1; the Latvian SSR - 24.6; the Ukrainian SSR - 21.1; the Moldavian SSR - 16.2; the Kazakh SSR - 16.6, whereas the lowest indices occur in the Uzbek SSR - 9.3; the Georgian SSR - 9.5 and the Turkmenian SSR - 9.4. Experimental documents indicate a comparatively high incidence of cancer and precancerous lesions of the skin and the lower lip among fishermen and seamen, which is probably due to long exposure to extreme fluctuations of air temperature, bright sunshine, strong winds. Among these occupational groups actinic keratoses localized on the face and hands frequently occur; in a number of cases epitheliomas are observed.

For studying the specific features in the distribution of tumours the c a n c e r o f t h e o r a l c a v i t y is of great interest. There are zones in the USSR with a relatively high morbidity of this form of tumour. These are the areas of Bukhara, Samarkand, Krasnovodsk and other cities in the Central Asian Republics, where a part of the population, instead of smoking tobacco, puts a mixture called 'nas', containing tobacco, ash, lime and some oils under the tongue. The recipe. of nas: 800 g of ash, 100-150 g of lime and some cotton oil are added to 1 kg of tobacco; sometimes cement is added instead lime. 80 % of users of this mixture are men and 20 % women. The examination have shown that persons using 'nas' have a great number of leukoplakias, papillomas and cracks on the mucosa of the oral cavity. The incidence of cancer of the oral cavity proved to be much higher in these areas than in any other parts of the country, reaching 15-21 per 100,000 population, whereas in the Baltic area this index did not exceed 9-10 per 100,000 population.

In several areas of the USSR there is a relatively high incidence of c a n c e r o f e s o p h a g u s /figures for 1974/, e.g., in the Yakut ASSR /49.4 per 100,000 population/, in a number of regions of the Kazakh SSR /Guryev - 86.4 per 100,000, Semipalatinsk - 47.0/, in the Karelian ASSR 15.3 per 100,000 and in some parts of the Far North while it is 2.8 per 100,000 population in Minsk. Low indices have been noted also in the Moldavian SSR /1.4 per 100,000/.

A comprehensive analysis of this complicated problem is now going on; a study of the ethnic and domestic habits and customs of the population has made it possible to reveal some differences in feeding habits which in some way apparently affect the high incidence of cancer of the esophagus, though they cannot fully explain it.

In zones where with the cancer of the esophagus, has a higher incidence its upper third is more frequently affected than in regions where it occurs comparatively seldom.

C a n c e r o f s t o m a c h. In the recent years

there has been a tendency towards reduction of the incidence
of cancer of the stomach for the whole of the USSR /42.3 in
1970, and 41.4 in 1974/; at the same time great differences
are found in the incidence rates of cancer of the stomach in
the individual republics.

Thus, these indices for Uzbekistan, Georgia, Tadzhikistan
and Turkmenia are 12.7, 13.8, 12.9, 16.0 per 100,000 population
respectively, whereas for the Russian Federation, Estonia,
Byelorussia they are 51.2, 50.5, 46.8 respectively. Such well-
-marked differences made it necessary to analyze the possible
etiological factors, influencing the incidence of this disease.
It is extremely important to study the feeding habits and their
effect on the development of precancerous diseases and cancer
of the stomach. The character and lack of protein in the .food,
or the abundance of food rich in carbohydrates, the quantity
and quality of the food taken, methods of cooking and preparation /the heavy consumption of smoked and canned food/,
regularity of meals, the use of hot food, spices, alcoholic
beverages and also smoking are significant here. Studies have
been published pointing to the association of cancer of the
stomach with various contents of salt in the soil and waters,
or with the presence of copper, iodine, magnesium, molybdenum
in them. Helminthic invasions are are considered to be important factors, too.

A recent tendency towards the reduction in the incidence
of cancer of the stomach is noted in the USSR, though this is
accompanied by an increase in the incidence of cancer of the
large intestine, including the rectum.

C a n c e r   o f   t h e   l i v e r. Primary cancer of
the liver occurs seldom in the USSR. Attention should be drawn
to the fact that the incidence of cancer of the liver is higher
in areas of Siberia where there is a higher incidence of
opisthorchiasis /Omsk, Tobolsk/. Among the etiological factors,
in addition to opisthorchiasis, other parasitic invasions may
be considered, particularly bilharziasis.

C a n c e r   o f   t h e   l u n g s. In the recent
years the incidence of the malignant tumours of the respiratory

organs increased considerably in men and slightly in women. The total morbidity index for lung cancer for the whole of the USSR increased from 20.8 in 1970 to 24.5 in 1974. There are clear-cut sexual differences in the morbidity of lung cancer; namely in 1974 in men the intensive morbidity index was 41.8, the standardized one 48.6, whereas in women indices were 9.6 and 6.7, respectively. There are definite differences between the lung cancer incidence of the individual republics. A positive relationship was established between the incidence of lung cancer and smoking. At zones where the smoking habit is absent or it is replaced by the habit of chewing tobacco or other mixtures, the incidence of lung cancer is relatively low. There are data pointing to the role of smoke pollution of the atmosphere and chronic pneumonias in the development of lung cancer.

M a m m a r y c a r c i n o m a. The growing incidence of mammary carcinoma among women is apparent. In 1970 the intensive and standardized indices were 18.6 and 15.2, respectively, whereas in 1974 they increased to 22.2 and 18.3. There are certain differences in the incidence of mammary carcinoma of the constituent republics; thus, the highest incidence of the disease is found in the Estonian and Latvian Republics /20.3 and 18.2/, whereas in the republics of Central Asia and the Transcaucasus these indices are not so high and fluctuate from 3.5 /Tadzhikistan/ to 13.6 /Azerbaijan/.

Investigations concerning the development of mammary carcinoma have revealed its dependence on certain living conditions, habits and customs of the woman concerned.

Mammary carcinoma develops mainly in women with functional deviations of the mammary gland and the ovaries. Its incidence is higher in unmarried women than in married ones. Rejection of breast feeding and very few pregnancies enhance the risk of developing mammary cancer. The ratio of mammary carcinoma incidence in women who had no children and those with six and more children is 2 to 1. There is practically no difference in the incidence of mammary carcinoma in unmarried and married women who had no children. The role of lasting breast feeding in the prevention of carcinoma and precancerous diseases of the mammary gland has been proved.

There is a definite connection between the number of abortions and the development of pretumourous diseases of the mammary gland. Abortions probably have a certain influence on the endocrine regulation of the mammary gland. Of certain interest is the question of the relationship between the duration of the menstrual period and the endocrine regulation of the mammary gland, on one hand, and the incidence of pretumourous diseases and carcinoma of the breast, on the other. According to preliminary data, patients with mammary carcinoma have a somewhat longer menstrual period than women in the control group. A reverse ratio was established between the incidence of mammary carcinoma and cervical carcinoma. In the majority of regions lowest incidence for mammary carcinoma coincides with a relatively high incidence of cervical carcinoma. This is due to the fact that a higher number of child births, while diminishing the threat of developing mammary carcinoma, somewhat raises that of contracting cervical carcinoma.

C a n c e r   o f   t h e   f e m a l e   r e p r o -
d u c t i v e   o r g a n s. During the recent years the incidence of cervical carcinoma has dropped /14.0 in 1970 and 12.9 in 1974/. The lowest incidence has been recorded in the republics of Central Asia and the Transcaucasus /4.5 in Tadzhikistan, 4.8 in Azerbaijan/ and the highest in the republics of the Baltic area, in the Ukrainian SSR /14.5/ and in the Russian Federation /14.6/.

It has been established that the incidence of cervical carcinoma is dependent upon the characteristics of sexual life and, in particular, the number of pregnancies and child births. Cervical carcinoma is observed exceptionally seldom in unmarried women who had no pregnancies or child births. Among the factors which play a role in the development of cervical carcinoma early sexual life, numerous marriages and promiscuity, low hygienic standards, early child birth inadequate obstetrical-gynecological care should be mentioned. Each of these factors or some of their combinations are characteristic

of different groups of the population and this doubtlessly determines a higher or lower cervical carcinoma incidence in
these groups.

In view of the state character of cancer control in the
USSR, it should be mentioned that data on tumour epidemiology
are of the greatest importance for planning a number of measures aimed at improving the oncological service to the population /network, training of personnel, the organization of
purposeful preventive and hygienic measures, etc./.

History of Cancer Control in the USSR

In Russia the first attempts at an active control of malignant neoplasms were made early in the 20th century. In 1907
a group of obstetricians and gynecologists in Petersburg discussed a project for organizing cancer control. A broad program
of medical and health education measures were outlined towards
controlling the tumours of the female reproductive organs;
however, lack of material assets prevented their implementation. In 1908 the Society for the Control of Cancer Diseases
was organized.

The aim of the Society was to study the causes of cancer,
the treatment and care of cancer patients and the realization
of the program outlined by the obstetrical-gynecological society. Beginning from 1909 the Society was called "All-Russian
Society for the Control of Cancer Diseases". The same year the
11th Pirogov Convention was held during which the attention of
the medical community was attracted to papers "On Cancer
Statistics and Symptoms of Cancer Patients in Russia" by A.E.
Gagen-Torn and "Cancer Control Measures" by N. M. Kakushkin.
A program paper "The Statistics of Cancer Diseases Throughout
Russia" was submitted to the 12th Pirogov Convention. In 1911
a private hospital for women suffering from cancer was opened
in Petersburg /before that an institute for the treatment of
tumour patients was opened in Moscow in 1903/. The First All-
-Russian Congress for the Control of Cancer Disease was held
in 1914 to which a paper was submitted by V.G. Korenevski and
F.K. Veber on "The Modern State of the Study and Control of
Malignant Neoplasms in Russia in View of the Need to Organize

such Control". In 1910 N.N. Petrov's book "The General Treatise on Tumours" was published, which was highly assessed by contemporary scientists and for many years served as a manual for physicians interested in the problem of cancer. It has to be admitted that in prerevolutionary Russia assistance to patients with malignant tumours was practically absent and only a few concerned physicians made attempts to tackle this problem and provide at least some medical aid for oncological patients.

Looking at the historical aspect of developing oncological service to the population in the USSR, one must note that from the very first years it was built up by the state as a specialized and independent branch of medicine; this largely determined the paths of its further development and improvement. As early as 1918 scientific research institutes of roentgenology, radiology and oncology were founded in Leningrad /then Petrograd/, Moscow and Kharkov, which launched studies and investigations into the problems of the pathogenesis, diagnostic and treatment of malignant tumours and tackled the most urgent tasks in organizing cancer control. In the following years the problem of organizing the control of malignant neoplasms was repeatedly brought to the attention of the medical community. Thus, in 1923 at the First Congress of Physicians of the Volga Region a decision was made on the organization of anticancer societies in the Union republics. At the All-Russian Congress of Roentgenologists and Radiologists in 1924 the diagnostics and treatment of malignant neoplasms were discussed as one of the program questions.

A year later, in 1925 an All-Russian Conference was held in Moscow on malignant tumour control. In 1931 the 1st All--Union Congress of Oncologists and Roentgenoligists was organized. The Congress recognized the necessity for the state and public control of cancer, mainly in the sphere of early detection, registration and treatment of patients with malignant tumours.

The participants of the congress gave wide support and approval to the proposal on applying the dispensary method in the practice of oncological institutions.

In 1933 the USSR joined the newly organized International Union Against Cancer. In 1934 the Soviet government issued a decree "On the organization for the Control of Cancer Diseases" which formulated the basic principles of a state system for services to oncological patients.

In 1938 the People's Commissariat of Public Health decreed the establishment of tumour-diagnostic rooms and oncological hospitals in 45 towns and cities of the country and introduced the obligatory registration of patients with malignant tumours in cities where oncological institutions were available.

Thus, already in the 20s and 40s the general principles of building up an oncological service were elaborated, a rather widespread network of oncological institutes, dispensaries and tumour-diagnostic rooms was set up and the general principles of organizing oncological care for the population were formulated.

The Great Patriotic War /Second World War/ delayed the further development of the country's oncological network, which started so vigorously in the prewar years. Nevertheless, already in April 1945 the government adopted a decision "On Measures to Improve Oncological Services to the Population", which marked an important stage in building up the oncological network and controlling malignant neoplasms. By this decision specialized oncological assistance to patients with malignant neoplasms was made obligatory throughout the territory of the Soviet Union; actually it was from this time that a new very important and significant period began in organizing cancer control in the USSR. It envisaged the establishment of 126 oncological dispensaries in the republics, regions, territories and large cities of the country.

At the same time the doctrine of oncological aid to the population of the USSR was formulated; the basic provisions of this doctrine are still valid and can be outlined as follows:

1. Cancer control is a nation-wide measure carried out under the guidance of the USSR Ministry of Health and its bodies in the republics. All the elements of this organization are interconnected and operate under a single plan and

by uniform methods.

2. All kinds of preventive measures and methods of treatment of oncological patients are free of charge and accessible to everybody.

3. The activities of specialized oncological institutions are based on the dispensary method, which permits to carry out the immediate registration of patients with primarily established diagnoses of malignant neoplasms, their special treatment, and follow-up medical supervision throughout the patient's lives and, lastly, the implementation of preventive measures on a nation-wide scale, aimed at the detection of tumourous and pretumourous diseases.

4. In addition to the specialized institutions, every general prophylactic institution of the country takes part in cancer control.

5. The training of physicians and paramedical personnel for work in oncological institutions and improving the oncological qualification of the physicians of the general medical network is carried out systematically.

6. Anticancer health education is carried out widely among the population.

The idea of implementing mass cancer-prophylactic measures on a nation-wide scale, as set forth by N.N. Petrov, found an expression in 1947-1948 in the organization of mass preventive screenings of the population aimed at detecting tumourous and pretumourous diseases.

The efficiency of these measures made it possible for the USSR Ministry of Health to issue a special order in 1948 which made it obligatory to carry out mass prophylactic screenings within the organized system of medical services to the population. Whereas during the first years 19-20 million people were screened every year, by 1960 36 million were examined, in 1963 more than 45 million, in 1967 83 million, and finally, in 1974 more than 100 million were screened.

From among the patients in whom a malignant neoplasm was diagnosed for the first time in their lives 7-10 % on an average were detected during the mass prophylactic screenings

512

of the population; in recent years it has become possible to raise the efficiency of the screenings by the wide introduction of suitable methods of examination.

In accordance with a government decision, beginning from 1953 the selective registration of oncological patients was replaced by overall and obligatory registration of the cancer morbidity and mortality of the population's and, in this way, the beginnings of a state oncological statistics in the USSR.

In 1956 the Minister of Public Health of the USSR issued an order "Improving Oncological Aid to the Population", which defined a system for organizing oncological aid, the pattern of the staff and functions of an oncological dispensary, tumour-diagnostic room, the functions of a district oncologist, the system of carrying out mass prophylactic screenings of the population, and also the role of oncological and roentgenological institutes in giving scientific and methodological guidance to the country's oncological network. The same year the USSR Ministry of Health published "A Collection of Instructions on the Questions of Organizing Oncological Aid, Prevention, Diagnosis and Treatment of Malignant Tumours". The publication of the Collection of Instructions was undertaken to familiarize physicians of the general medical network with the principles of registration, prophylactic examinations, diagnosis and treatment of patients with tumourous and pretumourous diseases. Besides, the Collection of Instructions included also registration forms for oncological patients, subject to filling in accordance with the state legislation. Experiences has shown that the volume has played an exceptionally important role to make the physicians of the general medical network and oncologists aware of their tasks in the sphere of organizing cancer control and improving oncological services to the population.

In 1968 the Central Committee of the Communist Party of the Soviet Union and the Council of Ministers of the USSR published a decision "Measures for the Further Improvement of Public Health and the Development of Medical Science in the Country" in accordance with which the construction of 22 major oncological dispensaries was launched with a total of 10,000 beds and specialized oncological boarding houses for 120 patients each.

The further development of oncological services to the population was regulated by a number of decisions of the USSR Council of Ministers and orders of the USSR Ministry of Public Health which envisaged important measures to strengthen the material and technical base of oncological institutions, the development of scientific research, the training of oncologists.

Scientific research in the field of oncology receives special support in the USSR. As already mentioned, in 1918-1920 roentgenological research institutes were founded in Leningrad, Kharkov and Kiev; in 1920 the Moscow institute for the treatment of tumours, as well as the N.A. Herzen Oncological Institute in Moscow under the Ministry of Health of the Russian Federation resumed their work.

In 1924 the Central Institute of Roentgenology and Radiology was opened in Moscow. In 1926 a scientific-practical institute of oncology was organized in Leningrad /at present the Oncological Research Institute named after Professor N.N. Petrov, under the USSR Ministry of Health/. A specialized journal Voprosy Onkologii /"Problems of Oncology"/ had been published in 1928, first in Kharkov and than in Moscow till 1937. Its publication was resumed in 1955.

The network of oncological, roentgenological and radiological research institutes steadily expanded in the postwar years as well. Its foundation and organization was based on the idea that every constituent Union Republic should have a centre for scientific research and organizational-methodological work in oncology. Therefore, in 1946 a research institute of roentgenology, radiology and oncology was founded in the Armenian SSR. In 1952 the Institute of Experimental Pathology and Therapy of Cancer, USSR Academy of Sciences, was organized in Moscow /at present the Oncological Research Centre, USSR Academy of Medical Sciences/, in 1957 an Oncological Institute was opened in the Lithuanian SSR, in 1958 an Oncological Institute was established in the Georgian SSR, and the Institute of Roentgenology, Radiology and Oncology in the Uzbek SSR. In

1959 the Institute of Oncology and Radiology was organized in the Kirghizian SSR. In 1960 the Institute of Experimental and Clinical Oncology was established in Kiev /today the Institute of Oncological Problems, under the Ukrainian SSR Ministry of Health/. In the same year the Institute of Oncology and Radiology in the Kazakh SSR, the Institute of Oncology and Medical Radiology in the Byelorussian SSR, and also the Institute of Oncology in the Moldavian SSR were established. In 1962 the Institute of Medical Radiology, USSR Academy of Medical Sciences, was established at Obninsk, and in 1963 the Oncological Institute was organized in the Turkmenian SSR.

Thus, at present the USSR has 20 scientific research oncological and radiological institutes which study problems of pathogenesis, diagnostics, treatment, and epidemiology of malignant tumours and the organization of cancer control. Besides, numerous medical institutes and institutes for postgraduate medical education, as well as a number of scientific research institutes and laboratiries contribute to the development of the comprehensive problem of malignant neoplasms.

In accordance with the order of the USSR Ministry of Health "Improving Oncological Services to the Population", the research institutes of oncology and radiology, beginning from 1956, provide scientific and methodological guidance to the oncological network of the country; this has led to a notable improvement in the standards of the medical and prophylactic work of the oncological network, to the more energetic introduction of scientific results into practice; the framework and possibilities for the advanced training and specialization of oncologists and for drawing them into research work have also expanded considerably.

Soviet scientists have made a great contribution to the development of the problem malignant neoplasms. Thus, N.N. Petrov, one of the major Soviet experts and clinicians, created the polyetiologic theory of tumour development, and greatly contributed to the development of clinical and experimental oncology, to well-established control system of the Soviet Union. The advance of clinical oncology is closely associated with the names of A.I. Savitsky, P.A. Gertsen, A.V. Melnikov, E.L. Berezov, S.S. Yudin, S.A. Kholdin, A.I. Rakov, B.V. Petrovsky, A.I. Serebrov, who substantiated questions pertaining to surgical radicalism and ablation in oncology, developed and improved a number of methods for treating malignant neoplasms. L.F. Larionov is justly considered one of the pioneers in the therapy of tumours in this country; a great contribution to the study of the viral origin of cancer has been made by L.A. Zilber, G.I. Abelev and others. Problems of the morphology and histogenesis of tumour are widely represented in the works of M.F. Glazunov, V.G. Garshin, N.G. Khlopin, I.V. Davydovsky, A.I. Timofeyevsky. Works by L.M. Shabad are devoted to studying carcinogenic agents in the environment and devising methods for their prophylaxis; works by R.A. Kavetski are devoted to the study of the complex interactions between the tumour and the organism. Among those who greatly contributed to the organization of oncological service for the population one must name N.N. Petrov, A.I. Serebrov, N.N. Blokhin, N.P. Napalkov, N.N. Alexandrov, E.G. Kudimova.

Thus, as a result of many years of joint work of the organizers of public health and scientists, a specialized oncological service has been built up in the USSR comprising 22 oncological research, roentgenologic and radiologic institutes, 249 oncological dispensaries, 3,133 oncological departments and tumour-diagnostic rooms, 50,300 specialized oncological beds in hospitals /1974/. 61.5 % of the 249 oncological dispensaries have at their disposal at least 100 beds each. The whole system of cancer control in the country is headed by the USSR Ministry of Health, which has an Oncological Services Board.

The leading oncological institution of the USSR Ministry of Health is the N.N. Petrov Oncological Research Institute, which coordinates scientific research in three main problems: /i/ Organization of cancer control and the prophylaxis of malignant tumours; /ii/ Diagnosis of malignant tumours, and /iii/ Clinical, surgical and comprehensive treatment of malignant tumours. Besides, the leading institute provides scientific and methodological guidance to the entire oncological

network of the country. The coordination of scientific research
in the sphere of theoretical oncological problems is entrusted
to the Oncological Research Centre of the USSR Academy of
Medical Sciences.

The realization of the basic principles of cancer control
and oncological services to the population is provided by a
widespread network of oncological institutions. The main structural unit of the oncological network is an oncological dispensary /republican, territorial, regional, city/, which is
subordinated to the appropriate Republican Ministry of Public
Health, regional, territorial or city health department. When
catering to several rural districts, a city oncological dispensary may have to fulfil the functions of an interregional
dispensary. The scope of activities of a dispensary is rather
wide and covers practically the whole range of questions involved in providing oncological services to patients. A good
idea of the duties of an oncological dispensary can be
revealed from the "Regulations Governing an Oncological Dispensary", which is as follows.

1. The oncological dispensary is a prophylactic institution, providing qualified specialized inpatient and outpatient
oncological services to the population of a certain territory
in which it is located /republic, territory, region, city/,
provides organizational and methodological guidance to prophylactic institutions in matters of oncology, specialization and
raising the qualification of physicians and paramedical personnel in the diagnosis and treatment of patients with malignant
tumours.

2. The structure of an oncological dispensary is determined
by the size of the population it serves, the level and pattern
of morbidity and the number of beds available. The structure
of oncological institutions must provide, first of all, for
surgical, gynecologic, radiological, roentgenologic, and out-
patient departments; highly specialized departments may also
be provided, such as for the tumours of the head and neck,
urological, pediatric departments.

3. The main tasks of the dispensary are as follows:

- to provide the full scope of qualified specialized in-patient and outpatient medical services to oncological patients;

- to provide organizational and methodological guidance to and to coordinate the activities of every oncological institution /oncological dispensaries, departments, tumour-diagnostic rooms/, organizational and methodological guidance to every prophylactic institution pertaining to questions of the early identification of malignant neoplasms and precancerous diseases, treatment and dispensary observation of patients;

- regular analysis of the data of morbidity and mortality due to malignant neoplasms;

- the drawing up of annual comprehensive plans for anti--cancer measures and submitting them for approval to the ministry of health of the republic, the territorial /regional, city/ departments of health;

- participation in drawing up long-term and annual plans for developing the network of oncological institutions and submitting them to the appropriate organizations;

- the timely development of prophylactic measures carrying out the diagnosis and treatment of malignant neoplasms, of modern methods and means of diagnosis and treatment of onco-logical diseases;

- to carry out methods for raising the oncological quali-fications of the paramedical personnel at prophylactic institutions by organizing ten-day courses, seminars and other forms of study;

- to analyse the causes of late diagnosis of patients with malignant neoplasms and to elaborate measures to remove them. Supervision of the drawing up and examination of negligence protocols;

- to work out proposals towards organizing and carrying out prophylactic screenings for detecting patients with malignant neoplasms and pretumourous diseases within the territory concerned;

- supervision over the carrying out of preventive screenings, aimed at detecting patients with malignant neoplasms and pretumourous diseases;

- to analyse the efficiency of preventive screenings of the population to detect malignant neoplasms and pretumourous diseases, and working out measures aimed at raising the efficiency of such screenings;

- to carry out accurate and complete registration of oncological patients to check up its organization at oncological dispensaries, departments and tumour-diagnostic rooms, and to carry out dispensary observation over oncological patients and of the state of such observation at dispensary departments and tumour-diagnostic rooms;

- to analyse the efficiency of treatment of oncological patients at medical and prophylactic institutions of the republic and to work out measures towards the most rational organization of medical services to these patients;

- to check up the timely hospitalization and beginning of treatment of oncological patients, to check up the complete and correct spending of assets for the free outpatient treatment of oncological patients;

- to check up the appropriateness of treating oncological patients at medical and prophylactic institutions;

- to organize and carry out broad health educational anticancerous campaign among the population, jointly with the houses of health education;

- to carry out the registration and submit performance reports according to forms, by the dates prescribed by the Ministry of Health of the USSR and the Central Statistical Board of the USSR.

4. The oncological dispensary /republican, territorial, regional, city/ is an independent unit of the public health system. It has at its disposal buildings with appropriate grounds, appropriate equipment, inventory and other property and enjoys the rights of a juridical person.

5. The oncological dispensary /republican, territorial, regional, city/ is subordinated directly to the Ministry of Public Health of the Republic, or to the territorial, regional or city health department.

The chief physician enjoys the rights prescribed for the

heads of republican, territorial, regional and city hospitals.

The chief physician of the oncological dispensary is, as a rule, the non-staff chief oncologist, and is responsible for the organization of oncological services in the republic /territory, region, city/.

6. The staff of the oncological dispensary /republican, territorial, regional, city/ is established according to patterns of current staffs.

7. The oncological dispensary may be a clinical /training/ centre for related chairs of a medical institute, of an institute for postgraduate medical education, or a scientific research institute, as well as a centre for the practical training of medical students and trainees of secondary medical schools.

8. For the purposes of widely involving the public and various organizations in the fulfilment of measures aimed at improving the performance of the oncological dispensary and the medical services to the population, a public council is organized at the oncological dispensary, which is guided by regulations endorsed by the USSR Ministry of Health and the All Union Central Council of Trade Unions /AUCCTU/ in 1965.

The overwhelming majority of oncological dispensaries are furnished with up-to-date diagnostic and therapeutic equipment enabling them to widely carry out X-ray, endoscopic, cytological examinations and also to provide comprehensive surgical and radiation therapy.

The construction of standard radiological buildings have made it possible to carry out comprehensive and combined methods of treatment and considerably improve the working conditions of the medical personnel.

At present concerted and purposeful work is currently going on towards consolidating the oncological dispensaries.

In the USSR the number of oncological beds is two per 10,000 population.

In the system of oncological service to the population an important role is played by the tumour-diagnostic rooms or departments of outpatient clinics and by the regional oncologist, whose tasks include bringing the oncological services as close to the population as possible. Their basic functions are determined by the following regulations:

1. Tumour-diagnostic rooms /departments/ are organized as parts of polyclinics /polyclinical departments/ of the general city and central, regional hospitals, in accordance with current patterns of staffs.

2. The physician of the tumour-diagnostic room /department/ is subordinated to the chief physician of the polyclinic, and the organizational-methodological aspect to the chief physician of the regional /territorial, republican, city/ oncological dispensary, and is responsible for the state of oncological services in his area;

- a physician having special training shall be appointed as the physician of the tumour-diagnostic room.

If oncological departments are organized at polyclinics, the head of the oncological department assumes the functions of the regional oncologist. When several tumour-diagnostic rooms are available in a region, one of the physicians is assigned the functions of the regional oncologist;

- the opening hours of the tumour-diagnostic room /department/ are kept in the prescribed manner;

- the tumour-diagnostic room /department/ works according to a plan approved by the head of the institution in which the room /department/ is organized. The plan should be coordinated with the oncological dispensary.

3. The main task of the tumour-diagnostic room /oncological department/ is the organization of anticancerous measures to be carried out by the general network, carrying out the registration and dispensary observation of oncological patients, outpatient examination and timely treatment of patients.

In accordance with the above, the physician of the tumour--diagnostic room /oncological department/ of the polyclinic carries out the following:

- primary and consultative examination of patients, visiting him with complaints of malignant and benign tumours, and also premalignant diseases;

- organizes the hospitalization of patients with malignant neoplasms for special treatment;

- analyzes the reasons of refusal of cancer patients to go into hospital for specialized or symptomatic treatment;

- carries out the registration of all patients with malignant neoplasms residing in the territory belonging to the room /department/ and sees to it that notification slips on their condition are sent to oncological dispensaries;

- carries out prophylactic examination of patients with malignant neoplasms and some forms of precancerous diseases;

- marks the dates of examinations, the time and duration of inpatient treatment, the treatment given in the control cards, etc.;

- visits all oncological patients needing such attention in their home, with the exception of patients of the 4th clinical group, who are visited in the home by the physicians and nurses of the polyclinic /outpatient department/ at the patients' place of residence;

- carries out outpatient hormonal and chemotherapy.

4. The physician of the tumour-diagnostic room /oncological department/ organizes and carries out methodological guidance for anticancerous measures in his area, which includes:

- carrying out prophylactic oncological screenings of the population by the personnel of prophylactic institutions;

- health educational work among the population;

- involvement of the public for carrying out anticancerous measures;

- regular analysis of diagnostic errors and an examination of the latter together with the physicians of the polyclinic responsible for these errors and mistakes, and the organization of conferences to analyse the causes of the late detection of cancer.

5. The oncological room /department/ is staffed according to current patterns of staffs.

In its activities the oncological service of the country

is closely connected to the entire system of institutions belonging to the general medical network. If one takes into account that a patient first of all turns, as a rule, to the polyclinic at the place of his residence of to the medical unit at the enterprise where he is employed, it is obvious that his further fate depends on the accessibility of medical aid and the qualification and training of the physicians of the general medical network. At present the Soviet public health service has a considerable material and technical base at its disposal. There are some 25,000 inpatient medical institutions in the country with 3,012 thousand hospital beds, and some 36,000 outpatient polyclinical isntitutions. More than 5 million people are employed in public health, including 832,000 physicians, 2,500,000 paramedical workers and paramedical staff and more than 160,000 pharmaceutists. There are 118 hospital beds, 32.5 physicians and 99 paramedical workers per every 10,000 population.[x]

The primary examination of patients suspected for malignant tumours is carried out, as a rule, in an institution of the general medical network /outpatient polyclinical network/; likewise, patients being treated in a hospital for other than oncological diseases are subjected to obligatory prophylactic examination to exclude malignant neoplasms of the basic sites. The equipment of the outpatient polyclinical network and hospitals makes it possible to use the basic diagnostic methods necessary for the early identification of malignant neoplasms.

Apart from the prophylaxis the general hospitals carry out also substantial therapeutic work in oncology, since about 50 % of oncological patients are hospitalized for treatment /predominantly surgical/ in the general medical network. It should also be mentioned that the outpatient polyclinical network carries out prophylactic examinations of patients with a whole number of pretumourous diseases and also mass prophylactic screenings of the population.

---

[x] S.P. Burenkov, Journ. "Sovetskoye Zdravookhraneniye", 1976, No. 6, pp. 3-10.

Thus, the general medical network plays an extremely important role in providing oncological service to the population.

THE SYSTEM OF REGISTRATION OF PATIENTS WITH PRIMARILY DIAGNOSED MALIGNANT NEOPLASMS IN THE USSR

N.N. Aleksandrov and Z.M. Gutman

The nation-wide registration of patients with malignant neoplasms is a component of the integrated system of statistical information on public health and organization of health service in the USSR. The system is primarily concerned not only with collecting data necessary for rendering expedient medical care or for current and long-term planning of measures aimed at providing oncological service for the population, but also with accumulating materials which may be useful for research in cancer epidemiology and statistics.

The large-scale system of registering patients with malignant neoplasms was introduced in the USSR in 1932, first in the Ukrainian SSR, then in 1939 in every Soviet city having oncological institutions. The implementation of the cancer control programme was interrupted by the war and continued in the postwar period. Since 1953 the compulsory registration of cancer patients has been practiced all over the territory of the USSR.

The first postwar census of the Soviet population in 1959 created favourable conditions for expanding the statistical research in oncology. The rapid development of oncological statistics in the country was due also to the establishment of a large-scale network of specialized cancer control institutions. In 1959 the network included 226 oncological dispensaries and more than 1,600 oncological departments and consulting rooms in hospitals and polyclinics of the general medical care system.

In the USSR the system of cancer registration is characterized by the following principles:

a/ it is an obligatory task of any physician to notify the oncological institution about every primarily diagnosed patient with a malignant tumour; this makes it possible to register all cancer patients, including outpatients;

b/ the expedient notification about primarily diagnosed cancer patients provides not only for a regular and continuous information flow on such patients, but also for timely calls for check-up; and

c/ the regional character of the statistical information system warrants that of all necessary data on cancer patients, including information on previous treatment are accumulated by the respective oncological institute.

The observation on the above-mentioned principles makes it possible to combine efforts involved in studying cancer morbidity rate with the organization of life-long observation of cancer patients. This can be done to a full extent only if there is a generally available, free and adequate medical care and well-established network of specialized oncological institutions.

Thus, the major source of information on patients with primarily diagnosed malignant neoplasms is a physician of a therapeutic and prophylactic institution, who sees the patient first. According to the existing regulation, the physician must compile and send a report to the respective regional oncological institution within three days; the form of this report has been approved by the USSR Ministry of Health and is obligatory for all medical institutions in the country. This standard document is designed to register several other diseases, too, and is called "Notification on a patient with primarily diagnosed active tuberculosis, venereal disease, trichophytosis, microsporia, favus, trachoma, cancer or other malignant tumours".

Rules for filling in the "Notification", like other medical documentation used for registration and follow-up of cancer cases by the oncological dispensaries, are compiled in special instructions approved by the USSR Ministry of Health.

The "Notification" is filled in in Russian or in the language of the Union republic where the patient lives. Taking into account the considerable migrational processes within the country and the desire of many patients to obtain treatment in

the major oncological centres, especially in the metropolitan
ones, the existing rules stipulate that the "Notification" must
contain information not on the temporary, but on the permanent
address of the patient. This facilitates the registration and
follow-up of cancer cases by the respective regional oncological institutions. At the same time, it makes possible to
analyse morbidity rates in each region, calculating them separately for the urban and rural population in all the Union republics and regions of the country. An important requirement
for physicians filling in the "Notification" is the indication
of the complete diagnosis fo the disease. It should include on
the type of tumour /cancer, sarcoma, leukosis, etc./, its exact
localization in the organ, and the size of the affected area
/degree of the disease/. Moreover, the "Notification" should
contain information on the diagnostic technique used and
whether the patient is recommended for special /radical/ treatment or not. In this connection, according to the existing instructions it is necessary to indicate beside the degree of
the tumour process /in cases when it can be determined/ also
the clinical group to which the primarily diagnosed or registered case should be assigned. To this end, the standard classification of oncological patients by clinical groups known
for all physicians, has been introduced. The groups are as
follows:

Ia - patients with suspected malignant tumours;
Ib - patients with precancerous diseases;
II - patients with malignant neoplasms amenable for special
     or radical treatment;
III - patients requiring no special treatment since they have
      already completed it and are practically healthy; and
IV - patients with advanced forms of cancer requiring
     symptomatic or palliative medical care.

Since the tasks of specialized medical service for patients with malignant tumours consist both in establishing an
accurate diagnosis and providing the cancer patients with a
timely treatment and subsequent control an oncological institution uses the notifications received for filling in a

"Control dispensary record" for each new patient irrespective
of the clinical group to which he was assigned. The detailed
information on the results of primary and annual follow-up of
a cancer patient, contained in such a record, makes it possible
to specify the data reported in the notification and serves as
an additional source of statistical information on cancer patients. If a malignant neoplasm was first diagnosed in an oncological institution, especially in patients sent there with
a suspected tumour, the "Notification" is filled in by oncologists working in this oncological institution.

All information pertaining to primary oncological cases
is stored and processed in the organizational and methodological rooms of the dispensary oncological departments of regional
and city hospitals. At the end of the year under review the
local oncological institutions verify the diagnosis and send
notifications to the regional cancer control centre /regional
oncological dispensary/ where the documents are used to prepare
an annual statistical summary. All dispensaries compare these
materials with the information contained in the card file to
know whether a given patient has been registered as a cancer
patient. In a number of cases a regional dispensary may carry
out an additional survey of recently registered patients on
its own initiative to specify the diagnosis and to plan medical care, the survey being done as a form of control or
methodological assistance.

Apart from the above-described main channel of obtaining
information on oncological patients, oncological services make
use of other information sources. Thus, in those isolated
cases when the notification on a primary cancer patient is not
received for some reasons, the necessary information may be
obtained from data contained in "Extract from a cancer patient
record". The form was approved by the USSR Ministry of Health
as early as 1956. It is supposed to be filled in and sent to
the corresponding oncological institutions of the area of the
patient's residence, by all inpatient departments in which
the patient was checked up or treated. Information contained
in the "Extract from a cancer patient record" makes it

possible to detail in most patients the diagnosis, histological form of the tumour, nature of treatment received, etc.

Additional information used to specify the available data or sometimes to report on a primary cancer case may be derived from the "Report on diagnosis of a patient with a neglected form of malignant tumour". At present such records are drawn up not only for patients of the clinical group IV, but also for patients in stage III of a cancer which can be determined by visual examination /cancer of skin, tongue, oral cavity, lower lip, thyroid gland, cervix uteri, mammary gland, and rectum/.

Nevertheless, even if this additional information is available, isolated cancer cases remain to be unregistered due to the inadequacy of the survey methods and diagnostic errors. These cases are recognized only at autopsy. Therefore, from 1961 onwards, all regional oncological institutions have compared their data on registered patients with those on patients died from malignant neoplasms and registered in registration certificates for the previous month on the basis of medical certificates of death. This approach makes possible not only to supplement information on cancer patients, but also to control the filling in of death certificates more strictly and to verify the validity of the diagnosis indicated.

As a result, the coverage of patients with primarily diagnosed malignant tumours is steadily increasing. Only in the past decade the proportion of patients died of malignant neoplasms and not registered during their life by an oncological institution decreased from 5.8 % in 1967 to 2.7 % in 1973 /of the total number of patients with primarily diagnosed malignant tumours/. In the Byelorussian SSR the number of such cases in 1975 was 0.6 % of the total number of deaths from cancer and 0.4 % of the total number of diagnosed cancer cases.

Information on annually registered cancer cases is included in standard state reports being prepared by oncological institutions. This provides basis for compiling summarizing reports for each region, Union republic and the USSR as a whole.

Report of regional oncological dispensaries prepared on the basis of their card files of verified notifications on primary cancer cases diagnosed during the year under review, contain information on the number of all patients grouped by their place of residence /city-dwellers, village-dwellers/, by isolated or grouped localizations of malignant tumours, and by sex and age groups.

All oncological services /dispensaries, departments, consulting rooms/ use their card files of control dispensary records and of other medical documents to prepare statistical reports on the number of registered cancer cases, annual changes in their composition /those primarily registered, those struck off the register, or deceased/, redistribution of patients with regard to clinical groups, methods of treatment, number of previously treated cases, and duration of their life. This information is given in the reports according to certain tumour localizations and to all malignant neoplasms as a whole.

The distribution of individual service areas within the region among city and district oncological dispensaries, department and consulting rooms was proved instrumental in covering all cancer patients registered in the region, to bring together all information available in different medical institutions on cancer cases and to provide thereby a relatively comprehensive coverage of such cases in statistical reports, eliminating duplication in registering the same patients by different cancer control institutions.

Information contained in the annual statistical reports of oncological institutions makes it possible to have an idea not only on cancer morbidity rates, but also on cancer distribution /prevalence of the disease in a given population/ in the territory of each region and Union republic.

The major source of information about deaths caused by malignant neoplasms is the statistics on the causes of death, which is distributed and studied by respective organs of the Central Statistical Board of the USSR and is based on medical information on the causes of death /"Medical certificates of death"/. At the same time, the aims of the above-mentioned reports of oncological institutions and differ from those of the statistical surveys of the causes of death, mainly in the degree of detailing the list of individual tumour localizations and distribution of cancer incidence by age groups.

As the many years' experience gained by the Soviet oncological services has shown, the timely detection, registration and adequate treatment of primary cancer cases can be possible only if there is a close cooperation among each part of the public health network to which the patients belong and oncological institutions in which the majority of such patients are subjected to additional examination and special treatment.

The heads of urban and rural health services of the general medical network are made responsible for supervising the work associated with the correct filling in of specified forms of primary documents on cancer patients and with prompt sending of such documents to the corresponding institutions.

The oncological institutions regularly control the correctness and completeness of the documents compiled. An important role in providing the efficient examination, registration and follow up of oncological patients by the local cancer control institution, especially in rural localities, is played by regional consulting rooms. In the districts, where such rooms have not yet been set up, their functions are being fulfilled by specially trained physicians of the central regional hospitals. The organizational and methodological guidance of their work is the responsibility of oncological dispensaries serving the given area.

By the end of 1975 oncological services in the USSR, consisting of 20 research institutes of oncology and radiology, 229 oncological dispensaries and about 3200 departments and consulting rooms, treated 1,856.4 thousand patients /726.5 patients per 100,000 population/ of which 1,576,000 were practically healthy /third clinical group/. In 1975 the total number of patients with primarily diagnosed malignant neoplasms amounted to 492,654 /193.7 patients per 100,000 population/.

As a whole the system of statistical reports used in the Soviet Union to keep track of primary cancer cases and registered cases is instrumental in obtaining important information necessary for evaluating the prevalence of malignant tumours in a given population group as well as for outlining the latest developments in the diagnosis and treatment of cancer. Nevertheless, owing to the decentralized nature of cancer data processing such a system excludes the possibility of a many-sided evaluation and analysis of the primary information available in oncological institutions, which is extremely important for expanding research concerned with cancer epidemiology, for improving the forms and methods of cancer control, for the purposeful planning of further development and for the efficient administration of oncological services on a nation-wide scale.

It is necessary to take into account the constantly increasing number of cancer patients in the country and, hence, the number of cancer cases registered by oncological dispensaries. Only for the decade from 1966 to 1975, cancer morbidity in the USSR increased by 12.9 %, and the total number of cancer patients registered at oncological institutions grew by almost 1.5 times. These facts manifested themselves in an increased amount of organizational and methodological work carried out by oncological institutions, which meet considerable difficulties in obtaining more complete information necessary for implementing comprehensive cancer control programmes, mainly because the existing system of data processing is not adequately mechanized.

The situation, already in the early 1960's urged the need for the elaboration and large-scale implementation of reliable, readily available and sufficiently large computerized data processing systems capable of providing a comprehensive information on cancer distribution and on the level of oncological service in each Union republic, region, and administrative district.

The search for new approaches to establish such systems designed to provide relatively complete and easy-to-analyse information on cancer patients with the help of a computer has been started in several Union republics of the USSR.

The experience gained by the Byelorussian SSR in developing such a system merited acknowledgement among the Soviet oncologists. There a centralized data processing system using the Minsk-32 computer has been successfully tested for several years at the Republican Institute of Oncology. The system, worked out by the Institute's scientists, makes it possible to obtain information on the cancer incidence rate, cancer mortality rate, and the state of dispensary care services for oncological patients, including information on diagnostic and therapeutic methods used in treating such patients as well as on the results of treatment. In 1975 the USSR Ministry of Health decided to introduce, beginning from 1977, the computerized data processing system in all oncological institutions of the Soviet Union.

This system is based on machine-readable versions of the standard form of primary documents, that is "Notification on a primary cancer patient", and "Control dispensary record" of such patient. Here we have to mention that the introduction of this system involved a considerable amount of work needed which was necessary to adjust the existing and, as the many years' experience has shown, efficient principles of registering oncological patients and monitoring the system of the dispensary-based observation of cancer cases.

On the other hand, the practical implementation of this system has permitted, Soviet oncologists to carry out these principles on a higher level.

The new form of the Notification is printed on standard forms and differs only insignificantly from the previous version with regard to its contents. The new form includes, in particular, data on circumstances under which the disease has been revealed /after visiting a doctor on the patient's own initiative, during prophylactic examination, at autopsy, etc./, the indication of the patient's nationality and occupation, the clinical group into which he was allocated after cancer diagnosis, and information on the medical institution which sent the patient for examination and treatment. This kind of information is particularly important in analysing those patients' records which for one reason or other have not been received by appropriate territorial oncological dispensary. The reverse side of the "Notification" bears instruction how it should be filled in by the physicians of the general and specialized health service network.

More significant changes have been made in the dispensary record form. As compared with the previous /standard/ form, the information contained in it has been considerably supplemented and the columns have been rearranged so as to facilitate coding and computer processing of data on results of examination and treatment of cancer patients. The inclusion of such information as deadlines for the patient's visits to a doctor, stage and the primarily diagnosed sites of cancer, the frequency and nature of repeated treatment of the patient, has made it possible to markedly increase the information capacity of the new record form.

During the testing period of the centralized computer--based data processing system, it has been revealed that the improved form of the "Control record" contains practically all data specified in the "Notification". This has facilitated the use of the former as the main report document, primary information carrier, for computer input. As a result, it became unnecessary to code the "Notification" for their subsequent computer-aided processing. At the same time, the completeness of information on the number of primary cancer cases is ascertained by the fact that at the end of the year under review, the entire file of control records assigned for computer processing is supplemented with a few similar records which have been compiled /on the basis of notifications and certificates of death/ only for those patients who have not been registered at an oncological dispensary. The "Notification" has retained its previous importance as a signalling and control document the filling in of which presents no difficulty for physicians of any medical institution and does not complicate their everyday work.

The machine processing of only one document, the "Control dispensary record", bears several other important advantages since the use of a computer decreases not only labour and time inputs required for processing the entire data base, but also eliminates the possibility of feeding the same data on the same patient more than once into the computer, which was often the case in manual data processing. Besides, the necessary machine time is reduced and the development and operation of a particular software is considerably facilitated.

The filling in of control records and their coding are carried out by respective oncological dispensaries only. Decoding of the records using a simple numerical code, requires a certain skill, but it can be performed by medium-level medical personnel under doctor's supervision. The work should be done during the whole year according to the rules envisaged by the respective methodological recommendations. The recommendations contain several classifiers for the personnel of organizational and methodological rooms as well as to physicians of oncological dispensaries; moreover, they include the necessary information on the norms and standards regulating the rules common for all the Union republics of filling in and coding of primary documents. In the instructions particular attention is given to developing a standardized approach for the evaluation of individual parameters such as nationality and occupation of patient, cancer morphology, type of treatment used, etc.

For revealing coding errors in the control records, the system's software envisages the use of several control algorithms taking into account the parameters of the coding signs and verifying their logical compatibility. If, by chance, wrongly coded information is entered into the computer, it is not recorded on the magnetic tape but is put onto the computer printing device that shows which document contains a coding error. When corrected, such documents are sent for repeated processing, and this eliminates practically every possibility of the input of wrong data. The software stipulates also a possibility of elucidating errors which may arise during transfer of data from control records to punched tape. The automatic control used in this case consists in calculating the arithmetic sum of all the numberical codes of the signs being coded in each of the primary documents assigned for processing. The results are recorded on punched tape and when the information is entered into the computer it calculates the coded data for the second time, if the results do not coincide with the control sum on the punched tape, this means an error which appeared during the transfer of information on the primary punched tape.

The software has provided also for a possibility of obtaining any combination of input data with the help of the computer and, at a later stage, this will make it possible to complete the list of output tables. At present, a standard set of such tables is recommended for practical use. It consists of 45 statistical forms for the administrative regions, each of the tables containing information on all 59 localizations of malignant tumours according to the headings of the International Classification of Diseases, 8th revision. The use of several other classification schemes and standardized indicators suggested by the World Health Organization has created favourable conditions for comparing statistical data obtained on an international level.

For the computer processing of coded information submitted by oncological institutions, plans have been worked out for using computer centres of the USSR Central Statistical Office, existing in all regional centres. In the remote areas the mailing of primary documents for computer processing over great distances presents certain difficulties. To overcome these, the use of special control cards for recoding the initial information, contained in a coded form in the control records, may be recommended.

The computer-aided processing of primary documents of oncological patients makes it possible to obtain a great amount of additional information exceeding many times the volume of data contained in the present-day annual statistical reports. As a result of the computer-aided processing of the data on the absolute number of cancer patients, as well as on their distribution by sex, nationality, and age group, it has become possible to calculate extensive, intensive, age and standardized morbidity rates for individual forms of tumours as specified in the unabridged nomenclature of the ICD, 8th revision. These indicators are calculated separately for males and females, for the urban and rural population of each Union republic, region, major city and district.

The computer processing of the "Control dispensary record" makes possible to obtain data important both from scientific and practical point of view such as frequency of morphological verification of the diagnosis, specific features of the histological structure of tumours, contribution of various medical institutions to the examination and treatment of cancer patients', causes of late diagnosis, efficiency of prophylactic examinations to diagnose early stages of cancer, frequency of refusal of curable patients to be treated for cancer, and number of patients untreated because of so-called general contraindications. A special group of information is represented by data on cancer mortality, being processed according to the programme similar to that of the morbidity data monitoring.

A great practical significance is attached also to data obtained during the comparative study of information contained in the new form of the "Control dispensary record" and pertaining to the nature, duration and results of applying a particular type of cancer treatment in different medical institutions.

The above-mentioned and other data of the centralized computer-aided processing of primary documents of oncological patients have provided a basis not only for the more adequate evaluation of diagnostic and therapeutic efficiency of the various medical institutions in each Union republic, region and district, but also for a rational monitoring of specialized cancer control programmes being implemented by oncological hospitals. At the same time the results discussed above have created conditions for a scientifically-based planning of cancer services, particularly in building new cancer centres, in training and efficient use of medical manpower, in increasing the number of hospital beds and in establishing highly specialized departments.

The many-sided information obtained with the help of a

computer has paved the way both for a large-scale evaluation of environmental factors responsible for cancer developing and conducting wide-ranging investigations into various problems in cancer epidemiology and into revealing groups of population with enhanced cancer incidence risk. All this is extremely important for developing improved forms of large-scale screening.

STATISTICS OF MALIGNANT NEOPLASMS IN THE USSR

N.P. Napalkov and V.M. Merabishvili

In accordance with the present-day requirements, oncological statistics must study the incidence of tumours among the entire population and its separate groups, the comparative frequency of tumours of different varieties and sites, the geographical, age, sex, occupational and other pecularities of the distribution of malignant neoplasms and mortality from them, as well as the efficiency of the cancer control system.

The main objectives of oncological statistics are:

/a/ determination of the present state and basic tendencies of the morbidity of, susceptibility to and mortality from malignant tumours;

/b/ evaluation of the efficiency of the measures aimed at prevention and early detection of malignant neoplasms, as well as of the treatment and rehabilitation of oncological patients;

/c/ provision of the health services with permanent information suitable for efficient supervision of the cancer control system.

In the USSR the service of oncological statistics functions in accordance of three main principles that ensure the efficiency of its work. These principles are:

1. Completeness of records of all patients with malignant neoplasms and those who died from them. This is ensured by the obligation of every physician to report to the oncological service each newly detected patient and by monthly collection of information on the recorded oncological patients and of that based on the death certificates from malignant tumours.

2. Signalling and operative character of obtaining, analysing and utilizing the information, which makes possible

the continuous supervision of the activities of the oncological network.

3. Regionality of the system of accumulation and operative utilization of the information on patients with malignant neoplasms with regard to their permanent residence.

To ensure the development of oncological statistics in accordance with these principles, all the records and operative documents of the therapeutic institutions containing information on oncological patients are constantly used as initial material. These documents are:

1. "Report on a patient with primarily diagnosed cancer or other malignant neoplasm /Record form No 281/.

2. "Control card of ambulatory observation" /Record form No 30/.

3. "Excerpt from the case history of a patient with malignant tumour" /Record form No 27-onco/.

4. "Record of detection of a patient with a neglected form of a malignant tumour" /clinical group IV/ /Record form No 248/.

5. "Report on patients with malignant neoplasms" /Inset report No 6 of form No 1/.

6. "Report on affection with cancer and other malignant neoplasms" /Report form No 61-zh/.

All the above initial documents of oncological statistics make possible, on the basis of the regional oncological dispensary, to set up an operative register of patients with malignant neoplasms.

Thus, the data on morbidity and incidence of malignant neoplasms collected from the health services on the level of regional oncological institutions together with the information on mortality which are, in their turn, concentrated by bodies of the USSR Central Statistical Office create optimal conditions for the completeness of the records. The efficiency of the regional oncological registers can be judged at least by the fact that in the USSR, on the whole, the proportion with malignant neoplasms registered only after death decreased from 5.8 % in 1967 to 2.7 % in 1976.

The principles by which the Soviet oncological statistical

service is guided in its activities are not fortuitous. Their
underestimation immediately reflected on the reliability of
the obtained material, is accompanied by considerable difficulties in its accumulation and analysis and prevents the
health services from completely utilizing the statistical data
for the efficient supervision of the cancer control organization.

The collection, elaboration and analysis of the information related to oncological statistics for the USSR as a whole
were assigned in 1974 to the Prof. N.N. Petrov /Order of the
Red Banner of Labour/ Research Institute of Oncology /USSR
Ministry of Health/. The work carried out since that time,
the incidence of malignant neoplasms and organization of medical aid to oncological patients in the USSR in 1971-1974,
shows that, if the existing tendencies persist, the number of
registered patients with malignant neoplasms will reach 2.2
million by 1980. Thus the rates of increase in the number of
patients with primarily diagnosed malignant neoplasms exceed
2-3-fold the rates of population growth in the country while
the increase in the rate of persons registered in oncological
institutions exceeds the latter fourfold.

Fig. 34 shows the dynamics of morbidity and mortality
from malignant neoplasms in the Soviet Union.

The steady increase in the morbidity rate of primarily
registered malignant neoplasms encountered by our country's
oncological network, must be taken into account in planning
the complex of cancer control measures.

From 1970 to 1974 the incidence of malignant neoplasms
in the USSR increased from 177.2 to 190.9 per 100,000 population, i.e., by 7.7 %; the mean annual increase in morbidity
during that period amounted to 1.9 %, and to 2.3 % in 1974
/Table 95/.

A higher incidence of malignant neoplasms in urban areas
has persisted all through those years. The mean annual increase
in morbidity in rural areas during the last 5 years exceeded
the incidence of malignant neoplasms in urban areas by 50 per
cent, which to a large extent is accounted for by the improved

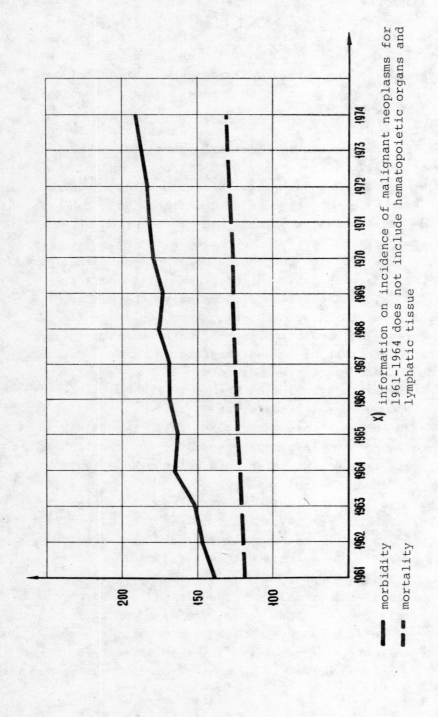

x) information on incidence of malignant neoplasms for
   1961-1964 does not include hematopoietic organs and
   lymphatic tissue

Fig. 34 Dynamics of the morbidity[x] and mortality from malignant neoplasms in the USSR
         per 100,000 population

540

Table 95

Morbidity from Malignant Neoplasms of the Population
of the USSR in 1970-1974

	Number of patients with primarily diagnosed malignant neoplasms, registered by oncologic institutions				
	1970	1971	1972	1973	1974
Total population					
Absolute number	430.172	445.402	455.139	466.295	481.225
per 100.000 population	177.2	181.7	183.9	186.7	190.9
Urban population					
Absolute number	263.037	273.786	283.068	292.433	305.735
per 100.000 population	191.4	194.5	196.1	197.8	202.0
Rural population					
Absolute number	167.135	171.616	172.071	173.862	175.490
per 100.000 population	158.7	164.5	166.8	170.6	174.2

registration in the rural areas. In the last year the increase in the incidence of malignant tumours was the same for both the urban and rural population.

A correlation analysis of the morbidity structures in the USSR in 1970 and 1974 has revealed their high degree of correspondence to $\rho = 0.99$ with a probability of $P < 0.01$. In 1974 changes in the distribution of malignant neoplasms occured only in two localizations: tumours of the rectum took the 8th place instead of lip tumours which were shifted to the 9th place. Now the leading localizations in oncological morbidity /Table 96/ are the stomach, trachea, bronchi, lungs and skin /Fig. 35/. These localizations account for about 46 % of all malignant tumours. During the last 5 years the incidence of malignant neoplasms of the stomach, oesophagus, lip and cervix uteri has decreased, while that of other localizations has increased, although to a different extent.

The highest mean annual rate of increase in malignant tumours is found in the rectum 7.3 %; in the last year the rate of this increase slowed down to 5. The second place in the mean annual rates of increase in malignant neoplasms is held by the oral cavity and pharynx /5.4/, while the third place by the mammae /4.7/.

A mean annual increase in morbidity has been found to be 4.1-4.4 for tumours of the lymphatic and hematopoietic tissue, the larynx, trachea, bronchi and lungs. In the last year the rates of increase in the incidence of malignant tumours of the mammary gland, as well as of the lymphatic and hematopoietic tissue slowed down, the incidence of cancer of the larynx did not change, while the rates of increase in the incidence of malignant tumours of the trachea, bronchi and lungs were somewhat higher.

The age and sex distribution of malignant neoplasms in the USSR during the 1970-1974 period has retained its main characteristics. As in the preceding years /Table 97 /, in 1974 the age with maximum morbidity in both men and women was 70 years and older. At the age of 40 the incidence of malignant tumours is higher in women than in men due to the tumours

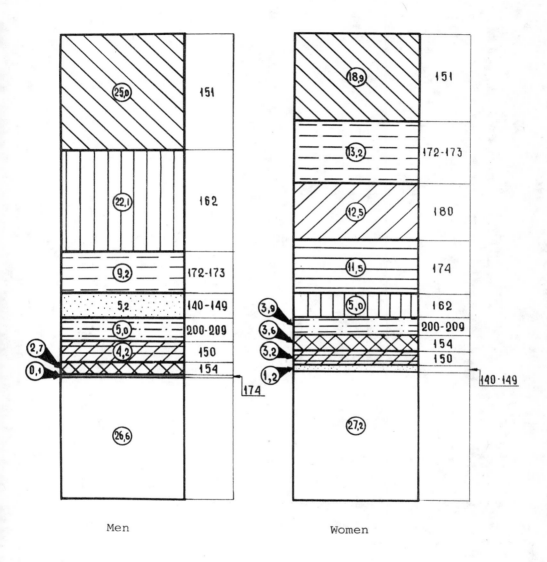

Men   Women

Fig. 35 Incidence of malignant neoplasms in the USSR in 1974
     /according to the main localizations, according to
     the International Classification of Diseases, 8th
     Revision/

Table 96

Number of New Cases and Morbidity /per 100.000 Population/ from Malignant Neoplasms of
Different Localization of the Population in the USSR from 1970 to 1974

Localization of malignant neoplasms	ICD Code Number 8th rev.	Absolute number					Incidence per 100.000 population				
		1970	1971	1972	1973	1974	1970	1971	1972	1973	1974
All malignant neoplasms	140-209	430.172	445.402	455.139	466.295	481.225	177.2	181.7	183.9	186.7	190.9
Oral cavity and throat, excluding lips	141-149	4.600	4.949	5.273	5.553	5.737	1.9	2.0	2.1	2.2	2.3
Lips	140	14.791	14.732	14.562	14.673	14.596	6.1	6.0	5.9	5.9	5.8
Esophagus	150	17.694	17.585	17.775	17.074	16.962	7.3	7.2	7.2	6.8	6.7
Stomach	151	102.697	103.335	103.812	103.812	104.432	42.3	42.2	41.9	41.6	41.4
Rectum	154	11.693	12.738	13.856	14.673	15.576	4.8	5.2	5.6	4.9	6.2
Larynx	161	6.890	7.469	7.821	8.198	8.409	2.8	3.0	3.2	3.3	3.3
Trachea, bronchi and lungs	162	50.389	53.228	55.746	58.215	61.820	20.8	21.7	22.5	23.3	24.5
Skin	172-173	48.705	51.221	51.404	52.056	54.678	20.1	20.9	20.8	20.8	21.7
Breast	174	24.593	26.301	27.539	28.824	30.299	10.1	10.7	11.1	11.5	12.0

Table 96 /cont'd/

Localization of malignant	ICD-Code Number 8th rev.	Absolute number					Incidencer per 100.000 population				
		1970	1971	1972	1973	1974	1970	1971	1972	1973	1974
Cervix uteri	180	33.960	33.992	33.464	32.669	32.611	14.0	13.8	13.5	13.1	12.9
Other organs	152–160 163,171 181–199	96.331	101.006	104.538	110.181	114.791	39.7	41.2	42.2	44.1	45.6
Lymphatic and hematopoietic tissues	200–209	17.029	10.046	19.603	20.367	21.314	7.3	7.7	7.9	8.2	8.5

Incidence of Malignant Neoplasms in the population

Localiza-tion and ICD Code Number 8th rev.	M a l e s						Total	
	Below 30	30--39	40--49	50--59	60--69	70 and more	Crude rate	Stand-ard-ized rate
All malig-nant neo-plasms 140-209								
1970	10.4	58.5	194.7	587.3	1.054.5	1.248.2	173.6	207.8
1971	10.7	56.3	201.0	593.2	1.074.6	1.264.6	177.8	210.9
1972	10.7	56.9	205.0	580.9	1.095.2	1.276.6	180.7	212.2
1973	11.1	59.1	213.7	591.3	1.094.7	1.204.0	184.8	215.0
1974	11.0	61.5	214.0	582.5	1.112.6	1.337.2	189.0	217.9
Lips 140								
1970	0.3	7.4	16.7	35.0	55.2	56.5	10.5	12.1
1971	0.2	6.2	16.3	35.3	53.2	58.4	10.3	11.8
1972	0.2	6.2	16.1	31.8	52.9	53.5	9.9	11.2
1973	0.2	6.1	16.3	31.8	53.8	56.5	10.1	11.3
1974	0.2	6.1	16.3	31.8	53.8	56.5	10.1	11.3
Esophagus 150								
1970	0.03	1.0	6.4	25.4	57.6	94.5	8.6	10.8
1971	0.04	0.9	6.5	24.8	55.6	94.0	8.5	10.6
1972	0.04	0.9	6.4	22.9	54.6	92.8	8.4	10.2
1973	0.03	0.9	6.1	22.8	52.6	84.7	8.1	9.7
1974	0.04	0.8	6.0	23.2	47.9	83.2	7.9	9.4
Stomach 151								
1970	0.5	13.6	53.4	164.9	305.7	358.1	47.5	57.4
1971	0.4	13.2	53.5	160.6	304.6	351.0	47.3	56.5
1972	0.5	12.8	53.9	152.3	303.4	346.8	47.1	55.6
1973	0.5	13.7	55.5	149.2	298.2	346.5	47.3	55.2
1974	0.5	14.0	55.0	143.1	292.8	352.1	47.2	54.7

of the USSR by Age and Sex from 1970 to 1974

						Total	
			F e m a l e s				
Below 30	30- -39	40- -49	50- -59	60- -69	70 and more	Crude rate	Stand- ard- ized rate
10.6	71.9	217.3	412.1	591.8	662.2	180.3	143.1
10.9	71.7	220.3	421.4	603.3	668.8	185.1	145.5
10.9	71.7	214.8	422.9	605.2	674.5	186.6	145.3
11.4	74.2	213.8	425.6	597.4	671.7	188.3	145.5
11.5	79.6	209.8	429.4	615.0	694.4	192.5	147.4
0.04	0.6	1.7	4.5	8.5	12.4	2.3	1.7
0.04	0.4	1.7	4.7	8.3	12.4	2.3	1.7
0.03	0.4	1.8	4.5	8.8	12.2	2.4	1.7
0.02	0.4	1.5	4.2	8.1	10.9	2.2	1.6
0.02	0.4	1.6	3.8	12.0	12.0	2.3	1.6
0.03	0.7	3.1	11.2	24.4	37.6	6.1	4.6
0.02	0.6	3.1	10.6	22.4	37.7	6.0	4.4
0.03	0.7	3.0	11.0	22.3	37.7	6.1	4.4
0.04	0.6	3.0	10.6	21.6	32.4	5.8	4.0
0.02	0.7	3.0	9.0	20.9	33.4	5.7	3.9
0.5	8.8	28.1	79.9	154.1	184.8	37.8	28.9
0.4	8.3	26.9	71.9	153.4	182.3	37.7	28.1
0.4	8.5	26.5	69.4	147.8	180.4	37.4	27.5
0.5	8.2	26.0	66.5	140.4	177.1	36.6	26.6
0.4	8.2	25.1	62.3	138.4	177.4	36.4	26.0

Table 97 /cont'd/

Localiza-tion and ICD Code Number 8th rev.	Males					Total		
	Below 30	30--39	40--49	50--59	60--69	70 and more	Crude rate	Stand-ard-ized rate
Rectum 154								
1970	0.2	1.6	3.6	12.6	24.2	34.5	4.0	4.7
1971	0.2	1.5	3.9	12.7	26.4	36.1	4.2	5.0
1972	0.1	1.6	4.3	12.8	29.4	39.5	4.6	5.4
1973	0.2	1.6	4.5	14.5	28.4	42.0	4.8	5.7
1974	0.2	1.8	4.7	14.7	33.0	42.1	5.2	6.1
Trachea, bronchi, lung 162								
1970	0.2	5.6	34.7	142.1	260.8	218.8	35.6	43.2
1971	0.2	5.2	37.5	146.6	267.1	223.0	37.0	45.4
1972	0.2	5.3	39.4	140.2	278.2	231.5	38.5	45.9
1973	0.2	5.7	42.9	151.1	280.7	237.0	40.1	46.9
1974	0.2	6.3	44.2	151.4	290.4	256.3	41.8	48.6
Skin 172,173								
1970	0.6	5.9	19.6	50.0	86.2	142.2	16.0	19.3
1971	0.6	6.3	20.2	50.9	89.5	149.0	16.8	19.9
1972	0.6	6.4	20.1	50.0	89.5	145.7	16.8	19.7
1973	0.6	6.4	21.1	50.5	87.5	144.0	16.9	19.7
1974	0.7	6.8	20.1	49.8	91.5	151.3	17.5	20.2
Breast 174								
1970		0.03	0.2	0.5	1.1	1.6	0.2	0.3
1971	0.03	0.08	0.3	0.5	1.1	1.4	0.2	0.2
1972	0.04	0.05	0.3	0.7	1.2	1.4	0.2	0.2
1973	0.004	0.05	0.3	0.6	1.2	1.8	0.2	0.2
1974	0.007	0.04	0.3	0.7	1.2	1.8	0.2	0.2

						Total	
			F e m a l e s				
Below 30	30- -39	40- -49	50- -59	60- -69	70 and more	Crude rate	Stand- ard- ized rate
0.1	1.8	5.0	11.6	20.2	25.4	5.5	4.3
0.2	2.2	5.1	13.0	21.7	25.9	6.0	4.6
0.2	2.0	5.7	13.5	22.6	28.9	6.5	4.9
0.2	2.2	5.9	14.1	24.7	27.4	6.8	5.0
0.2	2.6	6.0	14.2	24.4	29.2	7.0	5.1
0.1	1.4	5.3	17.2	34.1	37.7	8.1	6.1
0.1	1.6	6.0	17.4	36.1	39.4	8.6	6.3
0.2	1.6	6.2	17.2	34.8	41.3	8.7	6.3
0.1	1.7	6.3	17.3	35.5	41.4	9.0	6.4
0.1	1.7	5.9	18.3	37.2	45.4	9.6	6.7
0.9	8.1	23.8	47.4	77.2	113.9	23.5	18.2
0.9	8.1	24.5	48.9	80.0	116.3	24.4	18.7
0.8	7.9	23.7	47.4	79.6	113.1	24.2	18.1
0.8	8.5	23.1	46.7	78.3	111.6	24.2	18.0
0.9	8.9	23.2	46.6	81.4	117.1	25.3	18.6
0.4	13.6	42.9	46.4	41.9	34.0	18.6	15.2
0.4	14.1	45.7	49.0	44.2	34.7	19.8	16.2
0.5	14.8	45.3	53.0	45.5	36.7	20.5	16.6
0.6	15.9	46.4	56.7	46.3	37.6	21.3	17.6
0.6	18.3	45.2	60.4	49.2	40.5	22.2	18.3

Table 97 /cont'd/

Localization and ICD Code Number 8th rev.	Males							
	Below 30	30--39	40--49	50--59	60--69	Total		
						70 and more	Crude rate	Stand-ard-ized rate
Cervix uteri 180								
1970								
1971								
1972								
1973								
1974								
Lymphatic and hemato-poietic tissues 200--209								
1970	4.2	5.6	9.3	19.8	29.3	28.0	8.2	8.9
1971	4.3	5.8	9.6	20.6	31.6	31.5	8.7	9.2
1972	4.4	6.1	9.5	20.7	32.6	33.1	8.9	9.5
1973	4.6	6.4	9.9	20.7	33.6	32.4	9.1	9.8
1974	4.5	6.4	10.4	22.5	35.9	35.4	9.5	10.2

					F e m a l e s		
Below 30	30- -39	40- -49	50- -59	60- -69	70 and more	Total Crude rate	Stand- ard- ized rate
0.5	13.5	50.8	85.8	66.0	34.5	26.0	21.4
0.6	12.7	49.0	85.9	66.7	36.0	25.7	21.2
0.5	12.2	44.6	82.3	70.2	36.8	25.1	20.5
0.5	11.5	41.4	81.4	69.3	35.7	24.3	19.8
0.5	12.3	39.8	76.0	72.4	36.8	24.1	19.4
3.3	5.1	6.5	11.6	15.8	14.3	6.6	5.8
3.2	5.0	7.2	12.1	16.8	14.3	6.8	6.0
3.3	5.1	7.2	11.1	17.0	15.0	7.1	6.2
3.4	5.3	7.4	12.7	17.9	15.5	7.3	6.4
3.4	5.6	7.3	13.2	18.3	16.2	7.5	6.5

of the mammary gland, cervix uteri and rectum; this difference
however, is not great /Fig. 36/. At 40-49 years of age the
levels of oncological morbidity in men and women are close to
each other. The incidence of malignant neoplasms in men at the
ages of 50-59, 60-69, 70 and older is higher than in women by
40, 80 and 90 % respectively, and is primarily due to malignant neoplasms of the trachea, bronchi, lungs, stomach and
esophagus.

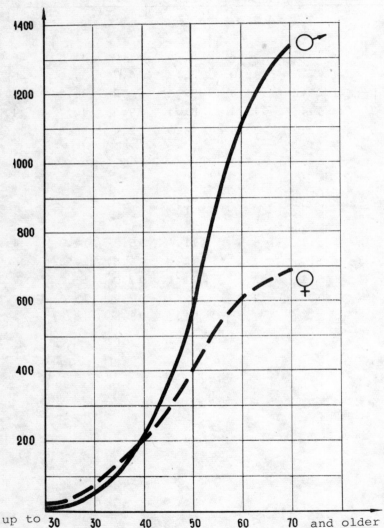

Fig. 36   Age and sex distribution of malignant neoplasms in
          the USSR in 1974 per 100,000 population

The general index of malignant neoplasms in women /192.5/ is higher than the corresponding index in men /189/ because of the larger number of middle-aged and old women, which is confirmed by the calculation of standard /Segi/ coefficients /147.4 in women and 217.9 in men/. Nevertheless, both the general and standard coefficients of incidence of malignant neoplasms have retained their tendency toward the increase in the recent years.

Now we shall consider the tendencies toward change in the morbidity indices of malignant tumours /Table 97/. Figs 37 and 38 show the morbidity indices in men and women according to the main localizations in 1974.

Against the background of gradual decrease in the incidence of cancer of the stomach the following main peculiarities of its dynamics are noted. From 1970 to 1974 the incidence of cancer of the stomach in men and women up to 30 years of age was practically stable. The women in other age groups exhibited a decrease in the incidence of cancer of the stomach, unlike the men, in the 30-39 and 40-49-year age groups of whom the incidence of cancer of the stomach has undoubtedly increased, while in the subsequent age groups /50-59 and 60-69 years/ it has decreased. Before 1973 this tendency was found also for persons 70 years of age and older; in 1974, however, the incidence of malignant neoplasms of the stomach increased in this group.

Although the incidence of cancer of the stomach in men of all ages is higher than in women, this difference is not the same for each of the age groups; in the age groups of 30-39, 40-49, 50-59, 60-69, 70 and older it is 70, 120, 130, 110 and 100 per cent higher, respectively, than in women.

The intensive coefficients of malignant tumours of the stomach in men are 30 per cent higher than the same indices in women, and the standard coefficients are 110 per cent higher, which reflects the existing difference in the intensity of the morbidity in the main age and sex groups.

Similar regularities of the incidence of cancer of the stomach have been noted by research workers of other countries.

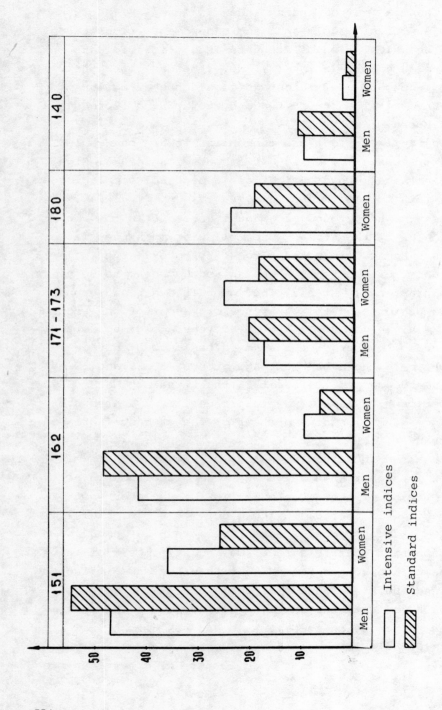

Fig. 37 Incidence of malignant neoplasms in the USSR in 1974 /according to the main localizations in conformity with the International Classification of Diseases, 8th
Revision/. 1.

554

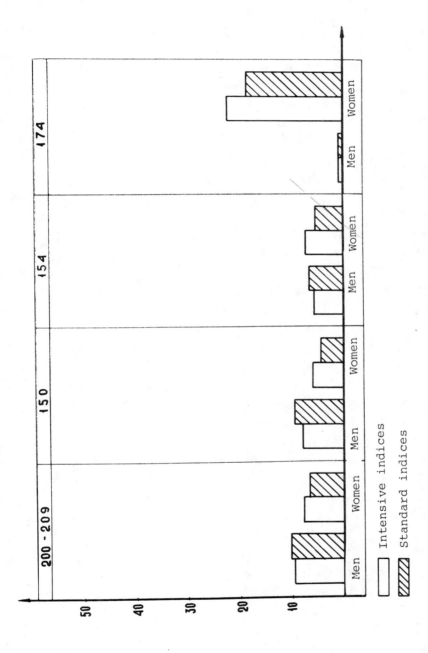

Fig. 38 Incidence of malignant neoplasms in the USSR in 1974 /according to the main localizations in conformity with the International Classification of Diseases, 8th
Revision/. 2.

555

This correlation was found to be 1.5 in 32 hospitals in Japan in 1974; in the USA /San Francisco, California, 1972/ it was 1.4, while in Czechoslovakia /1972/ 1.5.

The incidence of malignant neoplasms of the trachea, bronchi and lungs has been steadily increasing in the last 5 years in all age and sex groups; moreover, it has retained the peculiarity that the index of morbidity in men is 180 % higher than in women. The minimum differences are noted up to 30 years of age, the indices of morbidity in men and women are 0.2^{o}/oooo and 0.1^{o}/oooo, respectively, the maximum contrast being at the age of 60-69 - 290.4^{o}/oooo and 37.2^{o}/oooo. The indices are greatly influenced by age; thus, in men the index of morbidity up to 30 years of age was about 1,500th that of the incidence of cancer of the trachea, bronchi and lungs for 60-69 years of age $/0.2^{o}$/oooo and 290.4^{o}/oooo/.

In 1974 the general index of the incidence of cancer of the lungs was 330 % higher in men than the corresponding index in women /42.1 and 9.6/. It should be noted that the same ratio /4.3:1/ was also found for the given localization by the national review of cancer incidence in the USA /1969-1971/, although the rough mean indices for these 3 years are much higher than in the Soviet Union for both men and women, namely 63 and 14.7. Still greater differences are characteristic of the standard indices of the incidence of cancer of the lungs in men and women in the USSR, namely 48.6 and 6.7, respectively.

Cancer of the breast is, as is well-known, the main cause of mortality of middle-aged women in western countries; an increase in its mortality and morbidity having been noted in many countries in the recent decades. A tendency of the standard age indices toward stabilization in older age groups is observed now only in countries of the Far East.

The incidence of breast cancer is also continuially increasing in all age groups in the USSR. The general index of morbidity increased in 1970 from 18.6^{o}/oooo to 22.2^{o}/oooo in 1974. Sharp differences are observed in the incidence of malignant neoplasms of the breast of the various age groups; thus, whereas this index in the group of women up to 30 years of age is $0.6^{o}/oooo$, in the group of 60-69 years of age it is $60.4^{o}/oooo$, i.e., there is more than a 100-fold increase.

The incidence of breast cancer in men has remained in-variable in the last few years - $0.2^{o}/oooo$, the maximum index of $1.8^{o}/oooo$ being characteristic of the age of 70 and older.

Between 1970 and 1974 the incidence of malignant neoplasms of the cervix uteri has been decreasing. This tendency is characteristic of all age groups except women in the age group of 60-69 years, in whom the index of morbidity has increased from 60 to $72^{o}/oooo$, and women older than 70 years in whom no clear trend in the changes in morbidity is observed.

The maximum incidence, $76^{o}/oooo$, of cancer of the cervix uteri in 1974 was observed at the age of 50-59, the mean age of the patients being 60.3 years.

According to the Finnish Institute of Statistical and Epidemiologic Cancer Research, the mean age of patients with cancer of the cervix uteri was 56.6 years; the analogous index calculated by N. Mourali for the countries of the Eastern Mediterranean ranged from 48.6 to 57.5 years.

Tumours of the skin take the third place in the incidence of malignant neoplasms in the USSR and annually affect more than 50,000 people. Between 1970 and 1974 the tumours of the skin were characterized by a certain increase, namely from $16^{o}/oooo$ to $17.7^{o}/oooo$ in men and from $23.5^{o}/oooo$ to $25.3^{o}/oooo$ in women. It has to be mentioned that, as a rule, up to 50 years of age malignant neoplasms of the skin affect women, while after 50 years' men.

It should be noted that the intensive coefficient of the incidence of malignant tumours of the skin in men - $17.5^{o}/oooo$ - is lower than the analogous index in women /$25.3^{o}/oooo$/, whereas the standard coefficients give an entirely different characteristic of $20.2^{o}/oooo$ of the morbidity in men and only $18.6^{o}/oooo$ in women. The higher general coefficient of the incidence of malignant tumours in women is due merely to the fact that in the Soviet Union there are more elderly women than men.

Exactly the same phenomenon is observed when analysing

the incidence of cancer of the rectum. Up to 50 years of age both the incidence and the general intensive coefficients are higher in women /7°/oooo for women and 5.2^{o}/oooo for men/, while the standard coefficients are higher in men, namely 6.1^{o}/oooo in men, as against the 5°/oooo in women.

The incidence of cancer of the esophagus has steadily decreased in the Soviet Union from 7.3^{o}/oooo in 1970 to 6.7^{o}/oooo in 1974.

The age and sex indices of the incidence of cancer of the esophagus in men are 100 %, and more, higher than the corresponding indices of morbidity in women, except the group of 30-39 years of age. With age the incidence of esophagus cancer sharply increases. The incidence in the group of 70 years of age and older is 1,500-2,000 times as high as in people under the age of 30.

91 % of women and 86 % of men affected by cancer of the esophagus in 1974 were older than 50 years.

The incidence of malignant neoplasms of the lymphatic and hematopoietic tissue in men was higher in all age groups than the analogous indices of morbidity in women. The differences in the incidence of morbidity are much smaller than those of many other localizations. As essential peculiarity of the incidence of malignant neoplasms of the lymphatic and hematopoietic tissue is its great extent at young ages. One-fourth of the patients are affected before 50 years of age.

The above are the general tendencies of the incidence of malignant neoplasms according to the main localizations in the USSR as a whole. They are generally characteristic also of the Union Republics, although in some of the Union Republics there are specific peculiarities in the extent and dynamics of oncological morbidity /Tables 98 and 99/. What are these peculiarities? They are, in the first place, the different extent of incidence of malignant tumours.

With the mean All-Union incidence of 190.9^{o}/oooo, the incidence of malignant tumours in two Republics - Uzbek and Tadzhik - is less than 100°/oooo, while in 5 Republics - Russian, Ukrainian, Latvian and Estonian SSRs - the incidence of malignant tumours exceeds $200^{\circ}/oooo$ with the highest index of morbidity - $274.9^{\circ}/oooo$ - in the Estonian SSR. As contrasting to the general tendency toward an increase in the incidence of malignant tumours in the USSR the incidence has been decreasing between 1970 and 1974 in 5 Republics /Kazakh, Uzbek, Kirghiz, Tadzhik and Latvian SSRs/. Various localizations of malignant tumours have predominant distribution in a number of Republics. The cancer of the esophagus is encountered respectively in the Uzbek, Kazakh and Turkmen SSR 2, 3 and 4 times as frequently as in the USSR on the whole, while cancer of the stomach occurs 66.7 % less frequently in the Uzbek, Tadzhik and Georgian SSR. The highest incidence of malignant tumours of the trachea, bronchi and lungs is in the Estonian, Latvian, Lithuanian, Russian and Ukrainian SSRs /$27-36^{\circ}/oooo$/, while the lowest incidence occurs in the Uzbek, Tadzhik and Turkmen SSRs /$6-7^{\circ}/oooo$/. A relatively low incidence of malignant neoplasms is registered in Kazakhstan and the Republics of Central Asia also in a number of other localizations.

An analysis of the age and sex incidence of malignant tumours /Table 99/ evidences the absence of sharp differences in its extents in the various Union Republics.

Table 100 presents the information on oncological patients with malignant tumours on the records of oncological institutions.

Between 1970 and 1974 alone the contingents of patients with malignant tumours have increased by 20.4 %, on an average of 4.1 % a year. The largest groups of patients in 1974 on the records of oncological institutions were the following: $191.8^{\circ}/oooo$ with malignant neoplasms of the skin, $118.9^{\circ}/oooo$ with malignant neoplasms of the cervix uteri, $71^{\circ}/oooo$ with cancer of the lower lip, $65.9^{\circ}/oooo$ with breast cancer, $60.5^{\circ}/oooo$ with cancer of the stomach, $23^{\circ}/oooo$ with malignant neoplasms of the bronchi and lungs, and $17.2^{\circ}/oooo$ with malignances of the lymphatic and hematopoietic tissue. In this period the order of distribution has, persisted mainly in the structure of the contingents according to the different localizations. The rates of increase in the contingents of patients

Table 98

New Cases and Incidence /per 100.000 Population/ of Malignant Neoplasms in the USSR and Union
Republics from 1970 to 1974

	Absolute number					Incidence per 100.000 population				
	1970	1971	1972	1973	1974	1970	1971	1972	1973	1974
USSR	430.172	445.402	455.139	466.295	481.225	177.2	181.7	183.9	186.7	190.9
Russian SFSR	250.057	265.777	270.867	277.172	286.091	197.9	202.8	205.5	209.1	214.6
Ukrainian SSR	87.234	92.288	94.859	96.699	101.231	184.4	193.5	197.4	199.9	208.0
Byelorussian SSR	13.996	14.167	14.544	15.551	15.965	154.9	155.5	158.6	168.4	171.7
Uzbek SSR	10.040	10.682	10.507	10.347	11.013	82.8	86.6	82.6	79.0	81.6
Kazakh SSR	20.430	20.456	21.463	22.193	21.689	157.7	153.2	158.0	160.7	154.4
Georgian SSR	4.950	4.864	4.961	5.034	5.098	150.1	102.1	99.8	103.6	104.0
Azerbaijan SSR	4.835	5.707	5.489	5.995	5.914	93.6	108.2	102.2	109.6	106.4
Lithuanian SSR	6.249	6.503	6.081	6.828	7.280	198.6	204.2	207.6	210.2	222.2
Moldavian SSR	4.283	4.623	4.481	4.814	4.944	119.2	126.8	121.2	128.6	130.5
Latvian SSR	5.796	5.721	5.769	6.002	5.979	244.1	238.6	238.3	245.8	242.5
Kirghiz SSR	3.691	3.796	3.838	3.962	3.897	124.5	125.0	123.4	124.5	119.6
Tadzhik SSR	2.161	2.018	2.411	2.428	2.423	73.5	66.4	76.8	75.0	72.6
Armenian SSR	2.759	2.818	2.919	3.122	3.211	109.6	109.4	110.7	115.7	116.5
Turkhmen SSR	2.206	2.473	2.738	2.372	2.577	100.7	109.5	117.7	99.1	104.4
Estonian SSR	3.486	3.529	3.616	3.776	3.913	255.5	255.3	258.6	267.5	274.9

Lips /140/

USSR	14.791	14.732	14.562	14.673	14.596	6.1	6.0	5.9	5.9	5.8
Russian SFSR	8.775	8.780	8.688	8.723	8.700	6.7	6.7	6.6	6.6	6.5
Ukrainian SSR	3.790	3.713	3.620	3.683	3.691	8.0	7.8	7.5	7.6	7.6
Byelorussian SSR	387	355	373	364	398	4.3	3.9	4.1	3.9	4.3
Uzbek SSR	188	210	211	219	214	1.6	1.7	1.6	1.7	1.6
Kazakh SSR	665	722	707	754	640	5.1	5.4	5.2	5.4	4.6
Georgian SSR	112	118	102	98	95	2.4	2.5	2.1	2.0	1.9
Azerbaijan SSR	101	130	127	108	126	2.0	2.5	2.4	2.0	2.3
Lithuanian SSR	187	122	161	158	146	5.9	3.0	5.0	4.9	.4.5
Moldavian SSR	156	174	160	160	188	4.3	4.8	4.3	4.3	5.0
Latvian SSR	107	87	107	107	95	4.5	3.6	4.4	4.4	3.8
Kirghiz SSR	100	110	119	99	105	3.4	3.6	3.8	3.1	3.2
Tadzhik SSR	75	48	55	52	51	2.6	1.6	1.7	1.6	1.5
Armenian SSR	55	63	64	69	71	2.2	2.4	2.4	2.6	2.6
Turkhmen SSR	45	59	28	36	34	2.1	2.6	1.2	1.5	1.4
Estonian SSR	48	41	40	43	42	3.5	3.0	2.9	3.0	2.9

Esophagus /150/

USSR	17.694	17.585	17.775	17.074	16.962	7.3	7.2	7.2	6.8	6.7
Russian SFSR	9.030	8.827	8.715	8.219	8.286	6.9	6.7	6.6	6.3	6.2
Ukrainian SSR	1.231	1.234	1.336	1.204	1.251	2.6	2.6	2.8	2.5	2.6
Byelorussian SSR	212	215	181	184	161	2.3	2.4	2.0	2.0	1.7

cont'd

Table 98 /cont'd/

	Absolute number					Incidence per 100.000 population				
	1970	1971	1972	1973	1974	1970	1971	1972	1973	1974
Uzbek SSR	1.943	2.020	1.928	2.010	1.951	16.0	16.4	15.2	15.4	14.4
Kazakh SSR	3.323	3.218	3.455	3.273	3.179	25.7	24.1	25.4	23.7	22.6
Georgian SSR	115	102	96	102	100	2.4	2.1	2.0	2.1	2.0
Azerbaijan SSR	481	507	503	515	475	9.3	9.6	9.4	9.4	8.5
Lithuanian SSR	58	61	74	61	57	1.8	1.9	2.3	1.9	1.7
Moldavian SSR	62	66	54	60	53	1.7	1.8	1.5	1.6	1.4
Latvian SSR	58	62	49	51	48	2.4	2.6	2.0	2.1	1.9
Kirghiz SSR	239	256	249	245	241	8.1	8.4	8.0	7.7	7.4
Tadzhik SSR	229	213	245	284	267	7.8	7.0	7.8	8.8	8.0
Armenian SSR	95	86	90	93	97	3.8	3.3	3.4	3.4	3.5
Turkmen SSR	582	679	775	677	765	29.6	30.1	33.3	28.3	31.0
Estonian SSR	36	39	25	26	31	2.6	2.8	1.8	1.8	2.2
Stomach /151/										
USSR	102.697	103.335	103.558	103.312	104.432	42.3	42.2	41.9	41.6	41.4
Russian SFSR	68.622	69.000	68.682	68.353	68.339	52.6	52.6	52.1	51.6	51.2
Ukrainian SSR	16.449	16.863	17.216	17.387	18.144	34.8	36.4	35.8	35.9	37.3
Byelorussian SSR	4.177	4.090	4.004	4.220	4.351	46.2	44.6	43.7	45.7	46.5
Uzbek SSR	1.664	1.679	1.669	1.592	1.708	13.7	13.6	13.1	12.2	12.7
Kazakh SSR	4.244	3.996	4.092	4.347	4.033	32.8	29.9	30.1	31.5	28.7

Georgian SSR	735	674	674	718	675	15.6	14.1	14.0	14.8	13.8
Azerbaijan SSR	1.005	1.304	1.088	1.318	1.143	19.5	24.7	20.2	24.1	20.5
Lithuanian SSR	1.353	1.388	1.427	1.374	1.438	43.0	43.6	44.3	42.3	43.9
Moldavian SSR	558	665	643	682	683	15.5	18.2	17.4	18.2	18.0
Latvian SSR	1.105	940	1.055	1.087	1.042	46.5	39.5	43.6	44.5	42.2
Kirghiz SSR	835	816	829	792	831	28.2	26.9	26.6	24.9	25.5
Tadzhik SSR	381	354	472	448	431	13.0	11.6	15.0	13.8	12.9
Armenian SSR	479	500	483	495	499	19.0	19.4	18.3	18.3	18.1
Turkmen SSR	398	440	530	315	394	18.2	19.5	22.8	13.1	16.0
Estonian SSR	692	626	694	684	719	50.7	45.3	49.6	48.4	50.5

Trachea, bronchi and lungs /162/

USSR	50.389	53.228	55.746	58.215	61.820	20.8	21.7	22.5	23.3	24.9
Russian SFSR	31.200	32.547	34.415	35.712	37.772	23.9	24.9	26.1	26.9	28.3
Ukrainian SSR	10.878	11.919	12.222	12.903	14.049	23.0	25.0	25.4	26.7	28.9
Byelorussian SSR	1.343	1.299	1.449	1.555	1.660	14.9	14.3	15.8	16.2	17.3
Uzbek SSR	691	768	774	726	881	5.7	6.2	6.1	5.5	6.5
Kazakh SSR	1.974	2.071	2.246	2.348	2.406	15.2	15.5	16.5	17.0	17.1
Georgian SSR	528	540	542	574	542	11.2	11.3	11.3	11.8	11.1
Azerbaijan SSR	520	616	533	606	607	10.1	11.7	9.9	11.1	10.9
Lithuanian SSR	698	767	854	862	895	22.2	24.1	26.5	26.5	27.3
Moldavian SSR	497	518	522	528	532	13.8	14.2	14.1	14.1	14.0

cont'd

563

Table 98 /cont'd/

	Absolute number					Incidence per 100.000 population				
	1970	1971	1972	1973	1974	1970	1971	1972	1973	1974
Latvian SSR	763	772	745	808	858	32.1	32.3	30.5	33.1	34.4
Kirghiz SSR	291	347	354	365	372	9.8	11.4	11.4	11.5	11.4
Tadzhik SSR	147	182	191	226	209	5.0	6.0	6.1	7.0	6.3
Armenian SSR	306	297	307	327	320	12.2	11.5	11.6	12.1	12.3
Turkhmen SSR	138	156	160	146	178	6.3	6.9	6.9	6.1	7.2
Estonian SSR	415	429	432	509	519	30.4	31.0	30.9	36.1	36.9
Skin /172-173/										
USSR	48.705	51.221	51.404	52.056	54.678	20.1	20.9	20.8	20.8	21.7
Russian SFSR	27.181	28.378	28.674	29.555	32.433	20.8	21.6	21.7	22.3	23.6
Ukrainian SSR	12.523	13.133	13.110	12.845	13.189	26.5	27.5	27.3	26.5	27.1
Byelorussian SSR	1.380	1.591	1.592	1.577	1.670	15.3	17.5	17.4	17.1	17.9
Uzbek SSR	1.135	1.299	1.234	1.178	1.253	9.4	10.5	9.7	9.0	9.3
Kazakh SSR	1.976	2.136	2.124	2.342	2.329	15.3	16.0	15.6	16.9	16.6
Georgian SSR	538	540	509	510	465	11.4	11.3	10.6	10.5	9.5
Azerbaijan SSR	457	498	609	527	610	8.8	9.4	11.3	9.6	11.0
Lithuanian SSR	589	581	590	628	608	18.7	18.6	18.8	19.2	18.6
Moldavian SSR	600	644	536	497	612	16.7	17.7	14.5	13.3	16.2
Latvian SSR	615	667	632	582	608	25.9	27.8	26.1	23.8	24.6

Kirghiz SSR	521	530	531	603	535	17.6	17.4	17.1	18.9	16.4
Tadzhik SSR	393	343	333	322	405	13.4	11.3	10.6	9.9	12.1
Armenian SSR	241	283	285	291	301	9.6	11.0	10.8	10.8	10.9
Turkhmen SSR	198	231	255	223	232	9.0	10.2	11.0	9.3	9.4
Estonian SSR	358	354	390	381	428	26.2	25.6	27.9	27.0	30.1

Breast /174/

USSR	24.593	26.301	27.539	28.824	30.299	10.1	10.7	11.1	11.5	12.0
Russian SFSR	13.988	14.915	15.870	16.500	17.352	10.7	11.4	12.0	12.4	13.0
Ukrainian SSR	5.798	6.382	6.521	6.744	7.023	12.3	13.4	13.6	13.9	14.4
Byelorussian SSR	775	816	852	1.012	1.076	8.6	8.9	9.3	11.0	11.6
Uzbek SSR	421	519	481	511	552	3.5	4.2	3.8	3.9	4.1
Kazakh SSR	825	806	918	925	1.009	6.4	6.0	6.7	6.7	7.2
Georgian SSR	551	541	511	599	665	11.7	11.4	10.6	12.3	13.6
Azerbaijan SSR	318	320	330	352	372	6.2	6.1	6.1	6.4	6.7
Lithuanian SSR	421	435	444	473	529	13.4	13.7	13.8	14.6	16.1
Moldavian SSR	256	351	309	360	375	7.1	9.6	8.4	9.6	9.9
Latvian SSR	430	422	444	485	450	18.1	17.6	18.3	19.9	18.2
Kirghiz SSR	176	158	166	172	158	5.9	5.2	5.3	5.4	4.8
Tadzhik SSR	83	98	103	93	116	2.8	3.2	3.3	2.9	3.5
Armenian SSR	203	197	210	226	239	8.1	7.6	8.6	8.4	8.7
Turkhmen SSR	82	85	87	97	95	3.7	3.8	3.7	4.0	3.8

cont'd

Table 98 /cont'd/

	Absolute number					Incidence per 100.000 population				
	1970	1971	1972	1973	1974	1970	1971	1972	1973	1974
Estonian SSR	266	256	293	275	288	19.5	18.5	21.0	19.5	20.2
Cervix uteri /180/										
USSR	33.960	33.992	33.464	32.669	32.611	14.0	13.8	13.5	13.1	12.9
Russian SFSR	29.485	20.626	19.980	19.600	19.442	15.7	15.7	15.2	14.8	14.6
Ukrainian SSR	7.781	7.185	7.232	6.911	7.034	15.3	15.1	15.0	14.3	14.5
Byelorussian SSR	858	861	859	828	900	9.5	9.4	9.4	9.0	9.7
Uzbek SSR	638	701	645	624	669	5.3	5.7	5.1	4.8	4.9
Kazakh SSR	1.644	1.583	1.597	1.638	1.617	12.7	11.9	11.7	11.8	11.5
Georgian SSR										
Azerbaijan SSR	311	332	355	284	268	6.0	6.3	6.6	5.2	4.8
Lithuanian SSR	426	401	414	396	392	13.5	12.6	12.9	12.2	12.0
Moldavian SSR	530	522	502	544	522	14.7	14.3	13.6	14.5	13.8
Latvian SSR	379	343	352	332	337	16.0	14.3	14.5	13.6	13.7
Kirghiz SSR	367	330	368	362	369	12.4	10.9	11.5	11.4	11.3
Tadzhik SSR	132	130	134	144	151	4.5	4.3	4.3	4.4	4.5
Armenian SSR	197	213	230	233	235	7.8	8.3	8.7	8.6	8.5
Turkmen SSR	185	183	208	206	153	8.4	8.3	9.8	8.6	6.2
Estonian SSR	173	200	200	203	169	12.7	14.5	14.3	14.4	11.9

Lymphatic and
hematopoietic
tissues

/200-209/

USSR	17.329	18.846	19.603	20.367	21.314	7.3	7.7	7.9	8.2	8.4
Russian SFSR	9.926	10.374	10.730	11.061	11.473	7.6	7.9	8.1	8.3	8.6
Ukrainian SSR	3.779	4.237	4.438	4.623	4.867	8.0	8.9	9.2	9.6	10.0
Byelorussian SSR	907	790	856	914	958	10.0	8.7	9.3	9.9	10.3
Uzbek SSR	448	423	423	429	543	3.7	3.4	3.4	3.2	4.0
Kazakh SSR	605	654	760	730	748	4.7	4.9	5.6	5.3	5.3
Georgian SSR	275	319	309	318	334	5.8	6.7	6.4	6.5	6.8
Azerbaijan SSR	198	301	263	358	340	3.8	5.7	4.9	6.5	6.1
Lithuanian SSR	283	356	343	363	428	9.0	11.2	10.7	11.2	13.1
Moldavian SSR	297	281	351	362	344	8.3	7.7	9.5	9.7	9.1
Latvian SSR	314	267	300	317	325	13.2	11.1	12.4	13.0	13.2
Kirghiz SSR	143	173	155	157	184	4.8	5.7	5.0	4.9	5.6
Tadzhik SSR	69	74	129	162	163	2.3	2.4	4.1	5.0	4.9
Armenian SSR	263	270	275	265	277	10.4	10.5	10.4	9.8	10.0
Turkmen SSR	95	89	85	67	95	4.3	3.9	3.6	3.0	3.8
Estonian SSR	227	238	180	250	235	16.6	17.2	12.9	17.7	16.5

Incidence of Malignant Neoplasms of the Population of

	M a l e s						
	Below 30	30-39	40-49	50-59	60-69	70 and more	Total
USSR							
1970							
1971	10.7	56.3	201.0	593.2	1.074.0	1.264.6	177.8
1972	10.7	56.9	20.50	580.9	1.095.2	1.276.6	180.7
1973	11.1	59.1	213.7	591.3	1.094.7	1.234.0	184.8
1974	11.0	61.5	214.0	582.5	1.112.6	1.337.2	189.0
Russian SFSR							
1970							
1971	10.9	58.9	219.8	659.8	1.220.8	1.531.0	197.5
1972	10.9	59.6	224.1	636.5	1.236.6	1.546.5	200.5
1973	11.3	61.5	232.0	650.7	1.229.0	1.552.4	205.4
1974	11.3	66.2	232.9	649.0	1.231.9	1.612.1	210.7
Ukrainian SSR							
1970							
1971	12.2	55.8	186.1	544.0	963.1	1.101.6	191.7
1972	12.4	55.4	192.7	534.2	1.003.5	1.133.8	197.6
1973	12.5	59.4	203.6	544.3	985.3	1.169.9	202.4
1974	12.6	60.3	207.4	532.7	1.041.2	1.257.2	211.6
Byelorussian SSR							
1970							
1971	11.3	49.0	165.0	420.4	895.7	963.3	155.5
1972	12.1	52.6	162.0	459.2	885.1	1.005.2	161.2
1973	12.0	48.5	183.3	478.3	927.2	1.046.6	170.8
1974	10.7	53.7	185.0	467.7	949.2	1.038.6	172.9
Uzbek SSR							
1970							
1971	7.4	43.3	133.3	398.6	652.4	644.0	86.1
1972	7.0	42.0	123.6	392.1	662.0	635.2	83.6
1973	8.0	42.7	129.9	342.2	630.7	607.2	79.9
1974	8.4	42.9	129.6	361.5	688.4	623.6	82.7

USSR and Union Republics by Age and Sex in 1970-1974

	F e m a l e s					
Below 30	30-39	40-49	50-59	60-69	70 and more	Total
10.9	71.7	220.3	421.4	603.3	668.8	185.1
10.9	71.7	214.8	422.9	605.2	674.5	186.6
11.4	74.2	213.8	425.6	597.4	671.7	188.3
11.5	79.6	209.9	420.4	615.0	694.4	192.5
11.8	73.9	226.5	438.0	646.9	756.7	207.2
11.5	74.6	221.4	436.2	647.7	769.9	113.8
12.4	77.4	219.9	438.5	644.8	766.5	212.2
12.4	84.8	217.7	435.8	657.0	789.2	217.8
12.5	73.1	225.9	408.0	569.9	553.7	194.9
12.1	71.4	219.4	417.0	569.4	566.3	197.2
12.7	73.3	217.9	418.1	551.2	573.3	197.8
12.9	72.3	212.8	415.5	580.6	601.0	204.9
12.0	66.8	176.4	358.8	514.0	476.2	155.6
11.9	59.3	169.9	378.7	506.2	482.4	156.3
14.3	67.7	186.5	379.9	517.4	504.2	166.3
13.2	69.4	188.3	368.5	539.7	522.5	170.6
6.3	50.2	174.2	338.1	403.2	402.0	86.0
6.7	56.1	158.4	334.6	390.4	343.4	81.7
6.1	52.5	158.8	314.7	378.0	330.6	78.1
6.9	58.7	148.2	322.2	411.4	342.5	80.6

Table 99 /cont'd/

	Below 30	30-39	40-49	50-59	60-69	70 and more	Total
				M a l e s			
Kazakh SSR							
1970							
1971	9.1	63.3	236.6	708.9	1.277.1	1.362.1	155.7
1972	9.3	61.8	241.9	718.7	1.265.8	1.421.9	158.4
1973	9.2	68.8	261.1	718.2	1.341.7	1.385.4	164.3
1974	9.9	61.2	249.7	673.5	1.251.1	1.300.3	155.6
Georgian SSR							
1970							
1971	8.1	40.1	106.4	299.5	549.9	598.2	100.6
1972	8.7	37.7	107.4	302.7	547.0	643.5	102.9
1973	9.6	34.0	105.3	313.9	550.7	583.7	101.4
1974	8.4	41.5	99.6	305.9	538.6	607.4	101.7
Azerbaijan SSR							
1970							
1971	8.9	55.2	170.6	495.8	870.1	1.209.2	112.9
1972	6.0	45.9	148.7	469.6	859.1	1.230.9	106.8
1973	10.2	55.6	143.4	510.6	950.9	1.342.9	118.4
1974	10.1	61.3	137.1	494.3	952.4	1.321.5	117.9
Lithuanian SSR							
1970							
1971	15.2	56.2	168.8	448.2	940.8	1.296.6	207.2
1972	16.5	64.5	197.9	532.4	960.6	1.134.1	213.3
1973	14.5	72.4	230.3	517.0	1.000.8	1.031.9	215.4
1974	13.4	48.6	222.2	460.3	1.062.6	1.410.9	231.4
Moldavian SSR							
1970							
1971	147.9	48.2	143.6	357.3	701.3	843.3	122.1
1972	12.4	45.8	148.1	360.5	686.6	742.6	120.7
1973	12.1	46.5	144.4	386.9	678.6	809.9	125.4
1974	12.8	43.0	145.2	412.1	693.0	720.1	126.8
Latvian SSR							
1970							
1971 cont'd	13.7	50.3	166.9	487.9	1.007.9	1.544.9	239.1

570

Below 30	30-39	40-49	50-59	60-69	70 and more	Total
		F e m a l e s				
8.3	71.0	228.5	498.9	701.7	740.0	152.8
9.5	70.1	239.9	506.4	714.2	754.8	157.7
9.0	73.4	230.5	517.7	737.8	693.6	157.3
10.0	74.9	228.1	470.1	695.3	704.0	153.3
8.4	61.6	153.7	260.3	317.7	332.2	103.5
8.2	54.5	142.4	268.4	317.9	346.5	103.3
8.0	68.1	146.5	278.5	312.9	322.2	105.6
8.6	57.2	143.4	287.9	321.1	318.1	106.1
6.5	66.8	186.4	361.6	441.9	612.2	103.8
6.1	57.5	101.0	322.:	477.0	512.7	97.7
6.9	58.2	157.5	322.2	432.1	675.5	101.3
6.3	58.8	145.4	307.2	406.8	612.9	95.4
17.1	77.3	228.5	437.3	602.3	723.0	201.6
17.3	83.3	241.0	443.0	623.7	645.0	202.6
18.9	106.0	258.2	437.1	688.1	570.9	205.7
13.2	78.6	220.0	415.6	689.3	748.3	214.0
9.6	55.3	202.1	383.9	503.7	477.2	131.0
10.5	70.5	175.8	349.2	452.6	409.0	121.7
12.9	63.7	195.7	377.2	471.1	442.5	131.5
13.4	70.9	180.0	388.0	503.9	412.4	133.8
11.9	90.0	237.9	443.8	591.0	733.9	238.2

Table 99 /cont'd/

	Below 30	30-39	40-49	50-59	60-69	70 and more	Total
				Males			
1972	13.8	49.6	161.1	50.49	959.6	1.500.0	234.7
1973	12.9	50.7	188.1	503.6	1.033.0	1.546.5	247.6
1974	11.4	40.1	177.4	485.5	965.7	1.535.9	236.9
Kirghiz SSR							
1970	9.4	68.4	190.2	513.7	867.2	759.7	115.3
1971	9.6	60.8	203.0	501.1	902.7	1.004.9	123.8
1972	10.8	56.6	199.8	502.2	983.9	820.9	120.0
1973	9.5	61.6	191.3	516.4	1.019.6	804.6	119.7
1974	10.4	57.7	203.8	433.0	965.1	807.2	114.8
Tadzhik SSR							
1970	7.5	40.8	132.7	377.7	559.1	569.7	74.4
1971	7.7	37.5	130.9	318.0	528.3	520.5	68.8
1972	9.2	55.4	142.7	354.6	692.2	599.1	82.2
1973	8.9	48.0	141.2	385.0	674.4	541.2	79.3
1974	7.1	47.8	126.4	343.8	682.2	599.0	76.3
Armenian SSR							
1970	13.1	56.1	194.7	417.2	708.1	957.0	110.4
1971	11.3	46.3	150.8	428.7	853.3	1.006.3	111.4
1972	10.1	55.9	172.5	517.1	753.8	984.2	113.4
1973	10.4	63.6	146.2	575.6	786.2	1.053.0	117.2
1974	10.1	71.6	150.4	505.1	809.9	1.036.1	116.9
Turkhmen SSR							
1970	6.5	50.8	169.6	521.3	791.3	908.5	99.9
1971	5.2	43.5	195.6	539.0	931.3	1.073.3	109.9
1972	6.6	53.4	181.1	573.3	904.5	1.139.3	112.0
1973	7.3	40.9	175.3	517.2	739.3	826.5	94.0
1974	6.4	41.3	168.3	467.9	938.7	1.012.9	101.8
Estonian SSR							
1970	15.5	50.1	143.6	549.8	1.223.2	1.694.2	249.8
1971	13.5	45.0	160.3	553.6	1.082.7	1.650.8	237.7
1972	12.6	55.1	180.9	530.1	1.195.0	1.649.8	249.1
1973	12.7	52.0	207.5	621.5	1.167.4	1.788.9	281.0
1974	15.6	67.1	231.3	635.5	1.249.2	1.798.1	281.0

		Females				
Below 30	30-39	40-49	50-59	60-69	70 and more	Total
15.1	76.9	227.6	429.9	607.8	766.8	241.3
16.2	72.1	210.4	447.3	678.6	712.5	244.2
10.5	80.9	221.1	410.0	658.4	764.3	247.2
8.6	62.6	280.9	497.7	576.3	568.5	132.9
8.3	70.7	230.1	426.1	529.5	570.7	126.0
8.8	72.5	216.1	456.1	598.1	535.9	126.9
8.1	75.5	240.3	469.4	546.5	530.5	128.9
12.1	75.9	224.2	420.8	549.8	484.9	124.0
5.3	46.3	171.7	310.3	369.6	355.8	72.7
4.7	50.7	152.3	246.3	326.1	323.3	64.1
7.6	64.7	147.8	296.6	351.4	333.9	71.4
6.9	46.4	151.2	305.2	357.8	363.9	70.9
5.1	70.6	135.7	305.1	346.7	341.6	69.1
12.3	73.3	231.1	392.1	447.9	437.0	108.8
9.6	75.3	202.7	336.3	470.7	533.4	107.5
12.1	75.9	207.1	389.7	456.4	433.1	108.1
9.2	81.0	182.1	451.2	511.3	508.3	114.3
8.8	78.5	205.1	417.1	495.5	540.9	116.1
7.3	59.6	199.3	392.2	504.2	587.9	101.6
4.9	64.5	223.3	415.6	529.7	693.9	109.2
5.9	63.0	216.4	486.5	655.1	785.3	123.7
6.2	53.0	216.0	428.8	562.7	508.3	104.0
6.9	51.2	192.1	440.0	558.1	644.8	105.9
16.1	82.5	218.4	429.9	671.2	924.3	260.3
13.9	79.5	257.2	485.2	659.4	925.8	270.1
16.5	83.4	241.8	499.2	697.5	888.0	266.7
17.0	82.1	242.2	473.3	686.3	879.0	269.6
15.5	80.7	237.0	450.7	693.6	896.9	269.6

Table 100

Absolute Number and Incidence of Malignant Neoplasms of Different Localizations as Reported by the Oncologic Institutions between 1970 and 1974

Localization	ICD Code Number 8th rev.	Absolute number					Incidence per 100.000 population				
		1970	1971	1972	1973	1974	1970	1971	1972	1973	1974
All malignant neoplasms	140-209	1.473.818	1.545.894	1.617.863	1.693.661	1.774.546	604.3	627.6	650.7	675.2	700.7
oral and pharyngeal cavities	140-149	180.280	185.935	190.860	196.862	201.712	73.9	75.5	76.8	78.5	79.6
Lips	140	162.669	167.286	171.438	176.067	179.826	66.7	67.9	69.0	70.2	71.0
Digestive organs and peritoneum	150-159	216.719	222.002	228.671	237.147	246.070	88.8	90.2	92.0	94.5	97.2
Esophagus	150	14.458	14.191	14.434	14.325	14.384	5.9	5.8	5.8	5.7	5.7
Stomach	151	144.666	145.436	147.351	150.072	153.155	59.3	59.0	59.3	59.8	60.5
Rectum	154	24.809	27.014	29.474	32.042	34.461	10.2	11.0	11.8	12.8	13.6
Respiratory organs	160-163	73.296	77.925	82.726	88.200	94.012	30.1	31.6	33.3	35.2	37.1

Site	Code										
Larynx	161	23.475	25.396	27.275	29.232	31.246	9.6	10.3	11.0	11.6	12.3
Trachea, bronchi, lungs	162	46.446	48.861	51.682	54.864	58.622	19.0	19.8	20.8	21.9	23.1
Bones and connecting tissue	170–171	23.742	25.183	26.345	27.790	29.084	9.7	10.2	10.6	11.1	11.5
Skin	172–173	399.353	422.408	443.490	463.321	485.906	163.7	171.5	178.3	184.7	101.8
Breast	174	129.627	138.251	147.115	156.674	166.939	53.1	56.1	59.2	62.4	65.9
Urogenital organs	180–189	393.561	413.536	433.465	453.064	474.189	161.4	167.9	174.3	180.6	187.2
Cervix uteri	180	260.724	270.848	281.189	291.261	301.115	106.9	110.0	119.1	116.1	118.9
Other genital organs	181, 183, 184	90.766	97.508	104.152	110.815	118.534	37.2	39.6	41.9	44.2	46.8
Urinary bladder and 189 other urinary organs	188,	28.902	31.273	34.010	36.127	38.730	11.9	12.7	13.7	14.4	15.2
Lymphatic and hemato- poietic tissues	200–209	30.850	33.591	36.817	40.031	43.713	12.7	13.6	14.8	16.0	17.2

with malignant tumours of the breast have sharply increased, thus advancing this localization to the fourth place instead of the malignant tumours of the stomach. An increase in the contingents of patients with malignant neoplasms has been noted in all the Union Republics without exception. However, the number of patients /per 100,000 population/ registered in the oncological institutions of the different Union Republics shows wide varieties. While the average All-Union index is $700.7^{o}/oooo$, the index of the patients with malignant neoplasms on records in Estonia is $1107.3^{o}/oooo$; close to this value are the indices of Latvia /$981.9^{o}/oooo$/, the Ukrainian /$875.5^{o}/oooo$/, Lithuanian /$795^{o}/oooo$/, and Russian SFSR /$783.2^{o}/oooo$/. The smallest are found in Tadzhikistan /$199.4^{o}/oooo$/, Uzbekistan /$200.1^{o}/oooo$/, Turkmenia /$207.7^{o}/oooo$/ and Azerbaijan /$260.8^{o}/oooo$/.

The distribution of patients with malignant neoplasms according to the period they have been on the records since the diagnosis was made /Table 101/, reveals a considerable positive shift which proves the efficiency of cancer control in the country.

Between 1970 and 1975 alone the contingents of patients with malignant tumours on the records of oncological institutions for a period of 10 years and longer have increased by 137,000 and now total 414,000 persons or 24 % of all the patients on the records.

In 1974 the USSR had 249 functioning oncological dispensaries, 3,133 oncological departments and 50,300 beds for patients with malignant tumours.

The provision of the population with oncological beds varies between wide limits; thus, whereas in the Latvian, Estonian, Kirghiz, Ukrainian, Russian and Byelorussian SSR there are 3.2, 2.7, 2.5, 2.1 and 2 oncological beds, respectively, Tadzhikistan and Armenia have 1 bed each, Georgia has 1.2 beds, Moldavia 1.5, and Turkmenia and Uzbekistan 1.6 beds each per 10,000 population.

Table 102 offers information on the treatment of patients with malignant neoplasms of the second clinical group who

576

received special treatment during the year under review. Considering the dynamics of the structural changes in the methods of treatment used between 1970 and 1974 we must note the stability of these methods. The first place has been retained by radiotherapy, the second by surgery, the third by cytostatic treatment, the fourth and fifth places by combined and general treatment. It should be noted that cytostatic therapy is still unjustified widely administered to patients of this group, especially in cases of malignant tumours of the respiratory organs /41.2 %/ and of the gastrointestinal organs system /23.2 %/. In some Republics these indices are still higher; thus in Turkmenia, the Ukraine and Moldavia, respectively, 65 %, 63 % and 54 % of the patients of the second clinical group with malignant neoplasms of the respiratory organs were administered only cytostatic therapy; this method of treating patients of the second clinical group with malignant tumours of the organs of digestion was used in Turkmenia in 74.5 % of all cases, in Kirghizia in 61.8 %, in Azerbaijan in 41.5 % and in Tajikistan in 36.9 % of the cases.

The surgery in treating patients with malignant neoplasms in the Uzbek, Turkmen and Kirghiz SSR is inadequate /17-19 %/; moreover, it is applied mainly in tumours of external localizations.

The USSR Ministry of Health devotes special attention to the development of a network of oncological institutions and large oncological dispensaries, and takes measures to re-equip oncological institutions with up-to-date diagnostic and therapeutic apparatus and to use electronic computers in summarizing and processing the statistical information on oncological patients on a country-wide scale.

All these measures will make it possible in a short period of time to enhance the efficiency of the therapeutic and prophylactic aid to patients with malignant neoplasms.

In the USSR mortality from malignant tumours holds second place among all the causes of death. /For the distribution of mortality from malignant neoplasms between the Union Republics in 1970 see Table 103/

Table

Distribution of Patients with Malignant Neoplasms by the Time

1970

Localization	ICD Code Number	Number of patients with malignant		
		Total Absolute Number	including patients less than 1 year	
			Absolute Number	% of the total number of patients
All malignant neoplasms	140-199	1.442.968	265.363	18.4
From this children up to 14 years /inclusive/	140-149	1.972	852	43.2
Lips	140	162.669	14.742	9.1
Esophagus	150	14.458	8.497	58.8
Stomach	151	144.666	48.650	33.6
Rectum	154	24.809	8.019	32.3
Larynx	161	23.475	5.464	23.3
Trachea, bronchi, and lungs	162	46.446	23.604	50.8
Skin	172-173	399.353	46.960	11.8
Breast	174	129.627	22.170	17.1
Cervix uteri	180	260.766	30.802	11.8
Other female genital organs	181, 183,184	90.766	17.143	18.9
Urinary bladder and other urinary organs	188, 189	28.902	7.808	27.0
Neoplasms of lymphatic and hematopoietic tissues	200-209	30.850	9.677	31.4
From which children up to 14 year /inclusive/		1.746	849	48.6

101

Elapsed from their Registration by an Oncologic Institution

neoplasms, registered by oncologic institutions; data are as of the end of the year.							
registered upon diagnosis							
Abso- lute number	% of the total num- ber of pat.	Abso- lute number	% of the total num- ber of pat.	Abso- lute number	% of the total num- ber of.pat	Abso- lute number	% of the total num- ber of p.
300.476	20.8	238.401	16.5	360.952	25.0	277.786	19.2
576	29.2	292	14.8	205	10.4	47	2.7
25.759	15.8	25.804	15.9	48.533	29.8	47.831	29.4
3.913	27.0	1.213	8.4	649	4.5	186	1.3
32.647	22.6	19.425	13.4	25.402	17.6	18.542	12.8
7.250	29.2	7.761	15.2	3.685	14.9	2.094	8.4
6.173	26.3	4.263	18.1	5.163	22.0	2.412	10.3
13.188	28.4	5.311	11.5	3.544	7.6	799	1.7
77.584	19.4	73.183	18.3	119.197	29.9	82.429	20.6
29.412	22.7	22.507	17.4	31.206	24.0	24.332	18.8
46.873	18.0	41.946	16.1	73.582	28.2	67.521	25.9
20.798	22.9	15.796	17.4	21.553	23.7	15.476	17.1
7.921	27.4	5.414	18.8	5.469	18.9	2.290	7.9
9.824	31.8	5.433	17.6	4.219	13.7	1.697	5.5
519	29.7	237	13.6	121	6.9	20	1.2

Table 101 /cont'd/

Localization	ICD Code Number	Number of patients with malignant		
		Total Absolute Number	less than 1 year	
			Absolute Number	% of the total number of patients
All malignant neoplasms	140--149	1.730.833	292.924	16.9
From which children up to 14 years /inclusive/	140--149	2.609	940	36.0
Lips		179.826	14.255	7.9
Esophagus	150	14.384	8.002	55.6
Stomach	151	153.155	49.070	32.0
Larynx	154	34.461	10.674	30.9
Rectum	161	31.246	6.539	20.9
Trachea, Bronchi and lungs	162	58.622	28.576	48.7
Skin	172--173	485.906	52.131	10.7
Breast	174	166.939	26.932	16.1
Cervix uteri	180	301.115	29.536	9.8
Other female genital organs	181, 183.184	56.712	11.070	19.5
Urinary bladder and other urinary organs	188, 189	38.730	9.420	24.3
Neoplasms of lymphatic and hematopoietic tissues	200--209	42.713	12.108	27.7
From which children up to 14 years /inclusive		2.256	947	41.9

neoplasms, registered by oncologic institutons; data are as
of the end of the year

registered upon diagnosis

Absolute number	% of the total number of p.	Absolute number	% of the total number of p.	Absolute number	% of the total number of p.	Absolute number	% of the total number of p.
337.894	19.5	279.207	16.1	405.989	23.5	414.819	24.0
768	29.4	470	18.0	343	13.1	88	3.4
25.993	14.4	27.480	15.3	47.911	26.6	64.187	35.7
3.838	26.7	1.402	9.7	823	5.7	319	2.2
33.007	21.5	19.368	13.0	24.972	16.3	26.238	17.1
9.678	28.1	5.360	15.6	5.260	15.3	3.489	10.1
7.681	24.6	5.796	1.9	6.965	22.3	4.265	13.6
16.435	28.0	7.090	12.1	4.837	8.3	1.684	2.9
86.561	17.8	85.293	17.6	135.788	27.9	126.133	25.9
37.155	22.2	29.528	17.7	37.222	22.3	36.102	21.6
46.473	15.4	44.919	14.9	78.272	26.0	101.915	33.8
12.401	21.8	9.555	16.8	12.743	22.5	10.943	19.3
10.291	26.6	7.335	18.9	7.509	19.4	4.175	10.8
13.048	29.8	8.140	18.6	7.310	16.7	3.107	7.1
700	31.0	358	15.9	219	9.7	32	1.4

Localization	ICD Code Number 8th revision	Number of Patients	
		Total	Type
			Surgical only
1 9 7 0			
All malignant neoplasms /excluding tumours of lymphatic and hematopoietic tissues/	140-199		
Absolute number		254.471	
% of the total number of patients completed treatment		100	23.2
For this children up to 14 years /inclusive/			
Absolute number		804	
% of the total number of patients completed treatment		100	28.1
Oral cavity and throat	140-149		
Absolute number		18.929	
% of the total number of patients completed treatment		100	7.3
Digestive organs and peritoneum	150-159		
Absolute number		59.489	
% of the total number of patients completed treatment		100	52.2
Respiratory organs			
Absolute number	160-163	30.216	
% of the total number of patients completed treatment		100	11.8
Tumours of lymphatic and hematopoietic tissues	200-209		
Absolute number		17.671	
% of the total number of patient completed treatment		100	2.0
cont'd			

102

Patients with Malignant Neoplasms

completed special treatment for malignant neoplasms								
of treatment								
radiotherapy only				Mixed /surgical and radiotherapy				
		c o m b i n e d						
Tele-gamma the-rapy	X-ray the-rapy	Contact and tele-gamma therapy	Contact gamma the-rapy	tele-gamma the-rapy	X-ray the-rapy com-bined	Com-bi-na-tion	Cyto-static	Compre-hen-sive
6.6	20.9	6.5	3.0	5.0	8.0	1.4	15.9	7.7
10.1	15.8	0.4	0.4	4.5	11.4	0.5	16.9	10.3
8.7	55.3	1.5	1.1	2.9	17.8	0.7	1.1	2.6
4.5	2.2	0.2	0.1	0.7	1.1	0.2	27.8	7.8
16.7	8.5	0.2	0.3	3.7	3.3	0.4	47.1	6.1
6.8	8.8	0.1	0.2	1.2	1.6	1.1	66.5	9.7

Table 102 /cont'd/

Localization	ICD Code Number 8th revision	Number of Patients	
		Total	Type Surgical only
From this in children up to 14 years /inclusive/			
Absolute number		1.317	
% of the total number of patient completed treatment		100	5.6
1 9 7 4			
All malignant neoplasms /excluding tumours of lymphatic and hematopoietic tissues/	140-199		
Absolute number		290.993	
% of the total number of patient completed treatment		100	25.1
For this children up to 14 years /inclusive/			
Absolute number		1.029	
% of the total number of patient completed treatment		100	33.2
Oral cavity and throat	140-149		
Absolute number		20.614	
% of the total number of patient completed treatment		100	7.0
Digestive organs and peritoneum	150-159		
Absolute number		69.324	
% of the total number of patient completed treatment		100	54.0
Respiratory organs	160-163		
Absolute number		37.371	
% of the total number of patient completed treatment		100	13.5

cont'd

completed special treatment for malignant neoplasms

of treatment

radiotherapy only		c o m b i n e d			Mixed /surgical and radiotherapy			
Tele-gamma the-rapy	X-ray the-rapy	Contact and tele-gamma therapy	Contact gamma the-rapy	tele-gamma the-rapy	X-ray the-rapy com-bined	Com-bi-na-tion	Cyto-static	Compre-hen-sive
8.1	8.7	–	–	0.5	1.0	0.2	62.9	12.2
7.8	19.0	6.7	2.2	7.6	5.3	1.5	14.4	10.4
13.1	6.5	0.2	1.0	8.6	8.4	0.6	11.8	16.6
11.9	52.7	2.7	2.1	5.6	12.7	1.0	1.7	2.6
5.8	1.2	0.2	0.1	2.0	0.9	0.4	23.3	12.1
20.7	6.0	0.4	0.4	5.9	2.6	0.3	41.2	9.0

Table 102 /cont'd/

Localization	ICD Code Number 8th rev- ision	Number of Patients	
			Type
		Total	Surgical only

Tumors of lymphatic and hematopoietic tissues   200-209

    Absolute number   23.193

    % of the total number of
    patients completed treatment   100   1.5

From this children up to 14 years
/inclusive/

    Absolute number   1.749

    % of the total number of
    patients completed treatment   100   2.3

completed special treatment for malignant neoplasms								
of treatment								
radiotherapy only				Mixed /surgical and radiotherapy				
		c o m b i n e d						
Tele-gamma the-rapy	X-ray the-rapy	Contact and tele-gamma therapy	Contact gamma the-rapy	tele-gamma the-rapy	X-ray the-rapy com-bined	Com-bi-na-tion	Cyto-static	Compre-hen-sive
9.4	3.7	0.1	0.2	1.1	1.2	0.2	70.7	11.9
9.5	3.5	0.2	0.1	1.5	1.3	-	69.7	11.9

Table 103

Number of Deaths and Mortality per 100.000 Population from Malignant Neoplasms of the Population of the USSR and Union Republics in 1970

1 4 0 - 2 0 9

	Absolute number	Mortality per 100.000 population
	1970	1970
USSR	308.724	127.2
Russian SFSR	188.226	144.4
Ukrainian SSR	59.816	126.4
Byelorussian SSR	9.487	105.0
Uzbek SSR	7.479	61.7
Lazakh SSR	14.318	110.5
Georgian SSR	3.725	79.1
Azerbaijan SSR	4.141	80.2
Lithuanian SSR	4.438	141.0
Moldavian SSR	2.893	80.5
Latvian SSR	4.040	170.1
Kirghiz SSR	2.289	77.2
Tadzhik	1.606	54.6
Armenian SSR	1.769	70.3
Turmen SSR	2.096	95.7
Estonian SSR	2.401	175.9

The increase in the proportion of mortality from malignant tumours among the causes of death has been characteristic of all countries, especially in the last decades. It may be caused primarily by the sharp decrease in mortality from infectious, parasitic and other diseases, as well as by the aging of the population.

An analysis of both the general intensive and the standard indices of mortality from oncological diseases shows that the rates of its increase have essentially slowed down in the USSR.

It is characteristic that the intensity of the process of the population's aging /an increase in the proportion of people over 60 years of age in the structure of the population/ and the dynamics of the general intensive indices of mortality from malignant tumours during the examined period have changed in the same direction and have increased almost simultaneously. At the same time the standard indices of mortality from malignant neoplasms in the USSR not only do not increase, but, on the contrary, noticeably decrease.

The somewhat permanent increase in the mortality indices may be explained not only by the continuous aging of the population but also by the improved diagnosis of tumours, as well as the existing tendency to ascribe the death of people outside of hospitals to the "main groups of causes", including malignant neoplasms. It is also possible that the increase in the general index is connected with some actual increase in mortality from malignant neoplasms of various localizations.

Despite the certain fluctuations of the mortality indices for some localizations from 1970 to 1974 the structure of mortality from malignant neoplasms of various localizations changes but slightly.

In the structure of mortality from malignant neoplasms for 1974 /Fig. 39/, the leading role is still played by tumours of the organs of digestion /48.9 %/, mainly of the stomach /28.8 %/; tumours of the respiratory organs come next /18.5 %/; tumours of the female genitals are on the third place /9.1 %/; an important role in mortality is played also by breast cancer /4.6 %/. The tumours of these localizations

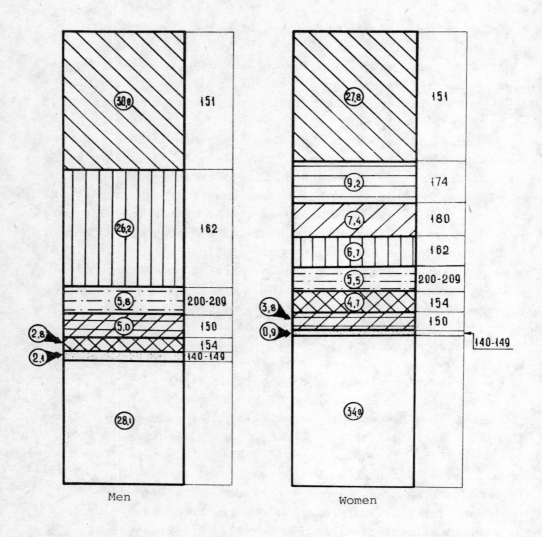

Men   Women

Fig. 39   The structure of mortality from malignant neoplasms
          of the population of the USSR in 1974 /according to
          the main localizations of the ICD, 8th revision/

altogether account for 81.1 % of the causes of death from malignant neoplasms. Of the remaining 18.9 %, 5.7 % of the
deaths are caused by neoplasms of the lymphatic and hemato-
poeitic tissues /Table 104/. Nevertheless, the dynamics of
the mortality indices of various localizations have undergone

Table 104

Structure of Mortality from Malignant tumours of the Population of the USSR

	ICD Code number	1970	1971	1972	1973	1974
All malignant tumours	140-209	100.0	100.0	100.0	100.0	100.0
Oral cavity and throat	141-149	1.3	1.3	1.4	1.5	1.5
Digestive organs	150-159	51.6	51.0	50.6	49.7	48.9
Esophagus	150	5.0	4.9	4.8	4.5	4.4
Stomach	151	32.0	31.0	30.4	29.5	28.8
Rectum	154	2.9	3.1	3.3	3.5	3.8
Respiratory organs	160-163	17.0	17.2	17.5	18.0	18.5
Trachea, bronchi, lungs	162	15.3	15.5	15.8	16.2	16.5
Bones and connective tissue	170-171	1.0	1.1	1.2	1.2	1.2
Skin	172-173	0.6	0.6	0.7	0.7	0.8
Breast	174	4.0	4.1	4.3	4.5	4.6
Female genital organs	180-184	9.4	9.3	9.2	9.2	9.1
Cervix uteri	180	3.9	4.0	3.9	3.8	3.6
Male genital organs	185-187	1.4	1.4	1.4	1.5	1.5
Urinary organs	188-189	3.2	3.2	3.2	3.3	3.3
Lymphatic and hematopoietic organs	200-209	5.8	5.8	5.8	5.7	5.7
Leukaemia and aleukaemia	204-207	2.9	2.9	3.0	3.1	3.2

certain changes. Thus the indices of mortality from tumours of the esophagus and stomach have noticeably decreased and a tendency toward their further decrease clearly manifests itself the indices for the few years between 1970 and 1974 are compared; on the other hand, the indices of mortality from tumours of the trachea, bronchi and lungs have appreciably increased and have shown a marked tendency toward their further increase. A certain increase is observed in the mortality from tumours of the oral cavity, pharynx, mammae and rectum, this increase being constant over the period of 1970-1974 /Table 105/.

The general, and especially the standard, indices of male mortality in the USSR, as a whole, are higher than those of female mortality during any of the examined years. This difference is becoming more and more obvious with each passing year.

An analysis of the age and sex indices of mortality does not confirm the current opinion that cancer "has grown younger", i.e., that its incidence has increased in young people. No increase in the indices of mortality form malignant neoplasms of people below 40 years of age, either men or women, has been revealed. Moreover, as in the preceding years, the special age indices of mortality sharply increase in both men and women; this difference is particularly noticeable in the age groups of 40-49 years.

Up to 40 years of age the indices of mortality among men and those among women do not essentially differ.

It is characteristic that the sharpest increase in mortality is observed for most localizations in the age groups of 40-49 years. The mortality indices in these groups are 3-5 times as high as in the age group of up to 30 years. This corresponds to the dynamics of morbidity and is a sufficient reason for raising the question of conducting mass prophylactic examinations first of all and most precisely from 35 years of age.

Table 105

Number of Deaths and Mortality /per 100.000 Population/ from Malignant Neoplasms of Different Localizations in the Population of the USSR

Localization	ICD Code Number 8th rev.	1 9 7 0		1 9 7 3		1 9 7 4	
		Abso lute number	Mortality per 100.000 popu- lation	Abso- lute number	Mortality per 100.000 popu- lation	Abso- lute number	Mortality per 100.000 popu- lation
All malignant neoplasms	140-209	308.724	127.2	327.853	131.3	334.585	132.7
Oral cavity and throat	141-149	3.958	1.6	5.858	1.9	4.968	2.0
Digestive organs	150-159	159.285	65.6	163.079	65.3	163.568	64.9
Esophagus	150	15.446	6.4	14.630	5.9	14.807	5.9
Stomach	151	98.789	40.7	96.908	38.8	96.323	38.2
Intestines	152-153	10.080	4.4	12.127	4.8	12.675	5.0
Rectum	154	9.169	3.8	11.461	4.6	12.570	5.0
Respiratory organs	160-163	52.569	21.6	59.205	23.7	61.890	24.5
Trachea, bronchi, lungs	162	47.240	19.5	53.226	21.3	55.215	21.9
Bones and connective tissue	170-171	3.203	1.3	3.933	1.6	3.935	1.6
Skin	172-173	2.015	0.8	2.341	0.9	2.582	1.0
Breast	174	12.329	5.1	14.643	5.9	15.444	6.1
Female genital organs	180-184	28.958	11.9	30.110	12.0	30.589	12.1

cont'd

Table 105/cont'd /

Localization	ICD Code Number 8th rev.	1 9 7 0		1 9 7 3		1 9 7 4	
		Abso-lute number	Mortality per 100.000 popu-lation	Abso-lute number	Mortality per 100.000 popu-lation	Abso-lute number	Mortality per 100.000 popu-lation
Cervix uteri	180	12.061	5.0	12.385	5.0	12.179	4,8
Male sex organs	185-187	4.383	1.8	4.849	1.9	4.996	2.0
Urinary organs	188-189	9.780	4.0	10.926	4.4	11.197	4.4
Lymphatic and haemato-poietic tissues	200-209	17.811	7.3	18.754	7.5	18.921	7.5
Leukaemia and aleukaemia	204-207	9.035	3.7	10.080	4.0	10.729	4.3

ORGANIZATION OF DETECTION AND EXAMINATION OF ONCOLOGICAL PATIENTS

N.N. Aleksandrov and Z.M. Gutman

It is one of the most important tasks of all the cancer control programs carried out in the USSR to create conditions for diagnosing malignant tumours early enough for the treatment to be most effective.

In order to solve this problem the public health organs carry out manifold work which includes measures to increase oncological knowledge of the practical physicians, to supply the prophylactic institutions with up-to-date diagnostic equipment, to expand the network of specialized tumour-diagnostic rooms and departments, health educational work among the population, etc. However, from among all the above-mentioned measures it is the organization of the early diagnosis of malignant tumours by active and timely detection of oncological patients that prevails.

For this purpose several programs have been drawn up and are functioning in the Soviet public health system which provide for the obligatory medical screening of the overwhelming majority of the country's population.

These programs can be roughly divided into two groups of measures. The first of them includes various forms of screening the population in the outpatient and inpatient institutions of the general medical network. The second one includes various forms of mass prophylactic screenings of the population. Outpatient polyclinics and hospitals of the general medical network are made responsible for the all-round examination aimed at detecting tumourous diseases of all persons older than 35 years, visiting the polyclinics and going into hospital for treatment, irrespective of the nature of the disease, for which they visit the doctor. The results of these examinations are recorded in the outpatient cards and case histories, indicating the date they were carried out, the results, and the name of the physician. Irrespective by of the character of the disease the cancer-oriented examinations of women older than 30 the equally obligatory at women's examination rooms of polyclinics for detecting tumours and pretumourous diseases of the reproductive organs, the mammary glands, the skin and the rectum. Such examinations are carried out by obstetricians who have had special training.

The methods and timing of these examinations are regulated by appropriate instructions and methodological directions of the Ministries of Health of the USSR and of the Union Republics. The physicians of territorial oncological dispensaries are responsible for checking up the quality and correctness of these examinations.

Taking into account that persons, who have for long been suffering from pretumourous diseases, encounter a higher risk of contracting malignant neoplasms particularly their obligate forms, all the outpatient and polyclinical institutions in the country carry out prophylactic examinations of such patients according to standardized methods, registration of detected patients, their regular examination and therapy, and also follow-up observation. The polyclinics of the general prophylactic examinations patients with atrophic gastritic, gastric ulcer and chronic nonspecific diseases of the lungs, including chronic relapsing pneumonias, with pretumourous processes in the oral cavity, while women with precancerous diseases of the female reproductive organs are under the observation at women's consultations.

The group of patients with pretumourous diseases subject to observation at oncological institutions is singled out /particularly persons suffering from polyps of the stomach and the intentines, callous ulcers of the stomach, focal-hyperplastic rigid gastritis, fibroadenoma of the breast, Kaposi's disease, dyskeratosis and papillomatosis of the lower lip/. According to the current regulations all patients with pretumourous diseases are taken off the register not earlier than a year after treatment, on the condition of their complete recovery.

Since every year at least two-thirds of the total population of the country turns for medical aid to the outpatient polyclinics, the described system of primary detection of patients with suspected cancer makes it possible to cover a considerable part of the entire adult population, including /and this is particularly important/ the overwhelming majority of persons of pension age, who, in distinction from the working population, are not so regularly subjected to mass prophylactic examinations. The institutions of the general medical network also follow uniform regulations for the examination of patients suspected for cancer. Whenever such patients are detected at a polyclinic and found in need of diagnostic confirmation, they are sent to the appropriate institutions and a Dispensary Observation Card is filled up /clinical group 1a/, which, together with the outpatient's card enables the district oncologist to carry out supervision of the quality and dates of their further examinations. This should be done within ten days and, depending on its results, the patient is either struck off the register, or, if the diagnosis of a malignant tumour is confirmed, sent for specialized treatment. When a disease suspected for being a malignant tumour is identified in a patient admitted to hospital, he is not discharged until the diagnosis is definitely established. If the given medical institution lacks the necessary diagnostic facilities, the patient must be promptly sent to a specialized /as a rule oncological/ institution.

Naturally enough, the timely detection of patients suspected for malignant tumours at institutions of the general medical network largely depends on the oncological awareness of the physicians, for they are the first who see the patient, moreover, on the localization of the tumour and the degree of the clinical manifestations of the disease at the moment of visiting the physician, as well as on a number of other factors.

Various patterns for the primary questioning and cancer--oriented examination of patients visiting the polyclinics have been developed and introduced into practice by the country's Central and some Republican Oncological Institutes intended for a fully adequate examination of patients suspected for malignant tumours and for raising the oncological awareness of physicians at the polyclinics of the general medical network.

In some of the Union Republics special "Preventive Examination Cards" are used for this purpose, which are printed on the back of the first sheet of the outpatient card and contain a number of questions facilitating the work of a physician of any specialty for detecting patients suspected for neoplasms of the most frequently affected organs. In other republics are examination patterns used for the same purpose, intended for identifying patients with tumours of certain localizations /the esophagus, the stomach, the lungs, the breast, the rectum/; such patterns, printed on standard forms, are used as inserts to outpatient cards.

The patterns for examining patients suspected for malignant tumours recommended for practical physicians are drawn up considering the need of reducing to the minimum the multiplicity of stages in carrying out such examinations as well as the real possibilities for using the entire complex of modern diagnostic means. Depending on the localization of the tumour, they include the following basic types of examination.

When discovering changes suspicious of cancer on the skin, the tongue, the mucosa of the oral cavity and the larynx, the disease is diagnosed finally by the physician on the basis of the findings of biopsy and subsequent histological examination of the obtained material. Patients suspected for malignant melanoma are sent, as a rule, for diagnosis to specialized institutions having every facility for a comprehensive examination, with the use of radio-isotopes, cytological, histochemical and laboratory diagnostic methods.

For patients suspected for cancer of the lung, a prompt X-ray examination in two projections is obligatory. In the majority of cases such an examination is supplemented with repeated cytological examinations of the sputum, or by bronchoscopy with cancer-oriented biopsy of tissues from the affected area. In connection with the expansion of the network of bronchial examination rooms at the polyclinics and pulmonary departments in the recent years there were the conditions for the broader application at general medical institutions of multipositional roentgenology of the lungs, tomography and bronchial examination methods including fibrobronchoscopy have been steadily improved. Nevertheless, when such facilities are lacking, the practical physician is recommended, in order to shorten the time of examination, to send patients suspected for cancer of the lungs to specialized institutions, without resorting to preliminary antiphlogistic therapy.

For the timely detection of cancer of the stomach in the conditions of a polyclinic in patients complaining of dyspeptic disorders or with clinical symptoms suspicious of this disease, clinical, laboratory, instrumental and X-ray examination methods are widely used. Roentgenoscopy of the stomach remains the basic method among them so far. The use of fibrogastroscopy in combination with cancer-oriented biopsy and cytological examination of gastric juice reliably provides for the detection of early forms of gastric carcinoma, particularly among persons with an increased risk of contracting the disease, placed under dispensary observation because of pretumourous diseases of the stomach.

The set of diagnostic examinations most widespread in clinical practice for patients suspected for cancer of the large intestine and the rectum includes obligatory palpation of the rectum, rectoromanoscopy and irrigoscopy which are supplemented, when necessary, by other kinds of roentgenological examination. The timely diagnosis of these tumours is considerably promoted today by the use of fibrocolonoscopy.

When mammary carcinoma is suspected the definite diagnosis is made in medical institutions of the general network on the basis of clinical and roentgenological /non-contrast mammography/ findings, and also by cytological examination of the discharge from the nipples and of material obtained during explorative puncture. Sectoral resection of the mammary gland in such patients is admissible only in those medical institutions which have facilities for carrying out rapid histological examination of the material obtained and /in case the diagnosis is confirmed/ for carrying out prompt radical therapy.

Examination of women suspected for cancer of the reproductive organs, found by the gynecologist at the polyclinic or the obstetrician at the women's examination room, is carried out in the majority of cases at women's consultations. In addition to the inspection of the cervix uteri with speculums and bimanual, including rectovaginal inspection, they are subjected to a more detailed examination, including colposcopy, cytological examination of vaginal smears and cancer-oriented biopsy. When more complicated diagnostic examinations are called for /curettage of the uterine cavity, conelike dissection of the cervix uteri, hysterosalpingo- and pelviography, etc./ the patients are sent to gynecological department of hospitals.

For ensuring continuity when examining oncological patients, they are sent for consultations, additional examinations and treatment to specialized institutions, as a rule by the heads of the regional tumour-diagnostic rooms or physicians responsible for the organization of oncological services to the population. An excerpt is attached to the referral slip from the medical /outpatient/ card or case history, and also the results of examinations carried out, including roentgenograms, cytological and histological preparations. The time allotted for examining patients suspected for malignant tumours /10 days/ and for their hospitalization for treatment after the diagnosis has been established /also 10 days/ serves as an important additional stimulus securing the timely diagnosis and start of therapy for such patients.

All the oncological institutions of the country have the task of carrying out constant supervision over the observance of the recommended patterns and dates of examination of patients suspected for malignant tumours, and also of the rules for sending them for further diagnosis and treatment. Medical errors made when examining such patients, cases when physicians ignore the available methods of examination, or violate existing instructions and methodological directions regarding such patients, are subject to obligatory discussions at medical conferences with the purpose of taking necessary organizational measures.

It goes without saying that the timely visit of an oncological patient for examination and for treatment largely depends on the awareness of the patient himself regarding the
seriousness of his disease. This question assumes particular
importance if the patient has to undergo complicated diagnostic
examination procedures or when it is necessary to solicit his
consent to surgery. Unfortunately, despite the wide-scale
propagation of information concerning modern achievements in
clinical oncology, some patients with malignant neoplasms detected during the curable stages of the disease, reject treatment either because of ignorance in regard to the seriousness
of the disease, or the erroneous idea that it is incurable.

The practice, as it exists in the USSR, of informing oncological patients or their relatives about the nature of the
disease is based on the observance of a number of principles
of medical deontology, obligatory for medical workers of all
medical institutions. In case of suspicion for cancer or the
presence of doubtless symptoms of this diagnosis, as a rule,
is not explained to the patient. The referral slip for examination or treatment given to the patient usually indicates the
diagnosis in a veiled form /"organic disease of the lungs",
"gastric ulcer", etc./, while the results of examinations
carried out are sent out by mail or handed over in a sealed
envelope. A similar entry is made in the final report of patients with established diagnosis of a malignant neoplasm. A
postal message goes to the medical institution which referred
the patient indicating the true diagnosis and all the data
necessary for subsequent dispensary observation of the patient.

The close relatives of an oncological patient and the
management of the place of his employment are entitled to
receive all the necessary information about him at any stage
of examination and treatment.

In cases when the patient refuses examination and treatment and the attending physician fails to convince him of the
necessity to promptly undergo such procedures, the patient
and his close relatives are invited for a talk by the head of

the department or chief physician. If the patient persists in his refusal of examination and treatment then he is informed on the true diagnosis of the disease and its prognosis.

On the whole, the system of organizing active detection and examination of patients suspected for cancer, as practised in the USSR, proved to be rather effective for the timely diagnosis of malignant neoplasms of many localizations, particularly such widespread tumours as cancer of the skin, the oral cavity, the lower lip, the breast, the cervix uteri and the rectum. Regarding tumours in these localizations, which are relatively easily accessible for examination /they make up more than 30 % of all malignant neoplasms annually registered in the USSR/, there are realistic prospects for the near-complete disappearance in the next few years of cases when patients are revealed with incurable forms of the disease.

The situation is much more complicated in case of tumours of the internal organs, the diagnosing of which at outpatient polyclinical institutions frequently presents serious difficulty even at rather advanced stages of the disease.

This is due to a number of reasons. One of them is the considerable gap between the attained level in the development of diagnostic equipment and its utilization in general medical practice. The experience shows that modern methods of examination of oncological patients - X-raying, clinical and laboratory endoscopic, morphological and radio-isotopic - given their comprehensive application, allow to correctly diagnose cancer in most of the cases already at the very early stages of the disease, even in patients who do not have complaints characteristic of the disease. Nevertheless, realistic opportunities for utilizing these methods are available mainly for large or specialized medical institutions, admitting patients needing further examination or definite diagnosis of the character of the tumour and the degree of its spread.

Particularly difficult is the early diagnosis of cancer in two categories of patients, namely patients who fail to request medical assistance despite the presence of symptoms of the disease and those in whom the initial period of the lesion proceeds without symptoms. According to the available data based on an analysis of cancer negligence protocols /clinical group 4/, such patients make up at least 40-50 % of all the patients in whom cancer is detected too late. A slight reduction of their number, particularly among patients of the first group, can be achieved by resorting to the above-mentioned organizational measures /improving health education among the population, expanding the network of medical institutions, particularly in the countryside, checking up the careful and vigorous collection of anamnestic data, etc./.

This problem can be solved to a certain extent by identifying such patients through mass prophylactic screenings of the population. The tasks of mass prophylactic screenings of the population are by no means limited to the detection of patients with tumour diseases; such screenings enable the detection of patients with pretumourous processes and chronic diseases requiring dispensary observation and treatment.

Mass prophylactic examinations of the population began to be carried out in the USSR in 1948. Such screenings, performed regularly by medical teams from the staffs of institutions belonging to the general medical network in the territories under their jurisdiction, have become one of the most important government measures in the field of public health.

The forms and methods of carrying out prophylactic screenings differ according to the economic, geographic and ethnic features of the administrative area, the occupations of the population in different branches of social production, the character of regional pathology and a number of other factors. The following forms have become most widespread in all the Union Republics: /1/ comprehensive examinations of organized groups of the population /workers and employees of large enterprises, construction sites, state farms, etc./, carried out at least once a year and /2/ periodical prophylactic examinations of certain occupational groups, within the framework of compulsory and regular /at least 2-4 times a year/ medical examination, in particular, workers of the enterprises of the food industry, of the public catering network, children's institutions, and persons getting into contact with occupational hazards.

Certain forms of specialized prophylactic screenings also became widespread, such as mass fluorography of the organs of the chest and screenings to detect gynecological disorders.

The number of people covered by prophylactic examinations in the USSR is steadily growing: in 1970 101,200,000 persons were subject to different kinds of examinations, in 1974 this number grew to 105,300,000.

In order to raise the effectivity of mass prophylactic screenings for the detection of cancer and pretumourous diseases oncological institutions organize special seminars for the physicians of the general medical network for carrying out such screenings. Special attention is given to methods of examination, the manner of registration of detected cancer patients and of referring them for dispensary observation and treatment.

At present intensive work is going on for ways and methods of improving the mass prophylactic screenings of the population. It is absolutely clear that their efficiency can be raised only at the maximal utilization of instrumental-laboratory diagnostic methods which considerably expand the range and possibilities for the early detection of tumourous and pretumourous diseases. At the same time it should be stressed that the successful utilization of instrumental-laboratory methods for examining large groups of the population is only possible under certain conditions, which may be formulated as follows:

1. High resolving power of the method.

2. Technical simplicity and rapid procedure.

3. The safety and atraumatism of the method for the examinee.

4. Suitability for the detection of tumours of the main localizations, which account for about 75 % of all malignant neoplasms.

The introduction of instrumental-laboratory diagnostic methods in the practice of mass prophylactic screenings calls for certain changes in the procedure of selecting persons eligible for examination. It is obvious that the whole group of persons subject to mass screenings /more than 100,000,000/ cannot be examined by instrumental-laboratory methods. The criteria for selecting persons needing such examinations are searched by different methods, among which the formation of a high-risk group occupies a dominant position. The concept of high cancer risk was formulated mainly in recent years.

By now a sufficiently large, though rather controversial body of material has been accumulated regarding the criteria and factors of high cancer risk, which requires further prospective study. The definition remains valid that in the high risk groups those categories of the population should be involved for whom, owing to a number of factors /age, genetical, occupational, way of life, the effect of environmental carcinogenic factors/, the danger of development of malignant tumours is higher than for other groups of the population, among whom the effect of these factors is either absent or small. Groups of persons with pretumourous diseases should be qualified as groups, in which factors of risk have already appeared and may lead to the development of some or other pathological process.

Among the numerous high-risk factors for individual localizations of malignant tumours one must specifically dwell on the significance of age in malignant tumour morbidity. It has been established that, irrespectively of the localization of the process and the patient's sex, a steep rise of the incidence rate is observed from the age of 40 upwards.

The above data lead to the conclusion that at present one can recommend the staging of prophylactic screenings beginning from as early as 35-40 years, which enables to considerably reduce the groups of the population eligible for examination and, consequently, carry out the screenings in greater detail, with the use of clinical and laboratory examination methods.

Thus, according to the materials pertaining to the age--sex structure of the population of the USSR /1973/, carrying out prophylactic screenings beginning from the age of 40 makes it possible to reduce the number of persons subject to examinations by nearly 32 per cent.

It should be stressed, however, that even with such a limitation of the number of persons eligible for examination, the groups of the population subject to oncological examinations still remain rather sizable and amount to /according to data for 1973/ 87,035,575 persons.

Before dealing with the organizational aspects of forming high cancer risk groups, some theoretical aspects of this complicated problem should be outlined. Numerous investigations have established that the factors of risk are very diverse and may refer to the environment, to the stereotyped habits. Some of these function constantly, stably and continuously, spreading their influence over large groups of the population. Others, on the contrary, exert their influence fortuitously.

By way of a critical approach to the assessment of the factors of risk, one may single out those that have been widely recognized /age, smoking and its connection with the increase in the incidence of lung cancer, the effect of diabetes, hypertension and obesity on the incidence of endometrial carcinoma and breast carcinoma/, and controversial factors /the character and rhythm of nutrition in cases of cancer of the large intestine and the rectum, of breast trauma/.

Probably it would be justified to determine the factors of risk which may be avoided /smoking, nutritional habits, a number of traditions/ and factors the influence of which practically cannot be eliminated /environmental pollution, hereditary predisposition/. It cannot be denied that the effect of the factors of risk on the organism in the majority of cases remains symptomless for a long period of time.

It must be admitted that the formation of high cancer risk groups involves certain difficulties, since the organizational forms of their screening have not been adequately elaborated. Besides, no clear-cut criteria of risk for the main localizations have been definitely determined yet, which makes the selection for the risk group more difficult. The study of these problems requires rather long prospective investigations.

In looking for ways to solve this problem two- and three-
-stage methods of conducting oncological examinations were put
to trial, involving the overall screening of the adult population, carried out by health workers or by paramedical personnel,
for selecting during the first stages persons with a higher
risk of contracting the disease. Such examinations proved rather effective when carrying out prophylactic oncological
examinations of the rural population. Studies conducted in the
Byelorussian SSR by a travelling specialist team have shown
that a two-stage examination of rural citizens after they themselves /or paramedical workers/ had filled in special Prophylactic Examination Cards, permits to notably improve the de-
tectability of patients with cancer /by more than 3 times/ and
pretumourous diseases /by 1.7 times/.

The experimental method of prophylactic oncological screenings is used for the same purpose in some of the Soviet Republics /Kazakhstan, Kirghizia, Estonia/. This method has proved
particularly valuable in Central Asia for screening the dwellers of highland areas, people engaged in nomadic stock-farm-
ing, etc. Nevertheless, the necessity of involving additional
personnel and assets for conducting such screenings as well as
the longer time inevitably required in these cases for examining the population, limit the possibilities for introducing
them into wide practice.

Taking into account that by now a number of highly effective methods, suitable for mass screenings /cytological methods, fluorography, mammography/ have been developed and
introduced in the public health practice, it seems to be advisable
to use them initially for the formation of groups, eligible for
further detailed examination and treatment.

In the country the availability of a broad network of
large-frame fluorographs, used earlier mainly for detecting
tuberculotic patients, is a realistic basis for organizing
annual mass prophylactic screenings of the organs of the chest
in a great number of people. By the help of this method patients
with pathological shadows in the lungs revealed by fluorography,
are directly sent to specialized institutions for definite

diagnosis, which allows to by-pass the numerous stages in their examination and to start their treatment earlier.

The use of large-frame fluorography considerably expands also the possibilities for realizing a program for the early detection of breast carcinoma.

Based on a representative study which has covered large groups of women and demonstrated the high solving power of the method, instructions have been worked out according to which all women aged above 35 years /with the exception of pregnant women/ are subject to such examination in whom individual prophylactic examination at the polyclinic by the physician or obstetrician of the examining room failed to identify any clinical symptoms of neoplasms of the breast. According to these instructions fluoromammography in women aged up to 45 years is carried out during the first phase of the menstrual cycle /from the 3rd to the 10th-12th day after the end of menstruation/, and in women older than 45 - irrespective of the phase of the menstrual cycle.

The method of large-frame fluorography may prove not less effective, particularly with the aid of a specially adapted apparatus to ensure visual control during the examination for detecting patients with early forms of gastric cancer. Since the routine X-ray examination of the stomach during mass prophylactic screenings, for obvious reasons, cannot be carried out, the use of large-frame fluorography under these conditions is practically the only way in which the roentgenological method can be used for this purpose.

Due to the high handling capacity of fluorographic installations, the simplicity and availability of the method permit the large-frame fluorography of the stomach belongs to the diagnostic methods which are fully suitable for mass prophylactic screenings. The advisability of using this method is confirmed also by its comparatively high resolving power. The results of large-frame fluorography of the stomach, carried out by staff members of the Byelorussian and the Rostov Oncological Institutes and covering nearly 20,000 persons, who complained of dyspeptic disorders or were under observation because of chronic diseases of the stomach, demonstrated that the method allows to select nearly all /90-95 %/ of the patients needing detailed examination for the definite diagnosing of the disease. It should be noted that among people over 40 years of age subjected to fluorographic examination, though they had no complaints of this kind /that is, they believed themselves to be practically healthy/, 0.2 % had cancer of the stomach and 0.6 % pretumourous diseases. Here, as the control X-ray examination revealed, no cases of cancer, ulcers and polyps of the stomach remained undetected by fluorography, while chronic gastritis went undetected only occasionally.

All this leaves no doubt that large-frame fluorography of the stomach makes possible to successfully select from among a great number of people subjected to prophylactic screenings persons needing further examination for detecting cancer of stomach. Such a selection, combined with the subsequent use of fibrogastroscopy, gastrobiopsy and cytological examination of gastric juices, renders possible to diagnose cancer of the stomach at very early stages of the disease, even in cases when it proceeds without any manifest symptoms.

It is obvious, though, that it is quite impossible to annually subject large numbers of people, who must be covered by mass prophylactic examinations, to large-frame fluorography and cytological examinations, or fiberogastroscopy. This makes it imperative to carry on the studies of criteria for forming groups of the population with a higher cancer risk, eligible for obligatory and regular examinations. So far this problem has been solved only partially by limiting the groups of the population subject to mass prophylactic screenings to the age groups older than 40 and by examining persons chiefly with pretumourous diseases.

It is especially interesting to examine large groups of organized population under conditions of industrial associations with the use of an automatized control system /ACS/, which permits to select groups subject to detailed examination. This method is now being introduced at some large industrial associations.

AUTOMATIZED PROPHYLACTIC ONCOLOGICAL SCREENINGS AT LARGE INDUSTRIAL ASSOCIATIONS

D.P. Berezkin and V.P. Nazarenko

Considering the existence of a great number of large industrial associations in the USSR, the creation of a special
form of prophylactic screenings at such enterprises is quite
justified, since it permits to involve a considerable group
of working people employed at these enterprises.

This section presents data on the creation of a model of
a new organizational form of mass prophylactic oncological
screenings of working people in production associations, aimed
at the timely detection of pretumourous and tumourous diseases
of the gastrointestinal tract.

The general program of developing the model may be
presented as follows:

Automation of the primary screening, i.e. providing for

1. the selection of persons subject to instrumental examination for the detection of diseases of the gastrointestinal
tract, including pretumourous and tumourous ones;

2. processing the information at every level required;

3. conducting the instrumental examination of the selected
groups;

4. the correct reporting on the conducted prophylactic
measures /documentation flow/.

In accordance with the above a number of concrete tasks
had to be solved:

1/ to develop a matrix /table of symptom-complex, see
Table 106/, allowing to carry out the primary mass screening
according to available symptoms /complaints/;

2/ to draw up a special questionnaire as the information
medium referring to each worker;

3/ to draw up programs for computerizing the information
aimed at singling out persons needing further detailed medical
examination, including instrumental examination;

4/ to draw up a well-balanced schedule for the examination of the detected persons at the medical unit of the
association;

5/ to provide for the closed flow of information by means of a developed documentation turnover system as an integral part of the association's Automatic Control System.

The elaboration of a model for a new organizational form of mass prophylactic oncological screenings for detecting pre-tumourous diseases of the gastrointestinal tract was based on the questionnaire method. The method essentially consists in filling out special questionnaires by all persons included in the group being examined.

Table 106

Table of Symptom-Complexes

Number	Symptoms and symptom-complexes	Category of urgency of the examination	Laboratory examination		Endoscopic examinations / X-ray examinations					Examination by the physician		
			Blood	Gastric content	Fiberogastroscopy	Esophagus	Stomach	Large intestine	Rectoromanoscopy	Otorhinolaryngologist	Surgeon	Internist
12	3.4+4.3+10.2	1			+							++
21	10.4+11.2	2					+				+	+
39	19.4+22.4+23.3	1							+		+	
62	1.3+5.2+7.2	3					+					+
104	3.4+2.4+12.4	3	+	+								+
173	20.3	2	+								+	
238	2.3+3.2+12.2	3	+			+						+

Notes: In the second column the first figures correspond to the number of a sign in the order of the questionnaire, and the second figures correspond to the number of this sign's manifestation.

For computer processing of the obtained information with the questionnaire method of prophylactic examination it was necessary to develop a test for the selection from among practically healthy individuals those eligible for instrumental examination. Such a test was a specially developed matrix /Table 106/ of symptom-complexes, which serves as the basic tool in implementing the primary screening with the aid of an electronic computer.

The matrix consists of a set of different combinations of diagnostic signs /symptoms/. In the ideal case one may presume that each disease /provided it is not absolutely symptomless/ has a corresponding definite type of clinical manifestations. Thus, for example, the diseases of the esophagus will be characterized by one set of diagnostic signs /here diagnostic signs are all sorts of complaints and a description of the state of one's health by the examinee himself/; cancer of the stomach will have another set of signs; diseases of the large intestine and the rectum will be characterized by a third set of symptoms, etc.

Hence, it was necessary to have at one's disposal such diagnostic signs that would make possible to formulate the necessary symptom-complexes. The selection of the most informative diagnostic signs and the formation of corresponding symptom-complexes has been carried out on the basis of studying data in the literature, analyzing the case histories of patients treated at the N.N. Petrov Oncological Research Institute, USSR Ministry of Health, and the experience of staff members of the Institute /expert evaluation/.

All this work has made it possible to create the above--mentioned matrix, containing 238 symptom-complexes.

Another important tool of primary screening is a questionnaire, fulfilling the role of a document carrying information concerning each particular person. Its content is intended to derive data warranting the formation of a set of diagnostic signs, contained in the matrix of symptom-complexes. In view of the fact that every worker fills out the questionnaire himself, the questionnaire must meet a number of requirements:

1/ the diagnostic signs contained in the questionnaire must be comprehensible to the questionees and at the same time be medically adequate;

2/ the questionnaire should not evoke any negative emotions in the questionees;

3/ the document should guarantee secrecy for the person who fills it out.

Resort to computer technology requires the observation of the following requirements:

1/ the arrangement of the signs in the questionnaire should be made with a view to subsequent machine processing;

2/ the form of the document should conform to the basic demands set to technical documentation in industry.

Other desirable features are the minimal size and cost of the questionnaire.

The structure of the questionnaire is based on the method of the selecting one out of several proposed replies to each question /diagnostic sign/. There are four such variants and each of them reflects four degrees of manifestation of the general condition or feelings of the questionee, which allows to differentiate various abnormalities in the functioning of the gastrointestinal tract.

The section of the questionnaire which concerns the set of diagnostic signs containing information about complaints and an evaluation of the state of the questionee's health was drawn up on the basis of studying the clinical symptomatology of malignant neoplasms of the gastrointestinal tract and expert evaluation of combination of diagnostic signs.

Signs reflecting the examinee's general condition as a result of his self-examination were united, for they may take place in different diseases, i.e. irrespective of the concrete localization of the pathological process /for example, general condition, body weight, appetite/. Such complaints as salivation, regurgitation, nausea, vomiting and changes in the attitude to food, as a rule contain information about disorders in the area of the esophagus and stomach. Obstructed

passage of food or pain during its passage are characteristic
in the majority of cases of diseases of the upper section of
the throat and esophagus. Unpleasant sensations following a
meal and pain in the upper part of the abdomen, occur mainly
in diseases of the stomach. Other signs may reflect serious disorders on the part of the large intestine and the rectum.

When studying the group under examination it seems very
important to reveal the presence of chronic disease, which
helps to determine whether the complaints refer to diseases of
which the examinee is unaware, or stem from diseases well known
to him. In this connection it is important to establish whether
the examinee is already placed under medical supervision for a
chronic disease of the organs of the gastrointestinal tract.

Let us return now to an examination of the "interaction"
process between the questionnaire and the above-mentioned
matrix of symptom-complexes. As a result of this process the
"decision" appears that the examinee may have some pathological
changes in the gastrointestinal tract, while the process itself
imitates the procedure of a primary screening.

The matrix of symptom-complexes is put in the computer's
memory.

The processing of the questionnaires, the information of
which is also put in the computer, takes place as follows.

The information contained in the questionnaires and consisting of n-diagnostic signs, is compared by the computer
with the symptom-complexes of the matrix, stored in the memory
/M/ of the computer. The analysis of symptom-complexes may
indicate the possible presence of one or another disease of
the gastrointestinal tract. Therefore the automated screening
procedure consists of designating the kind of laboratory-in-
strumental examination, an appointment with a specialist and
the determination of the category of the urgency of examination. This, in turn means that according to each symptom-
-complex of the matrix /or a group of symptom-complexes/ a
program of examination is prescribed to the person who filled
up the questionnaire, the information of which provides a set
of diagnostic signs permitting to formulate the symptom-

-complex coinciding with the corresponding symptom-complex of the matrix.

The category of urgency is determined by the severity of pathological signs. Here the entire group of persons subject to examination divided into three groups:

1st category of urgency - examination within one week on receiving the computerized conclusion.

2nd category of urgency - examination within two weeks.

3rd category of urgency - examination within three weeks.[x]

And, finally, as a result of the screening there is a considerable group of so-called practically healthy persons, who either have no complaints, or their character and manifestation do not indicate any serious disorder.

No concrete disease is diagnosed on the basis of the assessment of a symptom-complex, only a decision is taken on the advisibility of examining the condition of some organ or system. In other words, the task to be solved is not to set a diagnosis, to select the way of examination through which such a diagnosis may be properly made.

Following the processing of the questionnaire information, the machine output is printed out, containing data on the necessity of carrying out instrumental and laboratory examinations and indicating the category of its urgency.

Composite print-outs - referral slips are sent to the medical unit of the assiciation for laboratories and roentgenologists, endoscopists, laryngologists, surgeons and internists. These print-outs allow to organize the work of the medical unit of the enterprise by timely planning diagnostic procedures. Similar print-outs are sent to the subdivisions of the production association where the inquiring was made. On the basis of these print-outs every worker in the subdivision to whom one or another examination is prescribed is given a referral slip which plays the role of a feed-back document between the medical unit of the enterprise and its computer centre with the purpose of subsequently receiving cumulative data on the results of the prophylactic screening held.

x These time periods may change depending on the concrete conditions of the automatized screening operation.

After passing the prescribed laboratory and instrumental examinations /entered on the referral slip/, the patient is sent to the physician, who establishes the diagnosis, also recorded in the appropriate section of the referral slip according to the code of International Classification of Diseases, Eighth Revision /1969/.

The organization of an automated system of mass oncological prophylactic screenings

The conditions which at present, may ensure an optimal effect of prophylactic screenings are as follows:

1. The maximal accessible concentration of population in a limited area of territory.

2. Uniting the population by some single factor /relation to production/.

3. The presence of a clearly organized production process with the clearcut assignment of definite groups of workers to its different stages, which finds expression in the automatic control system /ACS/ and the automated technological production control system /ATPCS/.

4. The availability of a computer complex, capable of carrying out the rapid processing of large information blocks.

5. The availability of a medical unit, adequately supplied with diagnostic facilities, well-staffed with qualified personnel and capable of conducting prophylactic examinations and public health measures among the detected groups of patients.

As it has been stressed above, the conditions approaching such an ideal case are those existing at production associations.

For the realization and maximum utilization of such favourable conditions a method of automated screening was suggested, intended for solving the task of selecting persons subject to instrumental examination from among all the screened population.

It goes without saying that, when developing the organizational forms of a mass prophylactic oncological screening in the setting of a production association, use was made of the general principles of organizing and conducting mass prophylactic screenings as practised in the USSR, however, with some changes and additions corresponding to the possibility of computerizing the obtained information.

The Automatized System of Mass Prophylactic Oncological Screenings /ASMPOS/ of the workers of production associations consists of the following main units:

1. Organizational and preparative measures.

2. The sending out, filling in and collecting the questionnaires.

3. The computerization of information of the questionnaire with the aim of forming groups subject to further /detailed/ instrumental examination.

4. Notification of the subdivisions of the association and the medical unit about the selected persons needing various kinds of examinations.

5. The organization of instrumental and medical examination of workers singled out by computer decision.

6. Providing the computer centre with information on the results of the prophylactic screening carried out.

7. Drawing up a report at the computer centre on the results of the prohylactic screening of the workers of the association.

When carrying out the above measures it is desirable that they should be integrated into the routine /production/ life of the enterprise, so as to minimize losses of working time.

The ASMPOS procedure begins with the drawing up of a schedule and general plan by the medical unit and the computer centre of the association for conducting the prophylactic screening /Fig. 40, 41/. This plan, after being confirmed by the director of the enterprise, becomes an obligatory order.

Along with this, the physicians at the medical unit carry out still another set of measures:

1. Instruction of the activists of the Red Cross Committee and the time-keepers of the subdivisions about the rules of filling in the questionnaires.

2. Delivery of lectures and talks with the workers of the corresponding subdivision /workshops, departments/ on the

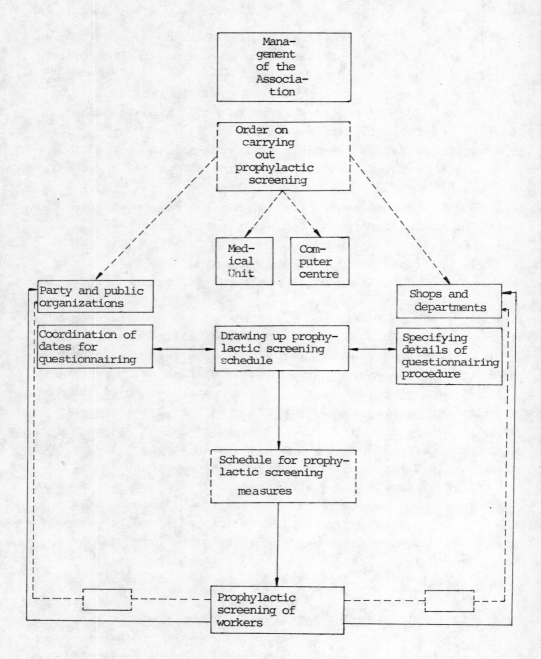

Fig. 40 Diagrammatic presentation of a mass prophylactic
screening of workers

618

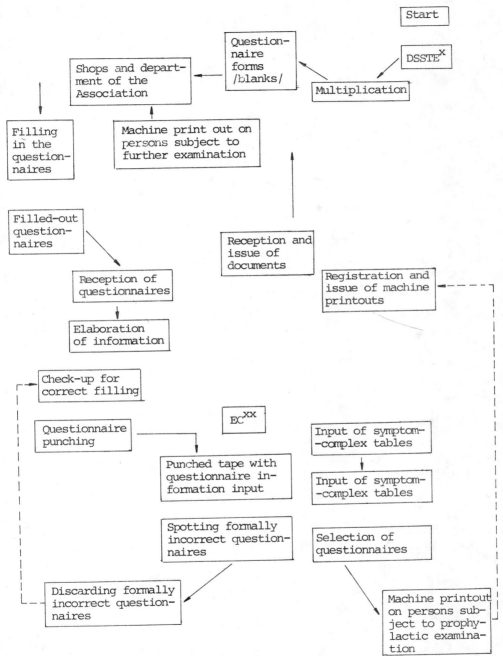

Fig. 41 Diagrammatic presentation of questionnaire movement
and processing
x Department for Standardization of Scientific and   xx electronic
  Technico-Economic Information   computer section

619

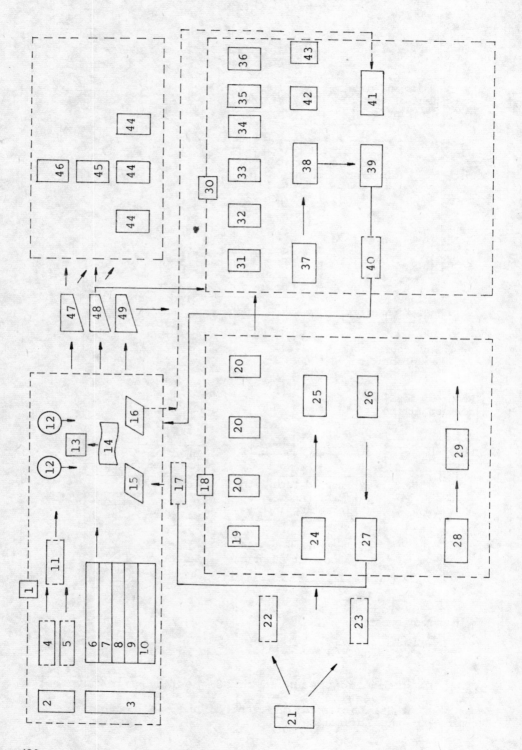

Fig. 42 Diagrammatic presentation of the flow of Documents when carrying out mass prophylactic screenings of workers at "Svetlana" Association, Leningrad.

SRI - standard reference information; MT - magnetic tape; PT - punched tape;
DSSTE - department for standardization of scientific and technico-economic information

1 - Computer centre, 2 - SRI, 3 - System programming, 4 - Employees, 5 - Programmed input and check-up of questionnaire information into EC, 7 - Programmed input of symptom-complex tables into EC, 8 - Programmed selection of questionnaires according to symptom-complexes in EC, 9 - Programmed input and check-up of Notification-slip information in EC, 10 - Programmed processing of prophylactic screening results in EC, 11 - Tables of symptom-complexes, 12 - magnetic tape, 13 - Electronic computer, 14 - p/t, 15 - Questionnaire punching, 16 - Notification-slip punching, 17 - Filled in questionnaires, 18 - Subdivisions of the Association, 19 - Time-board room, 20 - Production sectors, 21 - DSSTEI, 22 - Questionnaire forms /blanks/, 23 - Notifica- tion-slip blanks, 24 - Reception of questionnaire blanks for distributing to workers in production sector, 25 - Filling in the questionnaires, 26 - Handling in the filled- -in questionnaires, 27 - Reception of questionnaires from production sectors for sending to computer centre, 28 - Filling in table-board number, urgency category and type of examination, 29 - Serving to worker for examination, 30 - Medical Unit of Association, 31 - Registration office, 32 - Internist, 33 - Surgeon, 34 - Otorhino- laryngologist, 35 - Endoscopic examination room, 36 - X-ray diagnostic room, 37 - Recording date of examination, 38 - Carrying out examination, 39 - Recording results of examination, 40 - Tear-off slip of Notification Slip with examination results, 41 - Storage of processed documents, 42 - Laboratory, 43 - Archive, 44 - Subdivisions of the Association /shops and departments/, 45 - Chief Physician of Medical Unit, 46 - Management of Association, 47 - Machine printout of prophylactic screening results, 48 - Machine printout on persons subject to further examination, 49 - Check- -up machine printouts /controls/.

621

purposes and tasks of the prophylactic screening.

3. Utilization the paper of the association and the local radio network for the same purpose.

The next stage is to send out of the questionnaires, which are issued /if done for the first time/ to every worker of the appropriate subdivisions. It should be noted that the filling out of the questionnaires may be done both at work and at home. The latter circumstance is of essential importance, since checkups conducted by us showed that filling in the question-naires in the presence of others, particularly, of several persons, frequently results in the distortion of the informa-tion, since the majority of questionees want to avoid looking "sick", moreover in this case a number of so-called "intimate" questions are not answered at all.

As soon as the questionnaires are filled in, they are handed over to the time-keepers, who send them to the computer centre by a date indicated in the schedule. A diagram of questionnaire movement is represented on Fig. 41.

The next stage is that of processing the questionnaire information at the computer centre, the technical details of which have been omitted here because of their special technical character.

A diagrammatic representation of the entire documentation flow is given in Fig. 42.

Assessing the efficiency of ASMPOS operation

The ASMPOS was carried out at one of the large industrial associations of the city of Leningrad, the "Svetlana" Leningrad Electronic Instrument-Producing Association 4,747 question-naires were received for processing at the computer centre of the Association.

The results of processing of this information are repre-sented in Table 107.

In other words, a quarter of all the questionees, accord-ing to the decision of the EC, were eligible for instrumental--laboratory and medical examination for the detection of possible diseases, including pretumourous and tumourous dis-eases of the gastrointestinal tract.

Table 107

Results of Computer Processing of Questionnaire Information

Number of questionees covered	Computer decision					
	Subject for further examination				No examination	
	Laboratory		Instrumental laboratory		Number of persons	in % of total number of questionees
	Number of persons	in % of the number of questionees.	Number of persons	in % of the number of questionees		
4,747	96	2.0	1,128	23.8	3,523	74.2

According to the plan of the experiment, a kind of check-out and inspection station was formed, represented by a group of doctors, which is further referred to as the check-up medical examination. As a matter of fact, according to the ASMPOS the persons needing it were to be directly sent for instrumental examination without preliminary medical examination, as is the usual practice when conducting mass prophylactic screenings. Therefore the purpose of the check-up medical examination was:

1. To avoid mistakes that might endanger the health of the examined persons.

2. To imitate normal conditions of prophylactic screenings, which in the overwhelming majority of cases begin with a medical examination.

3. To make a comparison of the validity of the decisions of the EC and of the physicians.

Only 52.7 per cent of the 1,045 persons who were subjected to ·the check-up medical examination and who, according to the EC decision, had been prescribed instrumental examination, were found by the physician to need it. The main reason of their rejection was what was referred to as "medical intuition". Let us note that further on, it was from this group of persons that a control group was formed for comparing the validity of the EC and the physician's decisions. And, lastly, another control group was introduced, consisting of persons found "practically healthy" according to the EC decision.

Thus, three groups were formed:

Group 1, consisting of 486 persons needing instrumental examination both according to the EC decision and according to the decision of the physicians;

Group 2, consisting of 100 persons who needed instrumental examination according to the EC decision, but not of the physicians;

Group 3, consisting of 100 persons who, the EC decided, did not need instrumental examination.

All in all 686 persons underwent 763 instrumental examinations, mainly fibrogastroscopy and rectoromanoscopy.

In 526 out of the 686 examined persons with identical age--sex structure, 566 diseases were detected. Of all these 0.7 % were malignant neoplasms; 6.4 % polyps; 2.9 % ulcers; 0.7 % benign tumours; 56.9 % gastrites; and 32.5 % other diseases.

Table 108 represents the comparative results of the instrumental examination of three groups of workers of the Association.

Table 108

Comparative Results of Instrumental Examination of Various Groups

Groups of examined persons	Number of examinees	Diseases detected					
		malignant neoplasms		pretumorous diseases		other diseases	
		Number of persons	% of all examinees	Number of persons	% of all examinees	Number of persons	% of all examinees
All groups	686	4	0.6	52	7.6	470	68.5
EC group	486	4	0.8	45	9.3	348	71.6
Medical group	100	–	–	6	6.0	85	85.0
Control group	100	–	–	1	1.0	37	37.0

An analysis of the data from Table 108 shows that, on the whole, the EC won in the competition with the physicians. And

though no malignant tumours were detected in persons who passed
the check-up medical examination, the proportion of other diseases was rather high.

On the whole, the proportion of detected patients compared
to all who filled out the questionnaires is represented in Table
109.

Table 109

Indices of the Efficiency of ASMPOS

All persons who filled in question-naire	Diseases detected					
	Malignant neoplasms		Pretumourous diseases		Other diseases	
	number of pa-tients	% of all question-nees	number of pa-tients	% of all question-nees	number of pa-tients	% of all question-nees
4,747	4	0.08	52	1.1	470	9.9

Keeping in mind that these comparisons are somewhat
relative, we have made calculations of these indices per 1,000
population of the city of Leningrad and per 1,000 persons examined according to the questionnaire method at the "Svetlana"
Electronic Instument Producing Association. The following
results were obtained: cancer of the esophagus 0.1 per 1,000
Leningrad population and 0.2 for "Svetlana"; cancer of the
stomach - 0.6 for Leningrad and 0.4 for "Svetlana"; cancer of
the rectum - 0.1 for Leningrad and 0.2 for "Svetlana". Theore-
tically one may presume that, on the whole, all the tumours of
the gastrointestinal tract which could be generally expected
at the "Svetlana", have, indeed, been detected there.

In conclusion, it should be said that the nation-wide
character of the prophylactic measures open great possibilities
for their further improvement first of all through the utilization of available reserves that may be realized precisely
because of the social features of our national economy. The
above-mentioned reserves may be utilized mainly in the sphere
of improving the organizational forms of the prophylactic
measures.

ORGANIZATION OF HOSPITALIZATION AND MEDICAL SERVICES
TO PATIENTS WITH MALIGNANT NEOPLASMS

D.P. Berezkin, N.Ya. Shabashova and K.S. Mirotvortseva

The hospitalization of patients with malignant tumours is a dynamic process which depends on a number of factors; the main ones are the type of the malignant neoplasms, the degree of its spread, the patient's age, the type and facilities of the medical institution concerned.

Nevertheless, irrespective of the above circumstances, terms for the hospitalization of oncological patients are stipulated strictly. According to regulations issued by the USSR Ministry of Health, the hospitalization and treatment of patients with malignant neoplasms must start not later than ten days from the day the diagnosis is set; this concerns also cases of suspected malignant tumours for detailed examination and treatment. The responsibility for the timely hospitalization and beginning of treatment of oncological patients is assigned to the oncological dispensaries.

A crucial moment in hospitalization is the decision on sending an oncological patient to a certain medical institution. Two types of the latter can be involved: specialized medical institutions - oncological dispensaries and oncological institutes - and the hospitals of the general medical network. The question where to send the patient assumes special importance in connection with the fact that at present the methods of treatment for the majority of oncological patients are rather sophisticated and require not only high qualification, but high professionalism, which can be provided only by oncologists under the conditions of a specialized /oncological/ medical institution.

According to data for 1974, the USSR had 50,300 hospital beds for patients with malignant neoplasms, 60 % of these in the inpatient departments of oncological dispensaries. It should be stressed that, according to data for 1970, the majority of patients who received a full course of specialized treatment received it under inpatient conditions /84.2 %/ and only 15.8 % as outpatients.

626

Of course, the ideal case would be if all patients with malignant neoplasms receive medical treatment under the conditions of an oncological institution, the structure of which envisages surgical, gynecological, radiological, X-ray, and outpatient department and also may have highly specialized departments /tumours of the head and neck, urological, pediatric/.

Today, however, the opportunities for implementing such a program are still lacking. This is why a part of the patients are hospitalized in the inpatient departments of the general medical network. On an average, one may say that this part makes up about half of all the oncological patients. In this connection it has to be pointed out that the control over the correctness of treatment of oncological patients at the prophylactic institutions of a republic, territory, region or city is carried out by the territorial oncological dispensary.

What groups of patients receive treatment in the general hospitals? These are, first of all, patients with forms of malignant tumours, which are mainly subject to surgical treatment only, for example, cancer of the stomach and, to a lesser degree, cancer of the large intestine and the rectum. As far as breast cancer, cervical carcinoma, systemic diseases, cancer of the larynx and a number of other forms of the malignant tumours are concerned, the hospitalization of these patients in specialized oncological institutions is not only desirable, but also obligatory, for it involves the application of combined methods of treatment, requiring the utilization of appropriate equipment.

However, wherever the patient is sent, the elaboration of plan of treatment must be regarded as the most important and crucial moment in the entire process of hospitalization. At oncological institutions this procedure is carried out by a special commission, comprising several specialists - a surgeon, an X-ray specialist, a chemotherapist, and others. In non-oncological institutions the plan of treatment for oncological patients takes place with the obligatory participation of an oncologist.

In the inpatient departments of both non-oncological and specialized medical institutions great attention is given to the control of complications arising in the process of treating and also of inter-hospital mortality. It is impossible, of course, to establish definite norms in this matter, but a deep and all-round study of the causes of complications and mortality is an essential link of the entire therapeutic process.

Special commissions exist in every medical institution of the USSR engaged in the analysis of these questions - medical control commissions /MCC/ and pathological conferences /PC/. Taken up at the sessions of the medical control commissions all cases are dealt with in which serious complications arise, with a possible lethal issue or leading to marked defects. Each physician of the given medical institution or clinic participates in the proceedings of the MCC chaired by an experienced and competent specialist or the chief physician. The pathological conferences are held with the participation of pathologists and clinicians and their aim is the detailed examination of cases with a lethal issue. It should be pointed out that the main task of these commissions and conferences is not to censure a physician who made a mistake, but rather to give an educative effect, so that such cases should not happen again.

As to the methods of treating patients with various forms of malignant neoplasms, in view of the organizational character of this paper, we shall dwell on their substantiation, but will limit ourselves to information on the respective proportion of different kinds of treatment.

Thus, according to data for 1973, the indicators characterizing the proportion of administering complex[x] and chemohormonal treatment in the overall structure of all treatment methods came to 9.8 and 14.9, respectively. If we analyse the methods of treatment for individual forms of malignant tumours, we find that chemotherapeutic methods of treatment are used most widely for tumours of the hemopoietic organs and lymphatic

---

x Complex treatment is such a method when two or more kinds of treatment are given. For example, surgery, irradiation and chemotherapy.

tissue /67.9 %/, for breast cancer the complex method is used in 30.3 of the cases, and in cervical carcinoma the combined radiological treatment predominates /66.8 %/. The rather high frequency of using chemotherapeutic methods for tumours of the abdominal cavity and respiratory organs is due to the use of chemotherapeutic drugs during the generalization of the process, i.e. in cases when radical treatment is impossible.

Even these few data testify to the great amount of work carried out in the country at all the medical institutions with the purpose of improving methods of treating patients with malignant tumours. This is confirmed by the numbers of oncological patients on the register which reaches 1,500,000 persons.

Planning Inpatient Services to Patients with Primarily Diagnosed Malignant Tumours

Planning hospital services and particularly the necessary number of hospital beds for oncological patients is made possible by the nation-wide character of public health which guarantees the optimal conditions for extending medical services to the population.

The planning is based on data of the primary morbidity of the population with malignant neoplasms /in this case data for 1973/. All in all, this study covers information about 466,295 patients /186.7 per 100,000 population/ with primarily diagnosed malignant neoplasms. Taking into account that the morbidity pattern largely predetermines such matters as hospitalization and inpatient treatment of patients, data of primary morbidity were elaborated according to the basic localizations of the tumours. At the same time calculations were made of morbidity indices and their pattern for all the Union Republics, which made possible to study the requirements of oncological hospital beds in accordance with the epidemiological features characteristic of each republic.

A study of the dynamics of morbidity indices shows that beginning from the 60s and particularly in the recent years the tendency of a "runaway" growth of morbidity, so typical of post-war years, has been replaced by tendencies toward a slowing down of the increment of morbidity indices. At the same

629

time tendencies of a drop in the morbidity indices of tumours of the stomach, esophagus and cervix uteri, have appeared, together with a growth of the morbidity indices for cancer of the trachea, bronchi and lungs, breast cancer and carcinoma of the rectum, which has to be taken into account when planning oncological hospital beds for patients with malignant tumours. The implementation of the necessary calculations was based on the specific features of hospitalizing patients with malignant tumours, a characteristic of which is the obligatory hospitalization of all patients with primarily diagnosed malignant neoplasms. It is obvious that a part of the patients start treatment as outpatient /pre-operative X-ray therapy, in a number of cases chemotherapy/, but this circumstance by no means excludes the necessity of their subsequent hospitalization for continuing treatment.

Turning now to the definition of the average bed-day we have carried out an expert assessment of the data on how long patients with malignant tumours stay in hospital both in oncological institutions and in the general medical network, which admits from 40 to 50 % of patients with malignant tumours. These calculations have shown that the average bed-day for patients with malignant tumours is 40 days. Parallel to this we have calculated the average bed-day for the basic localizations of malignant tumours:

- cancer of the stomach - 29.6
- cancer of the esophagus - 40.0
- cancer of the rectum - 48.6
- breast cancer - 36.6
- cancer of the lung - 30.6
- cervical carcinoma - 36.2

G.A. Popov's formula was used for the calculations:

$$B = \frac{M \times P \times A}{D \times 100},$$

where B is the required number of hospital beds;

M - morbidity index;

P - percentage of selection per hospital bed /100 %/;

A - average bed-day;

D - average number of days when the bed is used a year, taken in accordance with official planning materials, equal to 340.

Thus, all the calculations of the requirements in hospital beds for patients with malignant tumours were carried out according to two basic bed-day indices /average for all patients and calculated for the basic localizations of malignant tumours/.

It must be kept in mind that here the requirement for oncological hospital beds is calculated for patients with primarily diagnosed malignant neoplasms only.

The forecasting of morbidity for the next five years indicates that the low rates of its increment /1.9 % a year/, will doubtlessly prevail. At the same time definite tendencies have appeared in the morbidity pattern, which must be taken into account when planning the number of hospital beds. It must be emphasized that these tendencies by no means change the pattern as a whole, where tumours of the gastrointenstinal tract occupy the first place; second are the tumours of the trachea, bronchi and lungs, the third place goes to tumours of the skin and, finally, on the fourth and fifth place are cervical carcinoma and breast cancer.

In the recent years there has been a slight drop in the incidence of cancer of the stomach /1962 - 41.6; 1974 - 41.4/, an increase in the incidence of cancer of the trachea, bronchi and the lung /1962 - 14.1; 1974 - 24.5/, breast cancer /1962 - 7.4; 1974 - 12.0/, cancer of the rectum /1962 - 3.0; 1974 - 6.2/, and lastly, a drop in the incidence of cervical carcinoma /1962 - 18.4; 1974 - 12.9/.[x] Taking into account that tumour localizations like cancer of the uterus and breast cancer are subject to treatment in the specialized oncological network, a differentiating approach is necessary when planning and distributing hospital beds. It should be noted that the existing considerable difference in the levels of morbidity of the different Union Republics is based on differences in the age--sex composition of their population and also on the quality of intravital diagnosis and registration of patients with

---

[x] Morbidity indices are given for 100,000 population.

primarily diagnosed malignant neoplasms. All these specific features must be taken into account when planning the hospital beds for the individual republics, thus, e.g., in the republics of Central Asia there are traditionally high morbidity indices for cancer of the esophagus, whereas in the Baltic area one sees high indices of morbidity for cancer of the stomach, the lung, breast cancer and cervical carcinoma.

As mentioned above, the calculation was made for the basic tumour localizations according to two indices: average duration of stay in the hospital, taken for 40 bed-days, and the average duration for the basic localizations, taken in accordance with the expert evaluation and calculations.

The results of the calculations showed that for providing inpatient treatment to all patients with primarily diagnosed malignant neoplasms it is necessary to plan a number of hospital beds equally to 54,858 beds, which is 22 beds per 100,000 population. The planning of the number of hospital beds according to tumour localization indicates that the greatest number of beds is required for patients with tumours of other localizations /5.2 per 100,000 population, which comes to 12,962 beds/. This group of tumours accounts for 23.9 per cent in the morbidity pattern, and it includes rarely occurring tumour localizations. Doubtlessly this group, due to the diversity of its composition, presents great difficulties for adequate hospitalization, since it includes tumours of the brain, of the head and neck, as well as tumours of the bones and soft tissues, etc. Most of them are subject to treatment in highly specialized medical institutions. In connection with the fact that these tumours are not registered by the oncological network according to nosologic forms, it is rather difficult to provide a detailed analysis of the number of beds for their hospitalization and inpatient treatment in the appropriate medical institutions. The distribution of the planned number of hospital beds, necessary for the hospitalization of patients with the basic forms of malignant tumours corresponds to the morbidity pattern in which cancer of the stomach, cancer of the lung, cancer of the skin, cervical carcinoma, breast cancer, cancer of the esophagus and cancer of the rectum appear in the following proportions - 22.3 %, 12.5 %, 7 %, 6.2 %, 3.7 % and 3.1 %.

A comparison of the necessary number of beds calculated according to the average bed-day and the bed-day for the above-listed localizations is of great interest, as it indicates very vividly the reserves of rational utilization of hospital beds, in case of some reduction of the average stay in hospital. Naturally, these reserves are first of all connected with the duration of time it takes to examine a patient in the hospital before starting treatment; for a number of medical institutions this period is obviously longer than necessary and may be considerably reduced by detailed and careful examination of the patient in outpatient conditions and by avoiding the repetition of the examinations in the hospital.

The introduction of complex and combined methods of treatment in practice, methods requiring the use of complicated equipment, a number of medicinal preparations, the wide combination of surgical, radiological, chemohormonal methods of treatment and, lastly, the availability of highly qualified oncological surgeons, X-ray specialists, radiologists and chemotherapeutists, which is possible only under the conditions of a specialized oncological institution - all this calls for a rather differential approach to the concept of "oncological hospital bed" and to the determination of the group of patients who need hospitalization in specialized institutions and in institutions of the general medical network. Thus, for instance, at present the complicated process of transition from purely surgical treatment of tumours of the above-mentioned localizations to combined methods of treatment is taking place. The latter include preoperative exposure to intensive courses of radiation followed by surgery also in short periods of time /within a week/ of completing X-ray therapy, which requires, in the long term, the hospitalization of such patients at specialized institutions, whereas at present at least 60-70 % of these patients receive treatment in the oncological wards of hospitals belonging to the general medical network. It is essential to take into account the above-mentioned factors when planning the required number of hospital beds in the republics, where morbidity indices for certain localizations essentially differ. Thus, for the USSR as a whole, hospital beds for patients with cancer of the stomach may be planned at institutions belonging to the general medical network, whereas the high incidence of breast cancer in the Latvian and Estonian Republics require the planning of hospital beds for treating breast cancer in the specialized oncological network, likewise, morbidity indices for cervical carcinoma in the Ukraine, in Kazakhstan, in Lithuania, Latvia and Estonia, which are not only above the average national index, but also above the indices for a number of other republics, indicate the need to plan the number of hospital beds for treating this kind of patients in the specialized network only.

Thus the planning of hospital beds for patients with primarily diagnosed malignant neoplasms calls for taking into account the morbidity levels not only in the country as a whole, but in each republic, and also the pattern of morbidity which makes possible a differentiated approach to the solution of this complicated question.

At the same time the planning of hospital beds, questions of hospitalization of patients with primarily diagnosed malignant neoplasms and the assessment of the immediate results of treatment by no means cover the entire problem of hospitalization of oncological patients.

The requirements for periodically repeated hospitalization for examination, for providing courses of supporting therapy /medical and X-ray treatment/ or for treating relapses and metastases makes necessary to plan an additional number of hospital beds for repeated hospitalization. For appropriate calculations questions pertaining to personal prognosis assume special importance; drawing up a personal prognosis for every patient discharged from hospital permits to predict the further course of the disease on a strictly scientific basis, and thereby, to determine his subsequent admission to an oncological ward with a considerable degree of probability.

It goes without saying that there are much wider possibilities for using personal prognostication; one must take into account the great importance of personal prognostication for the dispensary observation of patients, for their occupational rehabilitation, for studying the efficiency of treatment, etc. At the same time, it is very important to work out methods of personal prognostication also for an objective assessment of the character of the tumour process.

At present the development of methods for personal prognosis assumes an ever greater importance due to a whole number of essential circumstances. First of all, there is the need to solve, a number of tasks in the organization of cancer control on the basis of scientifically-based prognostication.

From among them first rational plans for complex and combined treatment must be drawn up.

Indeed, the rapid development of drug therapy opens new and substantial prospects regarding the treatment of patients with malignant tumours in general and particularly in cases when other methods of affecting the tumour prove inadequate. Success along these lines depends not only on the efficiency of the drugs, but also on the strictly personal treatment plan, which can hardly be imagined without a scientifically based prediction of the course of the developing tumourous process.

The personal prognosis is not less important for the organization of dispensary observation of patients with malignant tumours, that would provide for the timely detection of relapses and tumour metastases. This becomes especially important from the viewpoint of the possibility of effectively influencing the latter and giving preventive treatment courses in a number of cases.

Occupational rehabilitation of an increasing number of patients with tumourous diseases also requires scientifically based prediction of the further fate of these patients, which would help to avoid the still frequently stereotype decisions of the medical and labour examination boards. Furthermore, one should not forget the essential medical-social significance of personal prognosis in connection with the need for tactful information of the patient's relatives.

Apart from its practical importance, the development of personal prognostic methods is of a certain theoretical interest as well, due to the need of a quantitative description of qualitative signs and phenomena, characterizing such a complicated biological process as tumourous growth.

Proceeding from the above, one may formulate the main task of this study as the task of developing a methodology of personal prognosis in patients with the main forms of malignant tumours and revealing certain regularities that would permit to determine the basic principles of such a methodology.

DISPENSARY SERVICES FOR PATIENTS WITH MALIGNANT NEOPLASMS

N.Ya. Shabashova, D.P. Berezkin and K.S. Mirotvortseva

In the Soviet Union the dispensary method is one of the basic elements of the state system for protecting the health of the population.

The soviet public health is advancing along the way of developing and improving methods of prophylactic medical examinations, with the purpose of synthetizing the therapeutic and prophylactic aspects of medical activities. There is no doubt that the prophylactic examination of certain groups of the population, now widely used, is the first and very important stage in the process of transition to the provision of dispensary services to the entire population of the USSR, as envisaged by the decisions of the 25th Congress of the CPSU.

For patients with tumourous and pretumourous diseases the dispensary method is the basis on which their treatment and observation rests, since it promotes first of all the prophylaxis and early diagnosis of malignant tumours, as well as their rapid examination and treatment. The idea of the necessity of dispensary services to oncological patients was put forth by N.N. Petrov as early as in 1921. Since then the oncological dispensary method has passed through a number of organizational stages.

636

In 1945 the dispensary method was made obligatory within the system of organized oncological services on the scale of the whole country; in 1949 the prophylactic examination of patients with pretumourous diseases was started. This was preceded by extensive research work by Soviet scientists who had made a great contribution to the development of the study on precancerous diseases /N.N. Petrov, A.N. Savitski, A.V. Melnikov, A.I. Rakov, S.A. Kholdin, A.I. Serebrov, L.M. Shabad, M.F. Glazunov and others/. They investigated chronic processes, which precede the development of malignant tumours, worked out principles for the classification of premalignant diseases, and singled out groups among which the risk of a malignant tumour is particularly high /obligate precancers/.

The experience of the oncological service indicated that the dispensary method alone made possible to provide for the correct organization of prevention and treatment, followed by observation of patients with malignant tumours.

The dispensary method for patients with malignant tumours and pretumourous diseases makes possible to detect them at an early stage of the disease, and carry out measures aimed at first of all, the prevention of malignant tumours, and also to provide comprehensive medical services to this group of patients, including their registration and observation. The dispensary method envisages active forms of controlling morbidity of malignant tumours, influencing the working and living conditions of people by investigating possible carcinogenic effects, by systematic observation of the state of health of certain groups of the population, by regularly conducting prophylactic examinations of the same groups of the population in the course of many years. Of no little importance is the systematic dispensary observation of patients with malignant tumours who underwent one or another method of surgical, combined or complex treatment. This observation leads to the early detection of relapses and metastases and, in turn, helps to start their timely prevention and treatment.

Both the specialized oncological and the prophylactic institutions take part in the implementation of such observations in the towns as well as on the countryside.

At present the basic principles of dispensary work in oncology may be represented as follows:

1. Active detection /at outpatient departments, hospitals, during mass prophylactic screenings of the population/ and registration of patients with tumourous and pretumourous diseases.

2. Treatment of tumourous and pretumourous diseases.

3. Regular observation of patients with tumourous and pretumourous diseases.

4. Examining the patients's working and living conditions.

5. Close contacts between the oncological network and the institutions of the general medical network.

It has to be pointed out here that the measures included in the dispensary system for patients with tumourous and pretumourous diseases consist not only in prophylactic examination, but also in controlling early aging, the introduction of hygienic habits in the everyday life, protecting the organism from the effect of blastomogenic factors and familiarizing the population with elements of cancer prevention.

The following groups of patients are eligible for dispensary services:

1. Patients with pretumourous diseases.

2. Patients subject to specialized and radical treatment for malignant tumours.

3. Those who have completed radical and specialized treatment for malignant tumours /practically healthy/.

4. Patients subject to symptomatic treatment alone.

For the purpose of carrying out the complete registration of and providing dispensary observation to all oncological patients and those with pretumourous diseases, a division of such patients into clinical groups has been adopted in the USSR since 1956.

The 1st clinical group is divided into two subgroups, 1a and 1b. 1a - persons, suspected for having a malignant tumour. Patients assigned to this group must be examined and consultations must be held in the shortest possible time /no longer than two weeks/. lb - patients with pretumourous diseases. The majority of persons in this group are subject to treatment and observation at the district hospital or outpatient department. A part of the patients /with obligate precancers/ must be treated and observed at oncological medical institutions.

The 2nd clinical group includes patients with the established diagnosis of a malignant tumour, subject ot radical treatment /cancer of the stomach, cancer of the uterus, breast cancer and others/. Besides, the 2nd group includes patients subject to specialized treatment /hematological diseases, such as leukoses, lymphogranulomatosis, myelomas, some types of sarcomas, etc./.

The 3rd clinical group consists of patients who have undergone radical treatment and have no relapses or metastases /practically healthy/.

The 4th clinical group includes patients with neglected cases of the disease, subject ot symptomatic treatment only.

These clinical groups by no means reflect the stage of the process, and serve merely for clinical /working/ information and registration. They determine the degree to which the process is neglected, or is amenable to radical treatment, the results of treatment, an evaluation of the dynamics in reducing neglect, the proportion of the group of patients subject to radical treatment.

After the patients' clinical group is determined they are subject to dispensary observation. Thus, first-group patients must be examined within two weeks with the purpose of making the diagnosis definite. In the absence of a malignant neoplasm the patients are taken off the register; if the diagnosis is confirmed, another clinical group must be determined and the patients are directed for treatment accordingly.

1st-group patients are subject to dispensary observation and necessary treatment and are not taken off the register earlier than a year after recovery.

2nd group patients, following radical treatment /surgical, combined, complex, X-ray/ are transferred into the 3rd clinical group.

Patients in the 3rd clinical group /practically healthy following radical treatment/ are subject to dynamic dispensary observation. In case relapses and metastases, amenable to specialized treatment, are detected in them, they are transformed into the 2nd clinical group. When only symptomatic treatment is possible, such patients are placed in the 4th clinical group.

The most important elements of dispensary services to patients with pretumourous diseases are as follows:

1/ dynamic and active control of their condition;

2/ timely and adequate treatment.

For patients of the la group /suspicion for malignant tumour/ most significant is:

1/ the careful and purposeful examination of the patient to decide on the presence or absence of a malignant neoplasm;

2/ when adequate examination of the patient is impossible under outpatient conditions, the patient shall be sent to an oncological dispensary or hospital of the general medical network for detailed examination.

The most important factors in the dispensary services to patients with tumourous diseases are as follows:

1/ active treatment of the patients;

2/ the earliest possible detection of relapses and metastases of the tumour and their timely treatment;

3/ the detection and treatment of functional disorders which may arise following surgical, X-ray, chemohormonal treatment;

4/ rational employment of the patients;

5/ registration of therapeutic results and an evaluation of their efficiency.

Dispensary services to patients with pretumourous diseases lb group are differentiated. Patients with obligate precancers are subject to observation at oncological institutions /dispensary, tumour-diagnostic room at an outpatient clinic, district oncologist/. Patients with facultative precancers are under the observation of the physicians of the general medical network.

Dispensary services to patients of the 2nd clinical group /subject to specialized and radical treatment/ are provided by republican, regional, territorial, city oncological dispensaries, the oncologists of the district polyclinics or physicians responsible for oncological services.

Supervision of patients with malignant tumours of the 3rd clinical group /following radical treatment/ is the responsibility of oncological dispensaries and tumour-diagnostic rooms.

When an oncologist is unavailable in the district of a patient's residence or when the patient' residence is far from an oncological dispensary, dispensary services may be provided by the specialists of the district or city outpatient department according to the localization of the tumour. Supervision of such patients in the countryside is the responsibility of the physicians of the rural medical district.

Patients not eligible to radical treatment - 4th clinical group /late detection, relapse or metastases following earlier treatment - are transferred for dispensary observation and symptomatic treatment to the physicians of the general medical network. It is considered most advisable to provide symptomatic treatment to patients of the 4th clinical group as inpatients in the hospitals of the general medical network. Oncologists, surgeons, gynecologists are enlisted for consultations and for working out a plan of symptomatic therapy /see in the section dealing with the organization of medical assistance to patients with advanced forms of tumours/.

An important matter is the duration of dispensary observation of patients with malignant neoplasms. Data from the literature convincingly indicate that no definite time can be set, after which stable recovery could be guaranteed, since even after 10-14 years from the moment of radical treatment, the possibility of the appearance of metastases cannot be ruled out /5-10 %/. It follows, therefore, that irrespective of the time that has elapsed since radical treatment, patients with malignant neoplasms are subject to permanent dispensary observation. This principle is confirmed by the results of analyzing the causes of morbidity of oncological patients, which indicates that only a part of the patients /10-12 %/ die of concurrent diseases /among which lesions of the cardiovascular system prevalent are/, whereas the rest of the patients die because of the progress of their main diseases or from metachronous primary-multiple tumours, whose appearance /4-5 %/ should be kept in mind when providing dispensary services to patients.

At present one can hardly speak about the permanent and stable recovery of patients if relapses and metastases had been detected in them, yet in a number of localizations /the breast, the uterus, the bladder and the prostate/ sufficiently lasting and stable remissions can be achieved and the patients' life can be prolonged. The treatment of relapses and metastases in patients with cancer of the lungs, the stomach and the intestine is much more difficult. However, by early detection of relapses of the tumour, in individual cases drug or X-ray therapy produce a certain, if not a lasting effect.

The dispensary observation of patients with malignant tumours must, of course, lean on the method of personal prognosis, which describes the general tendencies in the further course of the disease. In such a prognosis the degree of the spread of the tumour /stage of the process, character of local metastases - singular or multiple metastases, their histological structure: highly differentiated, undifferentiated/ and rational treatment are the dominating factors.

According to the regulations adopted in the oncological network of the Soviet Union, patients of the 3rd clinical group, having been subjected to radical /combined, complex, surgical or X-ray/ treatment must be observed in the following periods of time:

During the 1st and 2nd years - every 3 months.

During the 3rd and 4th years - every 6 months.

In subsequent years - once every 12 months, irrespective of the time that has elapsed since the onset of the disease.

Nevertheless, it is a differentiated approach essential for providing dispensary services to the patients with various stages of the process. During the first three years after radical treatment stage 3 patients need particularly close observation /at least 4 times a year/, for it is precisely during this period that from 70 to 75 % of relapses and metastases occur. Patients of the stages 1 and 2 who have survived for 3 years, require very careful observation in the subsequent years since the incidence of relapses and metastases comes to not less than 30 to 35 % in this period.

A differentiated approach must be observed when urgent dispensary services are found necessary for different localizations of malignant tumours.

Cancer of the lung

The dispensary observation of a patient with cancer of the lung is based on the factors characterizing the properties of the tumour. Patients with undifferentiated forms of tumour and with adenocarcinoma, irrespective of its localization, patients with peripheral cancer and those who had regional metastases must be examined during the first half year not less than once a month, and subsequently once every three months.

Patients with a complex of relatively favourable factors /squamous cell forms, central localization and absence of regional metastases/ must be examined not less than once every 3 months over a period of 4-5 years.

The appearance of metastases in the medastinum, in the supraclavicular lymph nodes or remote, most frequently in the liver or skeletal bones, is possible throughout the life of the patient following radical surgery. Most often they appear during the first two years following surgery. The frequency in the appearance of metastases increases gradually over 3, 6, 12 months and achieves the maximum level about one and a half years following surgery, gradually diminishing again. This must be taken into account when observing patients during the immediate and more remote period.

Breast cancer

A five-year term of observation for patients with breast cancer cannot be regarded as a criterion of stable recovery. In 89 % of cases the death of patients with breast cancer, who died after different periods following radical treatment was caused by the progress of the main disease.

Patients with breast cancer are subject to active regular dispensary observation /at least 3-4 times a year/ irrespective of the time that has elapsed since the moment of treatment.

Cancer of the stomach

46.8 % of patients who undergo radical surgery live for 5 and more years; nearly half of the patients live for more than 5 years and some 25 % of all the operated patients live for more than ten years.

In these patients the main cause of death was the further progress of the process /the development of metastases and the emergence of relapses/. 68.3 % of all the relapses and metastases appear in the period of up to 2 years following radical treatment for cancer of the stomach. In about one third /31.7%/ of all the patients metastases and relapses are detected at a later period /14 % - from 2 to 5 years; 12.6 % - from 5 to 10 years; 4.5 % - after 10 years/. Therefore even a ten-year period of life without relapses and metastases does not guarantee absolute recovery, all the more so that all the patients in whom they are detected die in the first two years after their appearance.

Patients who have had radical surgery for cancer of the stomach must report for dispensary observation 3 times a year during the first two years, twice a year in the period from three to 10 years and once a year after a period of 10 years.

Cancer of the large intestine

During the first three years the patient must report for examination once every 4 months /three times a year/, since 67.4 to 80 % of metastases and relapses appear in this period. 17 % of relapses and metastases occur after a period of five years, this is why dispensary observation of such patients should be continued for at least 10 years after surgery. Besides, in 3 % of the patients metachronous tumours of other localizations appear.

Cervical carcinoma

The greatest number of relapses and metastases /79.0 %/

is detected during the first two years. In the subsequent years the number of relapses and metastases drops; after 5 years they are detected in 11.5 % of patients, therefore even a 5-year term of life following radical treatment does not guarantee clinical recovery.

Examination of women treated for cervical carcinoma must be conducted at least 3 times a year; this observation must be particularly active during the first two years following treatment.

Tumours of other localizations appear in 3.8 % of cases. The most frequent localization is the gastrointenstinal tract, tumours of the breast and the skin.

Oncological urological patients /tumours of the bladder, of the prostate and the ovary/.

In cases of tumours of the bladder 54.7 % of relapses appear during the first year following surgery owing to which cystoscopic examination in this period must be carried out at least once every 3 months, during the subsequent two years once every six months and later once a year.

In cases of tumours of the prostate gland 62.0 % of metastases are detected during 3 years from the beginning of treatment, which is a reason for constant observation of patients during this time, including X-ray control of the lungs and the skeletal system.

Most of the metastases of the tumours of the testis are detected during the first 2 years from the beginning of treatment, therefore in this period check-up examinations of patients /with laboratory and X-ray examination/ must be conducted not less than once every 3 months.

In the subsequent years examinations are carried out once every 6 months and after a period of 5 years once a year.

The overall dispensary observation must not be restricted to 5 years, since the appearance of relapses and metastases is possible even later.

Melanoblastomas of the skin

A particularly close observation of patients with melanoblastomas of the skin must be maintained during the first 2 years following the primary treatment, since relapses and metastases appear most frequently in this period. Dispensary observation must be differentiated according to the type of earlier treatment.

Patients subjected to dissection of the primary tumour only, require particularly close observation by the oncologist and must be examined not less than once every 4-6 weeks during the first two years and every 3 months in subsequent years.

Patients subjected to dissection of the primary tumour and regional lymphadenectomy should be examined during the first two years once every 3 months, then once every 6 months.

In the dispensary services recording and registering the results of dispensary observation are of great importance. To provide for complete registration and dynamic observation of patients the following special documents are filled in for every newly detected patient, irrespective of the clinical group:

1/ patients with a primarily diagnosed malignant neoplasm have a notification drawn up /see addenda/;

2/ a dispensary observation card form F-30 is filled in for patients with pretumourous diseases, with suspicion of a malignant tumour;

3/ a card of dispensary observation /form "U-30-6"/ is filled in for patients after the completion of radical or specialized treatment, which serves as a control document for checking up on the patient's condition, the date of specifying the diagnosis, dates of hospitalization and treatment.

All institutions providing dispensary services and observation of patients with tumourous and pretumourous diseases /oncological dispensaries, departments, consultation rooms, city and rural hospitals, outpatient departments of the general medical network, women's consultations, etc./ maintain control cards. Of these control cards two files are formed: one for patients with malignant neoplasms, the other for patients with suspicion of cancer and patients with pretumourous diseases.

The dispensary observation of patients allows to carry

out wide-scale continuous control of the patients' state of
health and to elaborate data on the survival of patients and
the efficiency of treatment. These data are presented in the
annual reports on the number of patients on the registry of
the oncological network and on the number of years they
survived. The documents providing this information are the
dispensary observation cards, form 30, which are summarized
and presented as reports, according to form 10 /in compliance
with clinical groups/.

STUDY OF EFFECTIVENESS OF TREATMENT IN PATIENTS WITH MALIGNANT TUMOURS

D.P. Berezkin, V.I. Yekimov and P.I. Yegorov

Until quite recently oncological service has used three
criteria characterizing the level of cancer control and the
common tendencies which could be determined in the dynamics of
malignant tumours:

1. Morbidity rate.
2. Mortality rate.
3. Susceptibility rate.

These circumstances have already been used for a long time
in carrying out organizational and therapeutic measures in the
field of cancer control. Nevertheless, at the present stage of
the development of oncology one more criterion has gained
importance: the evaluation of the effectiveness of treatment
in patients with malignant neoplasms. Besides the study of the
remote results of treatment, the tasks connected with analyzing
the level of treatment given at different oncological institutions of the country, revealing the reasons for the absence of
radical treatment, as well as with the problems of psychological, social and occupational rehabilitation of oncological
patients, constitute an integral part of this problem. It
should be also remembered that in recent years the possibilities
for the treatment of patients with malignant neoplasms have
considerably increased due to the fact that the combined methods of therapy, new sources of radiant energy and medicinal
preparations are now extensively used in medicine.

The health service of every country has already accumulated extensive material concerning the character of therapeutic measures and the remote results of the treatment of oncological patients. This information, however, though of great
scientific and practical value, is far from being always
available for deep analysis the results of which could provide
an answer to many urgent problems of the health service. At
the same time modern organizational and clinical oncology is
in urgent need of information on various methods for the treatment of oncological patients and their effectivity on a large
scale. If this information is analysed scientifically, it makes
possible to choose the most rational and promising kinds of
treatment which have been checked in a sufficient number of
observations of different medical institutions. It is quite
obvious that the processing of these data must be strictly
standardized and based on the modern methods of mathematical
statistical analysis with the use of the means of computing
technology.

It seems that this aim can be achieved only by using the
identical methods of collecting, processing and analyzing both
the primary information on the oncological patients and the
information on the remote results of their treatment.

In order to observe the above-mentioned conditions a
system should be organized for the study of the effectivity
of treatment in patients with malignant tumours. Such a system may be realized in one country, in a group of countries
or within international organizations.

In the USSR the All-Union Centre for Studying the Effectivity of Treatment in Patients with Malignant Tumours has been
organized, and functions at present located at the Prof. N.N.
Petrov Research Institute of Oncology /Leningrad/.

The main task of this Centre is not only to study the
character of therapeutic measures and the remote results of
treatment of patients with malignant tumours on the basis of
individual statistical reports, but mainly to organize and
control the system for studying treatment effectivity in oncological patients, together with the necessary number of

oncological institutions.

For organizing the system of this kind a number of conditions should be observed:

1. Document forms must be developed which are adapted for machine processing and at the same time suitable for filling in by physicians or medical assistants.

2. The process of filling in the document forms and the technology of information processing must fit the existing state system of medical assistance and the organization of the dispensary observation of the patients.

3. An effectively organized archive, easily available for repeated reference, must be created; such an archive is necessary for a long-term /5-10 years/ dynamic observation of the patients.

4. The internal system for the retrieval and processing of information must be organized.

5. The mathematical and technical provision of this system msut be ensured.

The unified form "Special Excerpt from Cancer Inpatient Record" /Supplement 22/, from which the necessary information is obtained, stipulates that the International Statistical Classification of Diseases, Lesions and Causes of Death, 8th Revision, 1965 /ICD, 1965/, should be used.

It should be pointed out that the main principle of the composition of this form, intended for subsequent machine processing, is the complete deciphering of each characteristic entered in the card. This system of the open decimal code is necessary not only for the subsequent processing of information by a computer. IA system introduces strict discipline in the process of filling-in the documents, thus also helps to overcome differences in the usage of terminology.

The use of electronic computers makes possible to process practically any number of documents containing information about patients with malignant neoplasms, as well as to supply all the information necessary for individual prognostication.

The document form consists of two parts.

The first part is intended for characterizing the treat-

Registration No.

Approved by USSR Ministry of Health,
Order No. 935 of 17 November 1972

All-Union Centre for Studying the Effectivity of Treatment in
Patients with Malignant Tumours

SPECIAL EXCERPT FORM CANCER INPATIENT RECORD

Diagnosis _____

Year _____ Month _____
of exact diagnosis

Year _____ month _____
of beginning treatment

Place of patient's residence
when he became ill: republic_

_____

region _____
county _____

Resident:

0. no data

1. townsman

2. countryman

Institution responsible for
patient's observation: _____

Nationality: _____
00. no data

Profession: _____
00. no data; 01 absent
02. has _____

Sex. 1. male; 2. female

Age _____ 00. no data

Number of bed-days _____

000. no data

Types of treatment:

1. no /examination/;
2. surgical only
3. radiation therapy only;

Reproductive function

0. no data; 1 no /for men/;

2. no sexual experience
/for women/;

3. has not become pregnant
/used contraceptives/;

4. primary sterility;

5. became pregnant but gave
no birth;

6. one delivery;

7. two deliveries;

8. three or more deliveries

Previous disease of organ
affected

0. no data; 1. absent

2. has: _____

Accompanying diseases:

    0. no data; 1. absent;

    2. tuberculosis;

    3. diabetes; 4. endocrinopathy

    5. other malignant tumours

    6. _____

    7. several

Duration of disease symptoms
/in months/ _____

00. no data; xx. symptomless

Number of tumours: 0. no data

1. solitary; 2. primary-
-multiple of the organ; 3.
3. primary-multiple of several

650

4. chemotherapy only;
5. hormonotherapy only;
6. mixed;
7. comprehensive;
8. symptomatic

Nature of treatment:
1. radical; 2. palliative;
3. no /examination/

Stage of disease:
0. no data; 1. O; 2. Ī;
3. II; 4. III; 5. IV

Stage of disease according to TNM scheme
0. no data; 1. T_o;

2. T_1; 3. T_2; 4. T_3;

5. T_4

0. no data; 1. N_o;

2. N_1; 3. N_2; 4. N_3.

0. no data; 1. M_o;

2. M_1

Rh-factor: 0. no data
1. positive
2. negative

ABO blood group: 0. no data;
1. O/1/; 2. A/I/; 3. B/III/;
4. AB/IV/

Menstrual and ovarian function:
0. no data; 1. absent /for males/; 2. reproductive period; 3. climacteric;
4. menopause up to 3 years;
5. menopause over 3 years

Type of growth: 0. no data;
1. exophytic /nodulous/;
2. mesophytic /intermediate, transitional, mixed/;
3. endophytic /infiltrative/;
4. _____

Tumour histology:
00. no data; 01. no examination; 02. malignant polyp /fibroadenomatosis, adenoma/; 03. well and moderately differentiated glandular carcinoma;

organs

Size of tumour /in cm/ _____
00. no data

Growth in adjoining structures:
0. no data; 1. no ingrowths;
2. ingrowth in _____

Localization of tumour in organ:

_____

0. no data

Regional metastases: 0. no data
1. absent; 2. solitary; 3. multiple; 4. no examination

Methods of determining regional metastases:
0. no data; 1. no metastases;
2. palpation; 3. lymphographic;
4. cytological; 5. histological;
6. _____

Remote metastases:
0. no data; 1. absent; 2. liver;
3. lungs; 4. bones; 5. brain;
6. retroperitoneal lymph nodes;
7. ovaries
8. _____
9. several

Complications after radiation:
0. no data, 1. no treatment;
2. absent; 3. leukopenia;
4. dermatitides; 5. cystitis, proctitis; 6. tissue necrosis;
7. _____ ; 8. several

Chemotherapy:
0. no data; 1. was not conducted;
2. chemotherapy only;
3. in combination with other methods of treatment;
4. _____

Preparation used:
0. no data; 1. did not take;
2. thio-TEPA; 3. 5-fluorouracil;
4. cyclophosphamide; 5. endoxane;
6. sarcolysine;
7. _____
8. several

Complications after chemotherapy: 0. no data; 1. no treatment; 2. absent;

04. solid carcinoma; 05. mucinous carcinoma; 06. scirrhous carcinoma; 07. mixed glandular carcinoma; 08. underdifferentiated cancer; 09. Paget's disease; 10. planocellular cancer; 11. carcinoid; 12. sarcoma; 13. melanoblastoma; 14. lymphogranulamatosis; 15. leukosis; 16. _____

Type of malignant tumours /for cases when disease was diagnosed without histological analysis/ 1. tumour was analysed histologically; 2. no tumour was diagnosed; 3. cancer; 4. sarcoma; 5. melanoblastoma; 6. carcinoid; 7. systemic disease; 8. _____

Type of surgical intervention:
0. no data; 1. no surgical intervention; 2. surgery performed: - _____

Complications in postoperative period: 0. no data; 1. no operation; 2. no complications; 3. suppuration of operative wound; 4. pyothorax; 5. pneumonia; 6. mediastinitis; 7. peritonitis; 8. thromboembolia; 9. ____;
10. several

Radiation therapy:
0. no data; 1. no radiation therapy was carried out; 2. radiation therapy only; 3. before surgery; 4. after surgery. 5. before and after surgery; 6. in combination with nonsurgical method of treatment;
7. _____

3. leukopenia; 4. thrombocytopenia; 5. panmyelophthisis; 6.
6. gastroenterologic;
7. _____; 8. several

Hormone therapy:
0. no data; 1. no hormone therapy was carried out; 2. hormone therapy only; 3. in combination with other therapeutic methods; 4. _____

Types of hormone therapy:
0. no data;
1. hormone therapy was not carried out;
2. androgens;
3. estrogens;
4. progestins;
5. ovariectomy;
6. _____;
7. several

Complications after hormone therapy:
0. no data;
1. no treatment was carried out;
2. absent;
3. disturbance of mineral metabolism;
4. hirsutism;
5. skin lesions;
6. _____;
7. several

Support of diagnosis:
0. no data;
1. histological;
2. cytological;
3. clinicoroentgenological;
4. _____

Resons why radical treatment was not carried out:

0. no data; 1. radical treatment was carried out. 2. process was too advanced;
3. patient's refusal of treatment; 4. accompanying diseases;
5. advanced age; 6. _____;
7. several

Types and sources of radiation therapy:

0. no data;
1. radiation therapy was not
   carried out;
2. X-ray therapy;
3. telegramus therapy;
4. Contact therapy /isotopes,
   needles, applicators/;
5. megavolt therapy /high-
   voltage energy sources/;
6. X-ray therapy + telegammatherapy;
7. X-ray therapy + contact
   therapy;
8. telegammatherapy + contact
   therapy;
9. Other types of combined
   treatment

Methods of radiation
therapy:
0. no data; 1. radiation
therapy was not carried
out; 2. external only;
3. intracavitary only; 4. interstitial only; 5. external
+ interstitial; 6. external
+ intracavitary; 7. _____

Immediate result of treatment:

0. no data;
1. recovery;
2. improvement;
3. no effect /or examination/;
4. aggravation;
5. died during surgery;
6. died due to complications
   in postoperative period;
7. died due to complications
   caused by chemotherapy;
8. died due to tumour growth;
9. died of intercurrent
   diseases;
10. _____

Supplement 22

Approved by USSR Ministry of Health,
Order No. 935 of 17 November 1972

Registration No.

CONTROL NOTIFICATIONS ON DYNAMIC OBSERVATION

Patient's surname _____ first name _____ patronymic ____

Sex: male, female. Year of birth _____ Patient's address_____
_____

Diagnosis _____

Date of exact diagnosis _____ year _____ month

Date of beginning of treatment _____ year _____ month

Special extract from cancer inpatient record and control notification on dynamic observation are sent to the All-Union
Centre for Studying Efficiency Treatment in Patients with Malignant Neoplasms at the address: Leningrad, 188646, Pesochnyj
2, ul. Leningradskaya 68, N.N. Petrov Research Institute of
Oncology, ACSETP

Notification on striking
patient off the register

Diagnosis _____

Date of exact diagnosis ___
____ year _____ month

Date or beginning of treatment _____ year _____ month

Date of death

_____ year _____ month

Institution responsible for
observation of the patient

_____

Cause of death:

0. no data; 1. cause of
death was not established;
2. died of malignant neo-
plasms at home; 3. died of
malignant neoplasm in hospital; 4. died of other
cause _____

Notification on striking patient
off the register

Registration No.

Control notification No. 7

Diagnosis _____

Date of exact diagnosis

_____ year _____ month

Date of beginning of treatment

_____ year _____ month

Observation year _____

month _____

Institution responsible for observation of the patient

_____

State of patient's health:

0. no data; 1. not established; 2. fit; 3. relapse or metastasis; 4. tumour does not grow; 5. patient disappeared; 6. moved to

_____

Additional treatment:

0. no data; 1. no additional treatment; 2. surgery only; 3. radiation therapy only; 4. chemotherapy only; 5. hormone therapy only; 6. mixed; 7. comprehensive; 8. Symptomatic

Invalidism due to disease:

0. no data; 1. absent; 2. group I; 3. group II; 4. group III; 5. _____

Patient's work status:

0. no data; 1. does not work; 2. returned to his previous work; 3. transferred to easier work

Control notification No. 6

Diagnosis _____

Date of exact diagnosis

_____ year _____ month

Date of beginning of treatment

_____ year _____ month

Observation year _____

month _____

Institution responsible for patient observation _____

State of patient's health:

0. no data; 1. not established; 2. fit; 3. relapse or metastasis; 4. tumour does not grow; 5. patient disappeared; 6. moved to _____

Additional treatment:

0. no data; 1. no additional treatment; 2. surgery only; 3. radiation therapy only; 4. chemotherapy only; 5. hormone therapy only; 6. mixed; 7. comprehensive; 8. symptomatic

Invalidism due to disease:

0. no data; 1. absent; 2. group I; 3. group II; 4. group III; 5. _____

Patient's work status:

0. no data; 1. does not work; 2. returned to his previous work; 3. transferred to easier work

Control notification No. 5

Diagnosis _____

Date of exact diagnosis

_____ year _____ month

Date of beginning of treatment

_____ year _____ month

Observation year _____

month _____

Institution responsible for
observation of the patient

_____

State of patient's health:

O. no data; 1. not established;
2. fit; 3. relapse or metastases; 4. tumour does not
grow; 5. patient disappeared;
6. moved ·to _____

Additional treatment:

O. no data; 1. no additional
treatment; 2. surgery only;
3. radiation therapy only;
4. chemotherapy only; 5.
hormone therapy only; 6.mixed;
7. comprehensive;
8. symptomatic

Invalidism due to disease:

O. no data; 1. absent; 2.
group I; 3. group II; 4.
group III; 5. _____

Patient's work status:

O. no data; 1. does not work;
2. returned to his previous
work; 3. transferred to
easier work

Control notification No. 4

Diagnosis _____

Date of exact diagnosis

_____ year _____ month

Date of beginning of treatment

_____ year _____ month

Observation year _____

month _____

Institution responsible for
observation of the patient

_____

State of patient's health:

O. no data; 1. not established;
2. fit; 3. relapse or metastases;
4. tumour does not grow; 5. patient disappeared; 6. moved to

_____

Additional treatment:

O. no data; 1. no additional
treatment; 2. surgery only;3.
radiation therapy only;
4. chemotherapy only; 5.
hormone therapy only;
6. mixed; 7. comprehensive;
8. symptomatic

Invalidism du to disease:

O. no data; 1. absent;
2. group I; 3. group II;
4. group III; 5. _____

Patient's work status:

O. no data; 1. does not work;
2. returned to his previous
work; 3. transferred to
easier work

Control notifications No. 3

Diagnosis _____

Date of exact diagnosis

_____ year _____ month

Date of beginning of treatment

_____ year _____ month

Observation year _____

month _____

Institution responsible for
observation of the patient

_____

State of patient's health:

0. no data; 1. not estab-
lished; 2. fit; 3. relapse or
metastasis; 4. tumour does
not grow; 5. patient dis-
appeared; 6. moved to _____

_____

Additional treatment:

0. no data; 1. no additional
treatment; 2. surgery only;
3. radiation therapy only;
4. chemotherapy only; 5.
hormone therapy only; 6.
mixed; 7. comprehensive;
8. symptomatic

Invalidism due to disease:

0. no data; 1. absent;
2. group I; 3. group II;
4. group III; 5. _____

Patient's work status:

0. no data; 1. does not work;
2. returned his previous work;
3. transferred to easier work

Control notification No. 2

Diagnosis _____

Date of exact diagnosis

_____ year _____ month

Date of beginning of treatment

_____ year _____ month

Observation year _____

month _____

Institution responsible for
observation of the patient

_____

State of patient's health:

0. no data; 1. not estab-
lished; 2. fit; 3. relapse or
metastases; 4. tumour does not
grow; 5. patient disappeared;
6. moved to _____

Additional treatment:

0. no data; 1. no additional
treatment; 2. surgery only;
3. radiation only; 4. chemotherapy only; 5. hormone
therapy only; 6. mixed;
7. comprehensive
8. symptomatic

Invalidism due to disease:

0. no data; 1. absent;
2. group I; 3. group II;
4. group III; 5. _____

Patient's work status:

0. data; 1. does not work;
2. returned to his previous
work; 3. transferred to
easier work

Control notification No. 1

Diagnosis _____

Date of exact diagnosis

_____ year _____ month

Date of beginning of treatment

_____ year _____ month

Observation year _____

month _____

Institution responsible for
observation of the patient

_____

State of patient's health:

0. no data; 1. not estab-
lished; 2. fit; 3. relapse or
metastasis; 4. tumour does
not grow; 5. patient dis-
appeared; 6. moved to

_____

Additional treatment:

0. no data; 1. no additional
treatment; 2. surgery only;
3. radiation therapy only;
4. chemotherapy only;
5. hormone therapy only;
6. mixed; 7. comprehensive;
8. symptomatic

Invalidism due to disease:

0. no data; 1. absent;
2. group I; 3. group II;
4. group III; 5. _____

Patient's work status:

0. no data; 1. does not work;
2. returned to his previous work
3. transferred to easier work

ment given to the patient and contains, besides indentification data, information on the properties of the tumour, the peculiarities of the patient's organism and the character of the treatment. The forms are filled in at an oncological institution and sent to the All-Union Centre for Studying Effectivity of Treatment in Patients with Malignant Tumours. The forms should be filled in by a physician or a sufficiently experienced medical assistant in accordance with the patient's medical history.

The second part comprises seven annual coupons of the dynamic observation of the patient and one notification of striking off the register. Information on the events occuring after the patient's discharge from the hospital /the data on the patient's state, additional treatment, rehabilitation/ is entered in each coupon for the corresponding year of observation. The coupons should be sent to the Centre once a year.

To ensure that the forms be filled in as correctly as possible the following instructions have been issued:

1. The All-Union Centre for Studying the Effectivity of Treatment in Patients with Malignant Tumours /Prof. N.N. Petrov Research Institute of Oncology/ must study the effectivity of treatment in patients with malignant neoplasms using the data contained in the statistical forms "Special Excerpts from Cancer Inpatient Record" with the control notifications of dynamic observation.

2. The proposed statistical form /approved by the Ministry of Health of the USSR, Order No. 935 of November 17, 1972/ must be filled in for all patients with primarily diagnosed malignant tumours who have been admitted to the hospital sponsored by any oncological dispensary /institute/ and afterwards placed under dispensary observation at this intitution.

Note: No Special Excerpt should be filled in for those patients who have been admitted to the hospital, but afterwards not placed under the observation at a given dispensary /institute/, nor for those patients who have been treated for relapses and metastases of malignant tumours diagnosed earlier.

3. The present statistical form consists of two parts:

The first part, "Special Excerpt from Cancer Inpatient Record", is intended for the collection of information on the immediate results of treatment and its transmission to the All-Union Centre for Studying the Effectivity of Treatment in Patients with Malignant Tumours. This part is filled in at the discharge of the patient from the hospital /or if the patient dies at the hospital/ in accordance with the patient's registry card /medical history/.

The second part, "Control Notifications on Dynamic Observation", is intended for studying the remote results of treatment, additional treatment and the working ability of the patients placed under dispensary observation. This part is filled in on the basis of information obtained during the observation of the patients.

The "Special Excerpt from Cancer Inpatient Record" should be filled in as follows:

4. All the characteristics contained in this statistical form are divided into 4 groups:

a/ the characteristics written in words and providing the following information: diagnosis, profession, exposure to professional hazards, earlier diseases of the affected organ, growth of the tumour into the adjecent structures, localization of the tumour in the organ, type of surgical intervention;

b/ the characteristics denoted by code numbers filled in against them: the patient's residence at the time of falling ill, the institution carrying out observation, nationality;

c/ the characteristics denoted by their absolute number: date of exact diagnosis, date of starting treatment, age, duration of hospitalization, duration of the symptoms of the diseases, size of the tumour;

d/ the characteristics denoted by numbers: residence, sex, kind of treatment, character of treatment, stage of the disease according to the TNM system, etc.

5. In the item "Diagnosis" the name of the tumour found in the patient must be written, and in the rectangle against this item the corresponding four-digit code number.

Example: If the diagnosis is cancer of the pyloric end of

the stomach, put code number 151.1 in the rectangle and write gastric cancer after the word "Diagnosis".

6. In the item "Localization of the tumour in the organ" the position of the neoplasm in the affected organ must be indicated, and in case of paired organs also the affected side.

Examples: The patient has tumour of the antral section of the stomach; in this case write as follows:

Localization of the tumour in the organ: Antral section of the stomach.

The patient has lung cancer. The tumour is located in the lower lobe of the right lung. This should be entered as follows:

Localization of the tumour in the organ: Lower lobe of the right lung.

When filling in the item "Diagnosis" and writing its code number the International Classification of Diseases, Lesions and Causes of Death, 8th Revision, 1965, should be used.

7. Besides diagnosis, the characteristics contained in item 4a should be filled in as follows: above the line placed against or under the name of the characteristic write its description.

Example: The patient has undergone subtotal resection of the stomach. This circumstance must be marked as follows:

Type of surgical intervention:

0 - no data

1 - no surgical intervention

②- Surgery performed: subtotal resection of the stomach

8. The characteristics to be registered by using a definite code number /item 4b/ are filled in as follows: the corresponding code must be written above the line against the characteristic.

Note: The oncological institutions collaborating with the All-Union Centre for Studying the Effectivity of Treatment in Patients with Malignant Tumours are provided with the code numbers used for filling in the characteristics in the forms /nationality, the institution carrying out observation, the patient's residence at the time of falling ill/.

9. The item "Institution carrying out observation" means the medical institution where the patient was hospitalized and which is carrying out the dispensary observation of the patient at present.

10. The characteristics contained in item 4c are denoted by filling in absolute numbers.

Example: Date of exact diagnosis: 1971, 3. Date of starting treatment: 1971, 4. Age: 45. Duration of the symptoms of the disease /months/: 6. Size of the tumour: /cm/ 10.

Note: If the hospitalized patient was given no treatment, the year and month of hospitalization should be entered in the item "Date of starting treatment".

11. If the characteristics are denoted by numbers /item 4d/, the number which corresponds to the actual characteristic of the patient must be circled.

Example: The patient was found to have multiple regional metastases. In this case the characteristic should be marked as follows:

Regional metastases:

0 - no data

1 - absent

2 - single

③ - multiple

4 - no investigation made

12. In the items which have an empty line besides the text additional data are written if necessary.

Example: Radiation therapy resulted in a rectovaginal fistula in the patient. This complication must be recorded by filling in the empty line /No. 7/ of the characteristic "Complications after radiation", and number 7 must be circled.

Complications after radiation:

0 - no data

1 - no radiation therapy

2 - none

3 - leucopenia

4 - dermatitides

5 - cystitis, proctitis

6 - necrosis of soft tissues

(7)- <u>rectovaginal fistula</u>

8 - several

13. If the patient was found to have several of the complications mentioned in the form, only the number corresponding to
the item "several" must be circled, and the names of the complications underlined.

Example: Chemotherapy resulted in the following complications: leucopenia, thrombocytopenia, which should be registered
as follows:

Complications after chemotherapy:

0 - no data

1 - no chemotherapy

2 - none

3 - <u>leucopenia</u>

4 - <u>thrombocytopenia</u>

5 - panmyelophthisis

6 - gastroenterological

7 - _____

(8)- several

14. When filling in the item "Types of treatment" the
directions "Clinical, Surgical and Combined Treatment of Malignant Tumours" issued by the Problem Commission /1972/ should be
followed in order to indicate the methods of treatment which
are used at present in clinical oncology:

<u>Treatment by a single method</u> is determined by the type of
therapeutic action used for both radical and palliative treatment.

Example: surgical intervention, radiation therapy /X-ray
therapy, telegamma therapy, high-energy radiation therapy/,
chemotherapy, hormonotherapy.

<u>Combined treatment</u> is the use of two kinds of therapeutic
action which are different in their character and affect local
and regional loci.

Example: surgical intervention + radiation therapy; radiation therapy + surgical intervention + radiation therapy.

<u>Complex treatment</u> is the use of a number of therapeutic

measures following in different succession and having a different effect on the tumour and the patient's body; their object may be local and regional lesions, as well as the whole body.

Example: 1/ preoperative radiation therapy + surgical interventions + chemotherapy; 2/ surgical intervention + radiation therapy + hormonotherapy; 3/ radiation therapy + chemotherapy + hormonotherapy; 4/ surgical intervention + chemotherapy + hormonotherapy.

Compound treatment is the use of two methods of treatment, similar in their biological action and affecting local and regional loci or the whole body.

Example: 1/ X-ray therapy + radiotherapy; 2/ chemotherapy with two or several preparations; 3/ overiectomy + administration of hormonal preparations.

15. When filling in the item "Nature of treatment" number 1 /"radical"/ must be circled if the primary focus of the tumour has been cured and the regional lymphatic nodes /in case of their lesion/ have been removed, and if no remote metastatic spreading occurred. In all other cases number 2 or 3 should be circled.

16. When filling in the item "Stage of the disease" it is necessary to follow the instructions contained in the "Collection of Instructions on the Problems of Oncological Assistance, Prophylaxis, Diagnostics and Treatment of Malignant Tumours and Pretumourous Diseases" /Moscow, 1956/, and when filling in the item "Stage of the disease according to the TNM system" the instructions in the methodological manual "Classification of Malignant Tumours According to the TNM System" /Leningrad, 1969/ must be followed.

The principles of this system are simple. The capital letters donete: T - tumour, N - regional lymph nodes, M - remote metastases. The figures added to these three categories /e.g., T1, T2, etc.; N0, N1, etc.; M0, M1/ indicate various degrees of the spread of the malignant tumour, which is, in fact, the stenographic description of any particular tumour.

Thus, a surgeon who is acquainted with the TNM system may

describe the tumour of the breast as T3N2MO. It means that the tumour has a definite size /more than 5 cm, but not exceeding 1O cm in diameter/, or causes the ulceration of the skin, or that the tumour is adhered to the pectoral fascia developed; at the same time immovable axillary lymph nodes can be palpated and the clinical signs of metastases are absent.

17. In the absence of the histological investigation of the tumour /in cases when there is no histological confirmation cf the diagnosis/ it is necessary to circle the number corresponding to the supposed diagnosis in the item "Type of malignant tumour".

The second part, "Control Notifications of Dynamic Observation" should be filled in as follows:

The dynamic observation coupons for each patient registered at the dispensary with the use of the Special Excerpt are one of the most important elements in studying the effectivity of treatment in patients with malignant tumours. Only if all the registered cases are closely followed up and the annual Control Notifications are available, can the All-Union Centre completely characterize the treatment given to tumour patients and indicate which of the present methods of treatment are most effective. In this connection the following should be observed:

18. In all the Control Notifications, as well as in the Notification of Striking Off the Register, the items "Diagnosis", "Date of exact diagnosis", "Date of starting treatment", "Institution carrying out observation" should be filled in simultaneously with filling in the first part of the form, as these items are important elements in the information retrieval system of the All-Union Centre for Studying the Effectivity of Treatment in Patients with Malignant Tumours.

19. In the characteristic "State of patient's health" the number of the item "not established" /1/ must be circled only if the patient has not come for examination at the oncological dispensary /institute/, and the information about this patient was obtained from a written communication or some other source indicating that the patient is alive. In case when

the tumour is localized number 4 must be circled.

20. On the reverse side of the coupon the items characterizing additional treatment and the occupational activity of the
patient must correspond to the given year of observation; these
items are filled in by circling the corresponding numbers /see
item 14/.

21. The control notification coupons should be filled in
for each calendar year during the whole period the patient is
under observation. The year which follows the year of the
treatment or hospitalization of the patient should be considered
the first year of observation.

Example: In May 1970 the patient underwent operation for
gastric cancer. In this case 1971 is the first year of observation, 1972 is the second year, etc.

For each year of observation only one control notification
coupon must be filled in during the first visit of the patient
to the oncological institution in the current year.

22. In case the patient dies, the Notification of Striking
Off the Register should be filled in, irrespective of the year
of observation.

23. To ensure timely processing of the data by the computer complex the forms and control notifications should be
sent to the All-Union Centre for Studying the Effectivity of
Treatment in Patients with Malignant Tumours at least quarter-
ly.

The work carried out by the All-Union Centre proves the
undeniable advantage of the machine processing of observation
results covering a large number of patients with malignant tumours.

The specially developed library of programmes for computers of different models /M-222, BESM-6, EC-1022/ makes
possible to carry out data processing with the aim to obtain
different amounts of tables with 1, 2 or 3 characteristics.
These can be divided into three main types, according to their
contents:

1. General characteristics of the contingent of patients.
2. Characteristics of treatment.

3. Remote results of treatment.

Age and sex characteristics, the stage of the disease, the degree of malignancy, the methods of surgical intervention, radiation therapy, chemotherapy, hormonotherapy and their combined variants, as well as some other characteristics, have been chosen as factors comparable with the remote results of treatment.

Considering the importance and complexity of the problem under study, the All-Union Centre for Studying the Effectivity of Treatment in Patients with Malignant Tumours, simultaneously with solving purely practical problems, works on the problems of creating the automated system of individual prognostication for all the main forms of malignant tumours.

The general technology of information processing in the All-Union Centre is outlined in Fig. 43.

The constant stage-by-stage analysis of results makes possible to timely correct operations of data processing, while the use of computer not only facilitates statistical analysis of clinical data, but it also enables one to evaluate the results of treatment in connection with many factors affecting all stages of the pathological process.

At present the All-Union Centre for Studying the Effectivity of Treatment in Patients with Malignant Tumours cooperates with 38 oncological institution in the USSR.

ORGANIZATION OF MEDICAL DETERMINATION OF DISABILITY AND REHABILITATION OF ONCOLOGICAL PATIENTS

V.N. Gerasimenko, V.V. Artyusenko and V.V. Lazo

In the last decade the introduction of complex methods of treating malignant neoplasms has resulted in wider possibilities to resort to radical treatment of tumours in a whole number of localizations, in longer life expectancy of oncological patients and in the emergence of a real possibility to carry out prophylactic and palliative therapy courses following treatment on a radical programme. In consequence of this, the contingents of patients followed up by the oncological institutions in our country are permanently increasing.

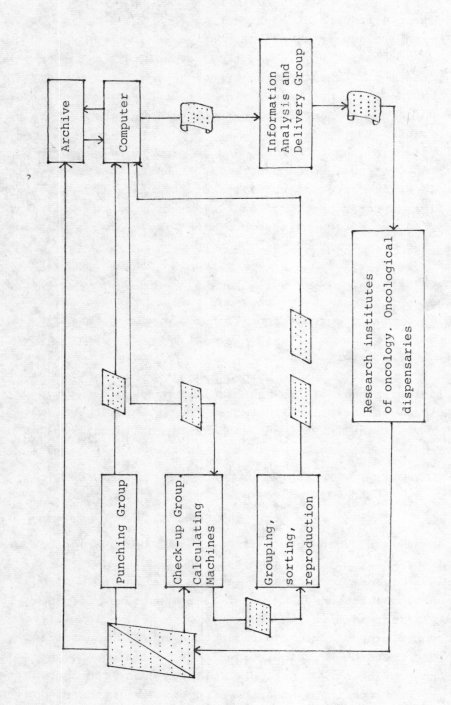

Fig. 43 Scheme of information processing in the All-Union Centre.

Thus, in 1965, the percentage of oncological patients who have been on the follow-up for 5 years and more was 39.2, in 1970 this figure increased to 44.2 while in 1974 it reached 47.5 /of which 24 per cent of patients had been on the follow-up for 10 years and more/. If one takes into account the fact that the ages most affected by malignant tumours are those of the active working life, it becomes clear that the increase of follow-up patients should be accompanied by a larger contingent of people subject to expert opinion concerning disability and to rehabilitation. According to statistical data for 1975, malignant neoplasms occupied the third place among the causes of disablement.

It should be noted that because of the skeptical attitude of oncologists towards rehabilitation of oncological patients, the study of this problem began only 10 to 15 years ago.

The possibilities inherent in the labour rehabilitation of oncological patients with malignant neoplasms following radical treatment have not yet been studied to an adequate extent.

The pecularities of the clinical course of the disease at different localizations, the specific features of its treatment and the functional impairments necessarily arising after a surgical intervention call for a highly differentiated approach to the question of the labour rehabilitation of these patients.

Though it is impossible to make an accurate prognosis of the disease in each particular case, already before the rehabilitation is decided upon, its objective should be determined and its plan drawn up. For this purpose, the physician should maximally take into account all the possible functional impairments which may be caused either by the disease or by the treatment and affect the patient's ability to work.

The process of rehabilitation represents practical implementation of the program which should be optimal for each patient and provide for the creation of conditions for him which are the most favourable both physiologically and physically.

The nature of such an individual program depends on the type of treatment, its scope, immediate and remote results of the treatment, the age of the patient, sex, occupation, his psychological stability, etc.

Depending on the patient's health status and the prospects of his rehabilitation or compensation of the functions lost as a result of the disease or treatment, the purposes of rehabilitation may be as follows:

1. Full rehabilitation of the patient's ability to work, which would enable him, after a period of reconvalescence, to resume his occupation or one similar to it;

2. The patient's recovery without a considerable loss of his capacity for work;

3. Partial recovery of the lost capacity for work through adequate treatment and training /supporting rehabilitation/;

4. Palliative rehabilitation - when a rational treatment is impossible but certain complications can be decreased /bed-sores, contractures, severe pain and psychological disorders/.

Depending on the course of the disease and effectivity of treatment, the objectives of the rehabilitation may be changed during the process of treatment. The rehabilitation program should aim at a maximal rehabilitation of the patient's ability to work, including physical, psychological, social and occupational adaptation.

In a resolution adopted by the ministers of health of the socialist countries at their IXth Meeting /Prague, 1967/, rehabilitation is defined as "a system of state, socio-economic, medical, occupational, psychological and other measures taken with a view to prevent the development of pathological processes which might result in a temporary or constant loss of capacity for work and to return the patients and the disabled to society and socially useful labour early and on an efficient basis".

In the socialist countries optimal conditions exist for a successful and comprehensive solution of the problem of rehabilitation. The prophylaxis, free qualified medical help, prophylactic examinations of the population, resort to

restorative treatment in sanatoria and health resorts on a
wide scale - all these measures create favourable prospects
for the development of measures of rehabilitation. In the
socialist system, rehabilitation gains state importance and is
extended to all persons with reduced capacity for work.
Specialized workshops are set up for people who are unable to
work at conventional enterprises and also reception - and -
distribution stations for people working at home. Within the
system of social security of the Russian Federation alone,
there are 200 specialized production enterprises and 51 workshops for disabled people. This has made possible to transfer
6.5 per cent of the disabled into the category of those able
to work in the year 1967. alone and thus reduce the expenditure
on pensions by about 30.5 million roubles.

In accordance with the above definition of rehabilitation
the main objective of rehabilitation in the socialist society
consists in preventing those diseases which cause temporary
or persistent loss of ability of work and in enabling the patients and invalids to return to society, to socially useful
labour, i.e. rehabilitation pursues, above all, human objectives.

It should be stressed that it is desirable and rational
that the patients return to work after treatment /if there are
no contraindications/, since their engagement in systematic
labour, especially in their former occupations creates confidence in recovery and in a favourable future.

The study of the economic aspect of the rehabilitation of
oncological patients convincingly demonstrates that, no matter
the duration of labour activities of the patient after radical
treatment, its economic efficiency for the state is beyond any
doubt.

The differentiated approach to the solution of the complex
problem of rehabilitation of oncological patients is ensured
in the USSR by the specialized system of organization of medical expertise, which allows for determining in which group
of invalidity the patient belongs and whether he can be
allowed to return to work under certain conditions.

The oncological Commissions of Medical Experts were set up in 1963 and belong to the organs of social security.

The Commission of Medical Experts is entrusted with the following task:

- establishment of permanent or prolonged loss of working capacity and invalidity group;

- establishment of the time of the onset of invalidity;

- establishment of causes of invalidity;

- determination of conditions and nature of work suitable for invalids;

- determination of measures which can promote restoration of working capacity of invalids /vocational training, retraining, restorative treatment, prostheses, and working devices/;

- the study of the conditions of work of invalids directly at enterprises and offices and in agriculture with a view to find out which jobs and occupations are suitable for particular invalids and to check on whether their job placement is correct.

The oncological Commission of Medical Experts functions on the basis of the oncological dispensaries and consists of three oncologists of different specialities /one of them is appointed chairman of the Commission/, as well as of a representative of a respective department of social security and the representative of the trade union of the enterprise where the patient worked. The latter, as a rule, takes part in the discussions regarding the possibilities of labour rehabilitation of the patient.

The organization of the oncological Commission of Medical Experts on the basis of the oncological dispensary considerably increases the possibilities of comprehensive investigations of patients through involvement of highly qualified oncologists in highly specialized fields and facilitates the utilization of laboratories and diagnostic departments of the dispensary.

In some cases, when during the determination of the degree of the loss of working ability has occured, it becomes necessary to investigate the functioning of the organism of the

patient more thoroughly, the commission can refer the patient
to the Institute for Expert Identification of Working Capacity
and Organization of Labour for Invalids.

The organization of the oncological commissions of medical
experts has, beyond doubt, promoted the solution of urgent
problems of rehabilitation of oncological patients. The annual
generalizations from highly representative data regarding the
dynamics of invalidity of patients and their occupational rehabilitation has made possible to work out specific methodological approaches to the assessment of the condition of the patient, the determination of the degree and duration of ability
to work and to elaborate certain criteria necessary for a
correct solution of the complex questions of medical, occupational and social rehabilitation for various forms of malignant tumours.

According to the Soviet legistlation, there are three invalidity groups. Invalidity is established on the basis of a
persistent loss of working capacity as a result of which the
patient has to discontinue his professional labour for a long
period of time or has to change the conditions of his work.
These changes or lighter conditions of work are necessary in
case of loss of qualification cr of a considerable reduction of
the volume of work. When deciding about the patient's ability
to work the Commission of Medical Experts proceeds from medical or social factors and in each particular case takes
account of the peculiarities of the condition of the patient,
the nature and course of the pathological process, the degree
of development of compensatory functions of the organism which
have been disturbed in consequence of the disease or in the
process of treatment, the concrete labour conditions, the
general and occupational background of the patient, his age
and professional line.

According to the existing legislation, the Commission
of Medical Experts periodically reexamines invalids with the
aim of checking on the pathological process in the patient
and his ability to work.

Invalids are assigned to group I if impairment of their

functions has incapacitated them so much that they are in need of constant daily or systematic assistance.

Those persons are assigned to invalidity group I, who have lost their ability to work permanently or for a long time. To this group belong patients with malignant neoplasms whose condition does not allow for radical treatment, patients with relapses and metastases which developed after treatment as well as patients whose communicability has become impaired as a result of surgical intervention.

The patient is assigned to invalidity group II if there are obvious functional impairments which, though not necessitating the constant care or observation of the patient, result in a complete permanent or temporary loss of ability to work or if the patient can be allowed to be engaged only in certain kinds of work and in specially created conditions.

Moreover, those are assigned to group II who are unable to work for a long period of time because the course of their disease may be adversely affected by the work. They are usually patients who have recently undergone radical treatment for malignant neoplasms of the main localizations /the breast, the lungs, the oesophagus, the stomach, the large intestine and the rectum, female genital organs/.

The invalidity group III consists of cases in which there is a considerable reduction of working capacity as a result of functional impairments after surgical intervention or application of other kinds of treatment /radiotherapy, pharmacotherapy/. Invalidity group III is established when it is necessary to find a job which requires a lower qualification for the patient. This occurs when the patient cannot continue his former occupation.

According to the existing legislation, group I invalids are reexamined every second year while group II and group III invalids are reexamined each year. If the state of health of the invalids is worsening /relapses and metastases, acute functional disturbances/, they can be reassigned into another group sooner.

Patients can be permanently assigned to an invalidity

group in cases: 1/ if they are affected with incurable forms
of malignant neoplasms, or if they have fistulas /fecal, uri-
nary/, which cannot be removed despite treatment, and which
cause unclearliness;

2/ if they have undergone surgical operation for removal
of tumours in the stomach, the lung, the larynx and other
localizations /the invalidity group is determined on the basis
of the degree of functional impairment of the organism; duration of observation of these invalids is no less than two
years/;

3/ invalid men aged sixty and more and women aged fifty
five and more, in regarding the fact that they have reached
pension age.

What is important for the Commission of Medical Experts
examining the patient for the first time for determining his
invalidity group, is the stage of the disease and the nature
of the medical intervention the patient has undergone. Later,
if relapses or metastases do not occur, primary importance is
attributed to anatomical-functional disturbances and decision
is made on the basis of the treatment the patient has received
and the possibilities of his rational job placement.

In the decision about returning the patient to work, his
occupation plays an important role. It should be observed that
such invalids are not overstrained physically or psychological-
ly and they are not engaged in work which is connected with
heavy physical load and occupational hazards. At the same time,
several investigations show that the possibilities of rehabilitation of patients with malignant neoplasms are wider than
it was thought before.

The study of the acitivities of the Commission of Medical
Experts has demonstrated that there are rather wide discrep-
ancies between the real working capacity of the patient and
decisions taken by this commission regarding the possibilities
of their work. It should be noted that many patients return
to work in spite of the decision of the Commission of Medical
Experts, and fulfil their duties splendidly. A number of
investigations have demonstrated that group II invalids who

do not work cope with the considerable volume of physical load in their lives at home without the deterioration of the state of their health.

It has also been established that a considerable number of patients who have undergone treatment for malignant tumours refuse to be examined by the Commission of Medical Experts and go to work upon expiration of time of their incapacity established in the medical certificate. This applies, in the first place, to intellectual workers, workers of high qualifications, or those employed in jobs not requiring any qualifications. More than 40 to 50 % of these patients return to work 4 months after radical treatment.

At present, in the Soviet Union the elaboration of the questions of rehabilitation is assigned to research institutes of oncology and to the large dispensaries. Sociologists, psychologists, psychiatrists and physiotherapists are extensively involved in the study of rehabilitation.

The extent research into rehabilitation of oncological patients, that has been carried out by large scientific research institutes /Oncological Centre of the Academy of Sciences of the USSR and the Professor N.N. Petrov Research Institute of Oncology of the Ministry of Public Health of the USSR, demonstrates that for the sake of successful rehabilitation one should adopt a complex of therapeutic and socio-psychological measures. It is evident that in order to fulfil the proposed program it is necessary to create rehabilitation departments and centres in the oncological institutes and dispensaries which work in a close contact with the oncological Commissions of Medical Experts. The pattern of relationship between the centres /departments/ of rehabilitation and other treatment institutions of the oncological network, between the Commission of Medical Experts, the family of the patient, and the enterprise where he works is given below is presented in Fig. 44.

The socio-psychological measures of rehabilitation include a number of questions concerning the personal and psychological features of the patient, determination of the

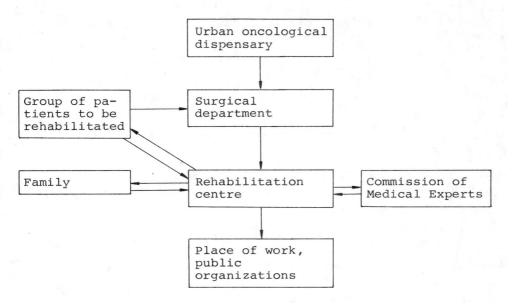

Fig. 44 Relationship between rehabilitation centres and other
institutions.

degree of the impairment and the methods of treatment necessary
to correct these impairments. At the same time, the socio-
-labour profile of the patient should be studied in its dynamic
aspect including the following:

    a/ feasibility and reasonability of his return to work;

    b/ the time of return to work;

    c/ degree of restoration of work capacity;

    d/ choice of an adequate occupation;

    e/ social position of the patients;

    f/ relations in the family /family rehabilitation/;

    g/ domestic conditions.

    Thus, the process of rehabilitation of the oncological
patient begins practically simultaneously with his treatment
and comprises the realization of a complex of comprehensive
measures the result of which is an optimal varian of readaptation of the patient to the family and to the society. The
implementation of these measures is realized by the following:

    1/ a wide network of oncological institutions each of
which provides up-to-date, high-quality treatment;

2/ a system of monitoring which gives a real opportunity for the timely detection of relapses and metastases, for the administration of courses of palliative therapy, for referral for treatment in sanatoria and rest-homes and for the adoption of other measures to improve the general health of the patient;

3/ a specialized oncological system for obtaining medical expertise which ensures a differentiated approach to deciding about the employment of invalids;

4/ a system of vocational retraining which makes possible for the patient to select a specialty adequate to his ability to work;

5/ a system of social assistance which ensures job placement for invalids and promotes the improvement of their material and domestic conditions.

In the USSR, in the large research oncological institutes rehabilitation departments are now being created. They are charged with the responsibility to improve rehabilitation of oncological patients.

ORGANIZATION OF MEDICAL ASSISTANCE TO PATIENTS
IN ADVANCED FORMS OF TUMOURS

N.Ya. Shabashova, K.S. Mirotvortseva and D.P. Berezkin

In the system of organization of cancer control the questions of medical assistance to patients in advanced stages of the disease are rather complicated and their solution cannot be other than manysided. There is no doubt that the many years of purposeful effort of the oncological network in the Soviet Union has resulted in a noticeable improvement in the indicators of oncological assistance to the population. The contingent of patients on register by the oncological network who have survived more than five years is steadily increasing /1965 - 39.2 %; 1970 - 44.2 %; 1974 - 47.5 %/. The number of patients who have undergone radical treatment is also growing. At the same time among the patients with newly detected malignant neoplasms each year a rather considerable group is identified in advanced stages of the disease /clinical group IV/, not subject to radical treatment. Thus, in 1960 this contingent

made up 21.3 %, in 1970 - 20.2 %; in 1973 - 21 % and in 1974
- 19.9 %. The fact that no definite reduction is observed in
the number of patients in advanced stages of the disease, makes
one to suppose that the indubitable improvement in the quality
of diagnoses of malignant neoplasms cannot result in a considerable increase of cases with early detected neoplasms because
there is a group of cases which show extreme malignancy at all
stages of the process. Such malignancy can result in the
generalization of the process already before the appearance of
symptoms of the primary tumour. It is evident that as the
quality of diagnosis is improved, the share of tumour cases of
high malignancy among the patients in clinical group IV will
increase.

In the course of time, apart from patients who were identified already in an advanced stage of the disease, clinical
group IV also comprises patients who either refuse treatment
or cannot be treated because of an accompanying disease. Those
patients also belong to clinical group IV, who have relapses
and metastases after radical treatment.

In accordance with the state legislation a "Protocol for
detection of a malignant neoplasm in an advanced stage
/clinical group IV/" has been introduced for each patient in
clinical group IV. The protocol is filled in in two copies;
one of them   is transmitted to the oncological dispensary
in the area of the patient's residence and the dispensary en-
rolls the patient in the register. The second copy remains in
the institution where the case was first detected. All the
cases of late diagnosis are discussed at medical conferences
where the physicians who observed or treated the patient also
participated. Special attention is paid to those cases which
reached an advanced stage because of inadequate examination
or because not all the methods necessary for making the diagnosis were used. When filling in the protocol one has to
describe chronologically all the stages of the examination of
the patient and the results of the examinations; special attention is paid to the causes of the onset of the advanced
stage, which are formulated as follows:

1. Incomplete examination of the patient;
2. Diagnostic error:
   a/ clinical, b/ roentgenological, c/ pathohistological.
3. A prolonged investigation of the patient;
4. Latent development of the disease;
5. Late application of the patient for medical assistance.

A profound analysis of the causes carried out by clinicians and organizers of public health has revealed that the dominant place among the causes of the appearance of incurable forms of tumours are latent development of the disease and the late application for medical assistance.

The analysis and generalization of the information contained in the protocols provide the basis for the elaboration of measures aimed to provide oncological assistance to the population and play an important role in the general system of organization of cancer control in the country.

The development of the oncological network and the improvement of the quality of the diagnosis of malignant neoplasms within the general medical services in recent years have made possible to raise the standards of examination of oncological patients. According to the order issued in 1976 by the Minister of Public Health of the USSR detection of malignant neoplasms in localizations available for visual examination /the skin, the tongue, the oral cavity, the lower lip, the thyroid gland, the cervix uteri, the breast and the rectum/ in the third stage of the disease is to be considered as equivalent to an advanced stage and calls for the filling in of the respective "Protocol for detection of a malignant neoplasm in an advanced stage". It should also be emphasized that the successes achieved by clinical oncology in the recent years have made possible to apply special treatment for a disseminated form of tumours, which allows the patients not only to survive longer but also to improve their conditions for a considerable period of time. In later stages, the possibilities for application of treatment are different from those in earlier cases. The more generalized the process, the less the indications for methods of local treatment - surgical and radiological and greater the indications for pharmacotherapy.

Surgical methods in advanced stages of the disease are also possible in some cases, more often in combination with pharmacotherapy and radiotherapy. Surgical interventions of palliative nature are resorted to in some cases as one of the phases of a complex treatment of disseminated cancer. In such cases removal of the primary tumour promotes the effect of chemotherapeutical preparations and radiotherapy of distant metastases. At the same time the approach the decision whether the patient can already be allocated in group IV should be approached very cautiously in the conditions of an outpatient clinic; if the case is doubtful or the application of every modern diagnostic method is not possible the patient should be referred to an inpatient department for examination and consultation with specialists.

The problem of care of patients in advanced stages of malignant tumours is rather complicated and calls for integrated measures. It should be borne in mind that the average life expectancy of such patients is from 1.5 to 2 years and that the last months of their life are marked, as a rule, by intense pain caused by the progression of the primary disease and the growing cachexia.

In a majority of cases such patients are in need of hospitalization, especially during the last months of their lives. In accordance with the Soviet legislation, they are admitted to the hospitals of the general medical services where they receive necessary care and symptomatic therapy.

Since some patients in advanced stages of the disease and their family refuse hospitalization, a system of home care is functioning for such patients. They are visited by a panel doctor, by the district oncologists, if necessary, and also by the local nurse who is in charge of making observing all the prescriptions of the physician. In the relations between the medical personnel and the incurable patients a special place is occupied by the questions of deontology or moral--ethical principles of the work of the physicians. It should be emphasized here that one of the founders of the Soviet oncology, N.N. Petrov, has promulgated his teaching about the duties of the physician in his classical work "The Principles of Surgical Deontology" and, in fact, has introduced the deontological principles as the ethical guidance for the oncologist in his relations with oncological patients. When visiting the patient, the physician should widely use psychotherapeutical methods. All the recommendations of the physician should be mandatory for the patient and the latter should observe them strictly. It is recommended to prescribe cycles of treatment of 1 to 2 months without avoiding popular means at the same time /infusion of plantain, aloe in combination with honey, etc./.

It is necessary to inspire confidence in the patient that such conditions are only stages in the course of the disease and will be followed by improvement, possible. When the patient feels that he is not abandoned, cared for, treated and is under observation, he acquires a mental equilibrium and follows the prescriptions of the physician. If pain is very intense, administration of opiates should not be restricted. An important component of the work of the district oncologist is his relations with the family of such patients. The truth should not be concealed from them and they should assist the physician in his hard struggle for the restoration of the patient's psychological condition.

The role of the local nurse is not less difficult, since the incurable patients are directly attended by her. She has to know what medical preparations have been recommended to the patient for improving his general condition and also for removing pain.

The nurse has to be able to demonstrate to the patient the techniques of the respiratory gymnastics which is an important means of prophylaxis against pneumonia and congestion in the lungs of bedridden patients. She has to observe also that the hygienic care of the patient is correct and has to demonstrate to the family the techniques of changing clothes and of making the bed over again, etc.

Nevertheless, the main task of the local nurse is to give

the patient moral support, to find words which would create in
him confidence in the possibility of recovery. Sometimes, the
patient knows the truth about his condition but hope never
leaves him and he seeks moral support, in the first place, from
medical workers. Such a patient is easily hurt and listens to
every word of the doctor or nurse.

The administration of the basic prescriptions of the physician /injections, dressings/ is entrusted to the local nurse
but the nurse of the oncological institution, who visited the
patient earlier, should in no case discontinue them in case
the patient develops relapses and metastases. Her visit is taken
by the patient as a sign that there is still hope and that he is
still under observation and treatment.

The humanistic principles of the Soviet medicine in relation to incurable patients can be formulated as follows:
chronic patients afflicted by malignant neoplasms need
symptomatic palliative treatment and have the right to receive
it /A.I. Serebrov/.

TEACHING OF ONCOLOGY, TRAINING OF ONCOLOGISTS AND
MIDDLE-LEVEL PERSONNEL FOR ONCOLOGICAL INSTITUTIONS
B.E. Peterson, Yu.V. Falilcev and R.M. Strelkova

Specialization of knowledge has been a characteristic
feature of the development of medicine during the last decades.
The successes achieved in the study of aetiology and pathogenesis of malignant neoplasm, the development and improvement
of the methods of prophylaxis, identification and treatment of
oncological diseases have made it imperative to separate oncology as a discipline in its own right, a discipline with many-
fold scientific and practical importance. The specific and
complicated nature of the process of the disease in patients
afflicted with malignant neoplasms, the difficulties involved
in early diagnosis and a wide use of combined and complex methods of treatment make necessary to provide for students of
medical universities, physicians and middle-level personnel a
special training in the field of oncology. It is obvious that
the fate of the patient stricken with a malignant neoplasm

depends to a large extent on the first physician who sees him. In a majority of cases, the patient seeks medical advice from a physician of the general medical services and thus training of undergraduates of medical institutes acquires a primary importance.

In the system of higher medical education in the USSR, there are 82 medical universities and 9 respective facultaties of the Universities. In 1975, as many as 43 thousand young physicians graduated from these establishments and went to work mainly into the general medical services. In the USSR, there are 32.5 physicians for every 10,000 population, a rate which is the highest in the world. Thus, improvement of the quality of oncological education in the medical institutes is of primary importance in the training of physicians for general medical services. At the same time, it should be recalled, that if in the future a graduated wishes to work in oncology, he should receive a more extensive oncological training. A future physician should adopt such a complex of knowledge in theoretical and clinical oncology which might enable him, irrespective of his future practical activities, to orient himself in the questions of diagnosis and clinical symptoms of malignant neoplasms, to carry out the purposeful examination of the patient on a modern level and to be familiar with the main methods of treatment of malignant neoplasms /surgical, radiological, pharmacotherapeutical/, indications and contraindications for their use and possible complications arising in the course of treatment.

Basically, the graduate of a medical institute should have knowledge on the major principles of organization of oncological assistance, the system of registration of primarily detected patients with malignant neoplasms and patients in advanced stages of the disease. And finally, the young physician should know the main features of symptomatic therapy of incurable diseases, since the problem of rendering them assistance is one which he will most surely encounter already at the first steps of his practical work. Therefore, one of the main tasks of a higher medical school consists in

improving the methods of oncological education of future physicians. Teaching of oncology according to a unified program,
which has been approved by the Ministry of Public Health of
the USSR and provides for 197 hours of theoretical and practical
studies, was introduced in the USSR already in 1970. At that
time the theoretical foundations of oncology are taught in the
third year by the staff of the chairs of pathology, patho-
physiology, general surgery, pharmacology /altogether 40 hours/.
The staff of other chairs was entrusted with teaching of the
clinical aspects of cancer, its roentgenological diagnosis,
treatment, including radiotherapy, and organization of cancer
control.

A logical sequel of the quest for an improved teaching of
oncology has been the appointment of docents in oncology at
the chairs of surgery in 20 medical universities and the creation of 2 chairs of oncology for teaching this subject in the
sixth year.

A radical solution of questions of oncological education
began in 1973; during the 1974-1975 period, chairs of oncology
were organized for teaching this subject in the sixth year in
73 medical universities of the country and in research institutes of oncology and oncological dispensaries, large regional,
district or republican hospitals. In accordance with the new
program, a total of 72 hours will be available to the newly
organized oncology chairs for a systematic course in oncology
in the sixth year when the students specialize in surgery,
internal medicine and obstetrics with gynecology, in addition
to the total of 197 hours still available to those chairs which
offer courses in theoretical and clinical oncology in the third,
fourth and fifth years. At present, a unified program has been
drawn up in oncology for students of therapeutic faculties of
the medical universities. Teaching of oncology begins in the
third year. The chairs of patho-physiology, pathology and
general surgery offer respective courses /in altogether 18
hours of lectures and 20 hours of practical studies/ in which
the students become familiarized with the modern state of
knowledge about the aetiology and pathogenesis of malignant

neoplasms, the role of carcinogenic agents of exogenic and endogenic origin, oncogenic viruses, biological features of tumour growth, the morphological characteristics of benign and malignant tumours, their histological and histochemical criteria, various classifications, regularities of metastasing and also about precancerous conditions. Thus, the students obtain information /mainly theoretical/ about malignant neoplasms. At the same time, still in the third year the clinical chairs familiarize the students with the general principles of early and timely diagnosis and treatment of oncological patients. The student receives an idea about cytostatics, radical, palliative, combined and extended operations, surgical interventions, as well as about the questions of oncological deontology.

Beginning from the fourth year, students are taught clinical oncology. Its presentation is based on the principle of the study of major nosologic forms of malignant neoplasms with which the students are familiarized at the chairs of surgery, internal medicine, urology and others. During the study of each form of neoplasms information is given about morbidity and mortality, aetiology and pathogenesis of pretumourous conditions, clinical aspects, diagnosis and principles of treatment of patients stricken with these types of tumours. At the same time, special clinical aspects of some forms of malignant neoplasms are taught by specialized chairs /ophthalmology, stomatology, otorhinolaryngology, etc./. The chairs of surgery and internal medicine /24 hours for each chair/ teach characteristics of development of the most common forms of malignant neoplasms, their diagnosis and treatment of patients with such neoplasms. Finally, in the sixth year, future physicians who specialize in major clinical disciplines /surgery, internal medicine, obstetrics and gynecology/ study in details the most important aspects of oncology at the chair of oncology /obligatory at a specialized oncological insitution/. Questions of aetiology and pathogenesis of malignant neoplasms are taught in the form of a theoretical course /12 hours, optional/. Special attention is paid to the basic features of the organization of anticancer service, methods of monitoring of oncological patients, the procedure of referring patients to specialized oncological institutions for consultation or treatment. In their sixth year, students study these questions at the reception of patients in the polyclinics of specialized oncological institutions /12 hours/. During these studies, the students familiarize themselves with the outpatient treatment of oncological patients and with their rehabilitation.

The practical studies which are conducted by the chair of oncology in the sixth year are related to the future specialty of physicians. The total of 60 hours is reserved for this purpose.

The radical changes in the system of oncological education at the medical universities should, no doubt, significantly raise the level of training of the students and also that of the physicians of the general medical services. It should also promote a higher level of diagnosis and treatment of patients with malignant neoplasms.

In the Soviet Union, over 40 chairs and courses in oncology have been organized which are charged with the implementation of methodological guidance over oncological education also at other chairs of the higher medical schools.

Training of teachers for the chairs of oncology of the medical institutes and improvement of their qualifications is done by the Central Postgraduate Medical School where a special chair of oncology has been offering special courses for teachers of medical institutes for a number of years. At the same time, the improvement of oncological education at the medical universities is only one of the stages in the training of an oncologist and it does not exhaust the question of training of highly proficient oncologists for the specialized oncological network.

The expansion of the network of oncological institutions /extension of the oncological dispensaries, the increase in the number of oncological departments, creation of the post of the district oncologist in outpatient clinics/ calls for training of qualified oncologists.

The permanent sophistication of the methods of diagnosis and treatment of patients with malignant neoplasms has already resulted in the fact that the concept "oncologist" has become, to a considerable extent, a collective term and that the complex treatment of the patient is carried out, as a rule, jointly by the surgeon, radiologist and chemotherapeutist those training is a complicated matter, with having specific features and requiring unified approach.

It should be noted that in the USSR the speciality of oncologist has been created more than 50 years ago, in 1926, when the first chair of oncology was organized in the Leningrad Postgraduate Medical School. It was organized and directed by one of the founders of national oncology, Professor N.N. Petrov. It should also be pointed out here that the cadres of oncologists were created in the Soviet Union by the specialization of surgeons, gynecologists and, to a lesser extent, radiologists.

An important role in the training of oncologists has been played by the chairs of oncology in the State Postgraduate Medical Schools. At present, chairs of oncology are in 11 such Postgraduate Schools /in Moscow, Leningrad, Kiev, Minsk, Kazan, Tbilisi, Zaporozhe, Kharkov, Baku, Alma-Ata, Tashkent/. These chairs offer courses for primary and postgraduate specialization. The courses of primary specialization /duration 4 to 6 months/ are organized for physicians who have practical experience of several years in surgery or gynecology. The objective of these courses is to train oncological surgeons or oncological gynecologists for work in special oncological institutions /oncological dispensaries, oncological departments, oncological rooms/. The program of specialization includes lectures in theoretical and clinical oncology as well as practical studies in the course of which the trainees learn skills for detection and treatment of patients with malignant neoplasms.

Apart from primary specialization, the chairs of oncology offer opportunities for improvement of knowledge to physicians

working in oncological institutions and also to physicians of
the general medical services. The system of improvement of
qualifications of oncologists consists of general and specialized courses. The general courses start with studies by correspondence /during 5 to 6 months/. Future trainees are required
to fulfil some assignments /writing of a paper/ on 2 or 3 topics
in theoretical and clinical oncology. The requirement to
complete the pre-course work makes it possible for the staff
of the chair to select the most proficient physicians and
create the atmosphere of competition. The day-time course
/lasting for one and a half to three months/ consists of lectures and practical studies. In the period of the day-time
course, the trainees obtain knowledge in the modern theoretical and clinical aspects of oncology and are given the opportunity to master new methods of diagnosis and treatment of oncological patients in practice.

During the last years, these specialized courses have
gained importance. Their organization has been urged by the
fact that a trend has emerged towards a higher specialization
in clinical oncology and also towards the creation of specialized departments in the oncological network. These courses are
intended for physicians who have been practicing their speciality for not less than 5 years.

One of the forms of providing refresher for oncologists
is a system of travelling lecture courses which are conducted
by the leading chairs of oncology and clinical radiology of
the postgraduate medical schools. These courses are organized
in various cities of the Soviet Union, at the large oncological dispensaries or scientific research institutes of oncology and radiology; they last for one to one and a half months.
Such travelling courses make possible to improve the knowledge
of physicians in oncology at places where they work and in the
conditions maximally approximating those in which some or other
oncological institution has to operate. The physicians of the
general medical services can also profit and improve their
knowledge in oncology through these courses.

Apart from the travelling courses, leading oncological

institutions conduct seminars for physicians of both the oncological institutions and the general medical services.

An important component of the system of training of highly qualified oncologists, including research oncologists, especially for scientific research institutes, is the postgraduate course /3 years/ and the clinical ordinatura /2 years/ which are organized in research institutes and by the chairs of oncology in medical schools and in medical institutes.

The candidates for admission to the postgraduate course intended for training research oncologists are selected from among persons who in their student years showed a propensity for scientific work participating in student circles and scientific associations. The experience demonstrates that it is more rational to select candidates for admission to the postgraduate course intended for training highly specialized clinical oncologists from among physicians who have been practising their line of specialization already for some years /surgery, gynecology, internal medicine, etc./.

A training period in actual service at outpatient clinics and laboratories of oncological research institutes is of great importance. The duration of such period may vary from 1 to 6 months. During this time, a future specialist has a good opportunity to master various methods of diagnosis and treatment of patients with malignant neoplasms. This form of training is widely used for specialization and improving the knowledge of cytologists, endoscopists, anesthesiologists, etc. This form is suitable for adoption within the framework of international cooperation in the field of oncology.

Training of middle-level personnel for the oncological network is, no doubt, necessary with regard to the special methods of treatment, possible complications and the specific requirements for care of oncological patients. It seems to be optimal to organize schools within the oncological and roentgenoradiological institutes and larger oncological dispensaries where teaching is focussed on the care of oncological patients. Schools of this kind have been created and are functioning in leading oncological institutes of the country; the positive

experience accumulated in this field proves that their further
development is justified.

HEALTH EDUCATION OF THE POPULATION
N.A. Tikhonova and L.V. Orlovsky

The health education of the USSR is organized centrally. It
is planned and subsidized by the State, is generally accessible
and free of charge. Many institutions /in the first place
medical ones/ take part in its organization. At the same time,
health education in the USSR is a social function: trade unions,
social organizations and activitists from among the population
take part in it. Its most important principal feature is that
it is mandatory for the entire network of medical services:
each physician and the middle-level medical personnel are
required to take part in this work.

For every physician, feldsher, midwife, nurse, health
education is honourary obligation and official duty.

Organization of education on cancer-control propaganda

Education on cancer control constitutes an integral part
of health education. Houses of Health Education are the base
for health education and these Houses play the role of methodological and coordination centres for propagation of knowledge
in medicine and hygiene. More than 500 such Houses exist, and
conduct their activities in anticancer propaganda in a close
contact with oncological institutions, mainly with oncological
dispensaries. The education on cancer control is included into
the plan of work of the Houses of Health Education and oncological dispensaries and forms an integral part of their activities. When drawing up the plan of work, the composition of
the audience, life-style of the listeners, the questions
pertaining to improving the qualifications of lectures and the
training of activists in public health are taken into account.

Generality is a characteristic peculiarity of the education on cancer-control because not only oncologists but also
medical workers of other specialities are required to participate in it. In accordance with the existing regulations, 4

hours per month are reserved from the working time of every
medical worker of any speciality for health education work including cancer-control propaganda.

The most active role in the cancer control work is played
by oncologists and it can be said that they are in the vanguard
of this struggle.

The Central Research Institute of Health Education acts
as the scientific methodological centre for health education.
The eminent oncologists of the country - N.N. Petrov, A.I.
Savitsky, N.N. Blokhin, A.I. Serebrov, L.F. Larionov, L.A.
Novikova, E.G. Kudimova, A.B. Chaklin and others - have taken
and do take an active part in the scientific development of the
methods of anticancer propaganda.

As an aid to physicians in mastering and applying unified
methods of publich health educaiton on cancer-control campaign,
the Central Research Institute of Health Education together
with the leading oncologists of the country compiles certain
materials - "Methodological manual for anticancer propaganda",
"Materials for lecturers", "Lecturers' collections" and other.
The Postgraduate Medical Schools present lectures for oncologists /oncological series/ in methodology of education on cancer control while the Central Research Institute of Health
Education organizes special seminars in which leading oncologists take part. For physicians working in the Houses of
Health Education, the Postgraduate Medical Schools annually
organize lecture courses and also ten-day periods, seminars and
methodological conferences on health education.

Physicians of the general medical services have the possibility to familiarize themselves with the methods of education on cancer control at the seminars organized by the Central
Research Institute of Health Education, Houses of Health Education, and also by the local branches of the "Knowledge" Society.
In some Union Republics they function as public services: one-
-year and two-year "Oncology Universities" for practising
physicians. In prophylactic· and treatment institutions, Houses
of Health Education, epidemiologic stations and also medical
sections of the "Knowledge" Society there are "Lecturers'

Groups" which are good schools for mastering of the methods of education on cancer control by physicians.

The Red Cross and Red Crescent Society, trade unions, and the "Knowledge" Society give a significant assistance to medical workers in their efforts aimed at enlisting an active cooperation of population in cancer control and at raising its health culture.

In the USSR considerable attention is paid to the training of the activists in public health - members of health stations, public health representatives, members of public councils at medical institutions. A significant role is played in this respect not only by the physicians of the oncological dispensaries and the Houses of Health Education but also by the Red Cross and Red Crescent society as well as by the trade unions. The public activists of public health assist medical workers and their practical activities, mainly in the organization of education of the population on cancer control. A preliminary training based on a deep understanding of their tasks is an important condition for the successful implementation of the activists duties in the field of cancer control.

The objectives, content and methods of propaganda

The anticancer propaganda should be directed, in the first place, towards enhancing the efficiency of treatment of oncological patients. In this respect, its objectives include education of the population to the need to seek treatment early and convincing them that persistent cure is possible provided the tumourous and pretumourous diseases are detected early.

The other main task of anticancer propaganda is the struggle for an active introduction into practice of simple, generally accessible and effective measures aimed at preventing malignant tumours.

Health education aimed at enhancing the efficiency of treatment of oncological patients

It has become evident that a persistent recovery of the patient is possible if treatment is started in time.

One of the main causes of the appearance of cancer cases in advanced stages of the disease is that the patient applies for medical help too late. To a certain extent, this depends on the quality of anti-cancer propaganda and can be explained by the inadequate knowledge of the population on cancer and its early symtoms.

The above determine the main target of education on cancer control, which is to convince the population that it is necessary to seek medical advice immediately upon the discovery of symptoms suspicious of cancer.

To achieve this purpose, the anticancer propaganda is intended to fulfil the following practical tasks:

- making people aware of early signs of cancer at the most common localizations;

- inspiring confidence in the possibility of cure, which can be more real, if the treatment is sought earlier;

- dispelling the fear of surgical treatment and convincing people in the danger of resorting to "domestic means" and seeking "treatment" from persons who are not qualified for it.

Great attention is given to a very detailed description of early signs of cancer, typical of certain localizations. It is explained that, as a rule, at the beginning of its development cancer does not manifest itself in pain or a higher body temperature, i.e. it is not accompanied by symptoms which might prompt the patient to immediately seek medical advice.

In describing the symptoms of malignant neoplasms, the attention of the audience should be focussed on early signs of cancer because from the viewpoint of deontology this is most appropriate and rational.

An integral part of the anticancer propaganda is the promulgation of the achievements of oncology concerning the main principles of modern diagnostics and treatment of malignant tumours.

By explaining the diagnostic possibilities of clinical oncology, the anticancer propaganda makes people understand that medical advice should be sought immediately upon the appearance of any signs suspicious of cancer and that one should see first not the oncologist, but the district physician or the polyclinic in the area where the patient resides, to a factory medical unit or a women's consultation clinic.

Moreover, the anticancer propaganda early warns people to the dangers of resorting to "domestic" means and emphasizes that it is a waste of valuable time and can bring nothing but harm, since it allows the disease to further develop unchecked.

Explanation of the essence and causes of cancer should not take up a large place in the propaganda work because it is of secondary importance: knowledge of these questions does not promote essentially in practice the early visit to the physician. Nevertheless, it is still necessary, because the awareness of the listeners of scientifically substantiated conceptions about cancer and the achievements of oncological science convince them of the possibility of an effective cure.

The role of health education in cancer prevention

This task can be achieved only if the population is constantly made aware about the effect that the evironmental factors exert upon the human organism, if people are informed of the means or methods of protection against these factors; if people are taught respective rules of behaviour which are in accordance with the requirements of hygiene and to follow these rules in their daily lives. It should be stressed here that this work should be conducted with a due consideration given to local conditions, to national habits, features and life-style of the population.

Due to the fact that cancer of the gastrointestinal tract, mainly, of the stomach is registered in the USSR more frequently than cancer in other localizations, a large part in the anticancer propaganda concerning prevention of pre-tumourous diseases is contributed to nutrition hygiene. It is explained that it is important to observe the rhythm of nutrition and a correct diet, to avoid overeating. Apart from that, the importance of a correct culinary processing of food and dangers of overconsumption of alcohol are emphasized.

In the propaganda aimed at prevention of the diseases

of the lung, antismoking propaganda is the most important. The carcinogenic properties of tobacco and cigarettes are explained and it is emphasized that smoking is harmful not only for the health of the smoker but also for people around him for they have to breathe the air polluted with smoke; means and methods helping to overcome the smoking habit are recommended, people are exhorted to fight against smoking especially among the miners and prevent it in the public places.

In schools, pupils are explained the harm that may be caused by smoking: in the curriculum of some disciplines such as nature studies, botany and anatomy and physiology of man.

In the propaganda the role played by great importance the pollution of air - by carcinogenic substances from factory and house chimneys; by automobile exhaust and by the bituminous dust raised as a result of the friction between the automobile tyres and the asphalt pavement - in the development of the diseases of the respiratiory organs is emphasized.

Concerning the prophylaxis of skin cancer, it is recommended to protect the skin, mainly the face, from the prolonged effect of the sun with wide-brimmed hats and for people who have to stay for long periods of time under the searing sun because of the nature of their work, especially in southern areas of the country, the observation of the usual rules of skin hygiene are recommended.

Prevention of the disease of the uterus and the breast calls for including the questions of female hygiene the educational work already in the childhood.

In the hygienic education on the prophylaxis of pretumourous diseases, the advantages of personal hygiene, of strengthening one's health, of physical exercises and sports are pointed out.

As a measure of preventing pretumourous occupational diseases at industrial enterprises and within the system of vocational training workers who get in contact with carcinogenic substances are systematically trained and educated on hygiene.

The modern level of oncology and organization of public health makes possible the successful prophylaxis of cancer based on a timely cure from pretumourous diseases.

To fulfil this task, the education on health control should be concentrated:

- on the explanation to the population that cancer can be prevented through treatment of pretumourous diseases;

- on making people aware of the signs of pretumourous diseases and explaining to them the importance of carrying out regular prophylactic examinations for the purpose of early detection of these diseases;

- on convincing people stricken with pretumourous diseases in the need to be followed up and to strictly observe all the prescriptions of the physicians regarding treatment, including surgical treatment and warning them against the attempts to resort to self-treatment and the use of substances not recommended by the physician.

By far the greatest part of educational work about prophylactic measures is represented by the information regarding those chronic diseases which, while existing for years or even decades, can provide a fertile ground for the development of malignant neoplasms. While explaining the realistic ways of cancer prophylaxis the physician should make people understand that cancer does not arise suddenly in healthy tissues and that some chronic diseases may be instrumental in its development and thus by their treatment cancer can be prevented.

In this connection, the importance of mass prophylactic examinations carried out in our country is widely explained and the significance of carrying out such examinations regularly and a 100 percent attendance of all strata of the population is emphasized.

Since the mass prohylactic examinations do not cover the entire adult population of the country yet, the importance of individual examinations is stressed. In particular, for each woman aged over 25 examination by a gynecologist every half a year should become the rule. In the polyclinics and outpatient clinics special examination rooms have been opened. Experience has proved that this measure has significantly contributed to the higher rate of detection of early stages of cancer and pretumourous diseases in women.

The education of women on cancer control includes also training in the methods of self-examination of the breast with a view to the timely detection of pathological changes in them. In the course of health education women are educated to the need to make such examinations regularly, each month and to see a doctor if they find any deviations from the normal condition.

The dispensary method should be widely propagated for it provides for a constant supervision and examination of patients with pretumourous diseases.

Among factory and office workers there may be some who, while stricken with a chronic disease, may not be under observation. For a timely detection of such patients, the physician conducts group talks with people newly employed by the given enterprise, in whom a chronic disease was detected in the course of their medical examination. Such talks are also conducted with the workers in the course of their studies within the frames of vocational training.

Methods and means of carrying out health education

The most diverse methods of health education are used in the anticancer propaganda. The selection of these methods depends on the concrete aims of the given cancer control measure, and also on the contingent of the population and the place where anticancer propaganda is carried out.

From among them the method of the spoken word is one of the most widespread and effective. Lectures by physicians are organized for various audiences. Many Houses of Health Education and the committees of the Red Cross and the Red Crescent Society have automobiles which are used for the purposes of health education. Thus lecturers can go to collective farms, field camps, timber exploitation stations, construction sites and other places which are located far from towns and villages. For this purpose, these automobiles are equipped with visual aids, small projector and literature for the population. As an aid to the lecturers, the Institute of Health Education publishes special literature: brochures and Lecturers' Collec-

tions. The content of the brochures includes the standard plan
of lectures and materials for it, methodological advice for
lecturers, lists of recommended literature, visual aids and
motion pictures on the topics of the lectures.

Moreover, the Central Institute of Health Education has
published a series of materials on the methods of the propaganda
of hygienic knowledge, with due consideration given to the pattern and incidence of pretumourous diseases in various climatic
and geographic zones of the country. In the anticancer propaganda
the method of talks conducted by medical workers is widely used.
Such talks create a more intimate atmosphere than a lecture.
Thus a closer connection is established between the medical
worker and his audience, which makes possible for the former
to unconstrainedly describe the basic rules for preventing of
cancer and the different methods of its diagnosis and treatment.
In rural localities, the talks are conducted by the middle-level
medical personnel. The content of the talks includes the usual
questions of anticancer propaganda - the importance of timely
attendance of prophylactic examinations, the importance of systematic self-examination of the breast, the procedures involved
in monitoring patients and other questions.

When seeing the patient, the physician talks to him individually, giving advice and using the most convincing argu-
mentation. Therefore, such person-to-person talks are considered to be the most effective method of using the spoken
word.

One of the forms of anticancer propaganda is a questions-
-and-answers evening organized with due consideration to the
background of the audience and the sphere of its interests.

Due to the fact that the entire population of the USSR
is literate, the spoken word method occupies a large place
in the anticancer propaganda: in the Union and Autonomous
Republics popular scientific brochures are published /in the
size of 3 to 5 pages/ intended to give a clear idea about the
seriousness of oncological diseases and to prevent substantiated, convincing and realistic recommendations with regard
to early detection and prophylaxis of cancer. Apart from the

brochures, leaflets are published which are distributed among the population. The regular publication of a health diary, each issue being devoted to one of the questions of cancer prophylaxis has been found to be effective.

An effective means aimed at promptly satisfying the interests of the population, and providing concrete answers is the Questions and Answers Board.

Articles in popular scientific magazines are very effective ways of education on cancer control. Visual propaganda is of lesser importance but the effect of a well-designed poster cannot be denied. The text that is written on the poster has to be brief and catching. The educational poster should make an impression lasting enough for the individual to make the necessary step.

At enterprises, local medical workers arrange exhibitions. The content of the exhibitions is determined by their purpose, which is to explain to the population the importance of a rational treatment of pretumourous diseases or educate them to the need of early detection of cancer and the real possibilities of its cure. Exhibitions devoted to cancer prophylaxis are usually arranged in such places where they can easily attract the attention of persons stricken with chronic diseases: in polyclinics, factory medical units.

Cinema, television and radio are of great importance in the education on cancer control. Very interesting films have been made on the subject of anticancer propaganda which are suitable for any audience.

Because of the short duration of these films and of the completeness of their story they can be shown in cinemas, workers' and rural clubs, in the parks of culture and recreation, over the television, and so on. Motion pictures are also projected after lectures, or, sometimes, their fragments are shown during the lecture. A questions-and-answers evening starts with projection. After the projection, the audience ask questions and the physician gives exhaustive answers.

The television serves the cause of anticancer propaganda by organizing talks by eminent scientists of oncology and by projecting films on special topics. Talks in the radio in the form of dialogues between the moderator and scientist are well received by the listeners.

The various means of anticancer education - lectures, films, brochures, posters are widely used by the People's Health Universities the number of which runs to several thousand. Their trainees include all who wish to receive useful information on medicine and hygiene. Such universities are organized at factories and offices, in the Palaces of Culture, in the collective and state farms. Scientists, physicians and other specialists teach in the universities as voluntary workers. Lessons are conducted usually once or twice per month with a curriculum designed for two years and cancer control is included there.

A strong impetus has been given to the development of the Health Schools. The curriculum of these schools is narrower in range. Both the Universities and the Health Schools represent a convenient form of the hygienic and anticancer education of the population.

The scale of education on cancer control carried out in the USSR is very large. For its organization and conduct, the most diverse methods and means of health education are used The improvement of knowledge of the population about cancer and anticancer measures has been observed, especially during last decades, and it is reflected in a higher efficiency of treatment of oncological patients. This depends to a large extent on the awareness of the population of the importance of timely seeking medical advice upon the appearance of the signs of tumourous or pretumourous diseases. If the population is not health-conscious, solution of such formidable problem as cancer control is impossible.

COORDINATION OF RESEARCH WORK ON THE PROBLEM:
"SCIENTIFIC PRINCIPLES OF THE ORGANIZATION OF CANCER CONTROL"
A.E. Zarubova, N.Ya. Shabashova and M.I. Buslaeva

Protection of health, treatment of diseases and prolongation of the life span constitutes one of the basic objectives of the State. In the Soviet Union the achievement of this objective in ensured by a system of socio-economic and medical measures. The principles on which the Soviet public health is based are its planned nature, the combination of prophylactic dispensary and curative services, availability of qualified medical assistance to the population free of charge.

It is on this basis that organization of oncological assistance to the population is built in the USSR. This system ensures wide possibilities in the field of prevention, diagnosis and treatment of diseases, monitoring and social and labour rehabilitation of patients with malignant tumours.

It should be recalled, however, that the growth and development of oncological network, its material-technical base and provision of personnel are not the only factors on which the further progress in the field of controlling malignant neoplasms depends.

The realization of large-scale measures in the organization of oncological assistance to the population necessitates first of all the development of scientifically substantiated criteria of their planning and implementation.

Since the social nature of the incidence of malignant neoplasms and mortality from them in the majority of countries, including the USSR, with a non-epidemic type of pathology is only too obvious, the organization of cancer control acquires enhanced importance.

Research, in its turn, can be effective only if scientific collectives, acting within a general program, combine their efforts. In this connection, coordination of scientific research acquires a special importance in the conditions of the scientific and technological revolution, since it makes possible to exercise a modern approach to the solution of the complex problems of cancer control. The origins of the system of coordination of scientific research date back to the 50-s; it was called into being by the development of a network of oncological institutions in the country in the postwar period and by the organization of a number of oncological and roentgeno-radiological institutes in the Union Republics.

It became obvious that there was a need to elaborate the
main directions for the future research and to pool the efforts
of both newly-created and older scientific research establishments in the interests of an effective solution of the tasks
they faced. In the course of its development the creation of
the system of coordination of scientific research has gone
through a number of stages and became more perfect and developed stage by stage. At present, the coordination of scientific research on the problem of malignant neoplasms is organized according to the following pattern: the entire work of
coordination belongs to the Ministry of the Public Health of
the USSR. Immediate responsibility for this work has been entrusted to a Scientific Council for the complex problem of
"Malignant Neoplasms", which is set up within the Presidium of
the Academy of Medical Sciences of the USSR. In its activities
the Scientific Council relies on two head scientific research
establishments - the Oncological Scientific Centre of the
Academy of Medical Sciences of the USSR which coordinates
fundamental research in oncology and the Scientific Research
Institute of Oncology, named after Professor N.N. Petrov and
decorated with the Order of Red Banner of Labour, of the
Ministry of Public Health of the USSR, which is entrusted with
the coordination of scientific research on three major problems of practical importance: diagnosis of malignant tumours,
clinical, surgical and comprehensive treatment of malignant
neoplasms and organization of cancer control and prophylaxis
of malignant tumours.

The Scientific Research Institute of Oncology named after
Professor N.N. Petrov is the head establishment of the Ministry
of Public Health of the USSR with regard to the above-mentioned
problems and is subordinated to the Administration for the
Oncological Assistance of the Ministry of Public Health of the
USSR.

In their activities the Scientific Council and the head
institutes rely on the so-called Problem Commissions, the membership of which is formed by the head institutes and is subject to approval by the Scientific Council for the complex

problem of "Malignant Neoplasms". Among the members of the Problem Commissions one can find eminent scientists, specialists in oncology, experimentators, clinicians, organizers of public health, specialists in the social hygiene, statisticians and also representatives of the practical field of the public health. Each Problem Commission exercises guidance over the work on one particular problem; its membership is formed in accordance with its objectives. It has to be mentioned that the Problem Commissions possess wide possibilities for involvement in their activities both individual scientists and scientific collectives. The head institutes and the Problem Commissions elaborate general directions and recommendation with regard to general directions of research on the existing problems, determine the most urgent tasks for the near future and for a 15-20-year period ahead, analyse research conducted in the country and generalize the results of the analysis, study the status of the given problem abroad and organize the cooperation between scientific research and various establishments in the practical field. The Problem Commissions also prepare an annual document which contains a description of every research conducted in the USSR in oncology, contributing thereby to the preparation of a major document which comprises a program of research in oncology for each five-year period and is called "Plan of Coordination of Scientific Research on the Problem of Malignant Neoplasms". The plan is broken down to particular problems, which in turn are divided into a number of generalized topics. The research institutes of oncology and roentgenoradiology of medical universities, Postgraduate Mecical Schools, allied scientific research establishments, problem laboratories, and so on take part in the execution of the topics. The executing institutions include the most significant and promising parts of their research in the coordination plan /within the framework of generalized thematic assignments/.

It has to be emphasized here that the coordination of scientific research allows for the republican institutes to select the topics of research on their own because the coordi-

nation plan provides only for the main directions and generalized topics of research.

At the same time, the Problem Commissions, the Head Institutes and the Scientific Council on the complex problem of
"Malignant Neoplasms" see to it that the institutes avoid duplication of work with regard to the selected topics and exercise
an integrated approach to topics and problems of major significance, thus ensuring the concentration of efforts and reducing the time required for research while attaining maximum efficiency.

The annual report, which is presented by the Head Institutes to the State Committee for Science and Technology under
the Council of Ministers of the USSR, provides for a thorough
supervision over the progress of research, its implementation
on schedule and over the results achieved.

In the recent years, special attention has been given to
the question of effective introduction of the results of scientific research into practice. Some of the topics of the Plan
of Coordination are so important that they are included in the
Plan of National Economic Development. And lastly, the State
Committee for Science and Technology under the Council of
Ministers of the USSR is empowered to carry out special financ-
ing of the most urgent and most promising lines of research.

It is necessary to emphasize here that within the general
system of coordination of scientific research the Problem
Commissions play an especially important role in actively coordinating the work of various research establishments. This
makes the elaboration of topics suggested by the given Problem
Commission highly effective, because its proposals are based
on a thorough study of the prospects of development and the
real possibilities of the executing institutes for introducing
the results into practice.

The Head institutes and the Problem Commissions have a
large volume of information in their possession which they
thoroughly analyse and annually prepare two documents; on this
basis one of them represents a summary of scientific research
on each problem in the USSR; the second one is devoted to the

analysis of the status of research both in the country and abroad. It is also the task of the Head Institute and the Problem Commissions to render scientific methodological assistance to the institutes working on the problem "Malignant Neoplasms", to maintain a close liaison with them, to involve them in cooperative research, to prepare joint publications and to arrange conferences and symposia.

The Head Institute constantly trains oncologists for republican oncological institutes and oncological dispensaries. The personnel for oncological institutes and dispensaries is trained in specialized postgraduate courses and ordinatura while practising physicians improve their qualifications in the departments and laboratories of the Institute; leading workers of the Head Institute offer consultations and supervise the preparation of theses by workers of the Republican oncological institutes and dispensaries. In the process of developing the principles of coordination of scientific research, another form of contact with the republican oncological institutes came into existence: leading specialists of the Head Scientific Research Institute of Oncology named after Professor N.N. Petrov have been appointed as supervisors of the work of the republican oncological institutes. This has resulted in very fruitful personal contacts, a more thorough familiarization with the status of scientific research work and improved the possibilities for rendering a scientific-methodological assistance to these institutes.

In the recent years, on the initiative on the Ministry of Public Health of the USSR, the Head Institute and the Problem Commissions have begun to convene annual meetings of directors of the Republican oncological institutes to discuss and work out cooperative research programs, which may be of principal importance for the further development of work in the organization of cancer control. The experience has shown that these meetings are very important and productive because they ensure the high effectivity in the implementation of the proposed research programs.

In the course of their activity in the coordination of

scientific research the Ministry of Public Health of the USSR,
the Scientific Council on the complex problem of "Malignant
Neoplasms", the Head Institute and the Problem Commissions
rely on the republican oncological and roentgenoradiological
institutes the majority of which was organized and began functioning in the postwar period /see the section on the History
of Cancer Control in the USSR/.

The organization of the republican and oncological and
roentgenoradiological institutes was necessitated by the need
to create special centres or branches in each Republic which
might be charged with the responsibility for the scientific-
-methodological guidance over the oncological network in each
Republic and over the development of scientific research in
oncology, with due consideration to the study and analysis of
local conditions and their importance in the incidence of, and
mortality from malignant neoplasms.

At present, republican oncological and roengenoradiologi-
cal institutes have been set up and are now effectively functioning in the twelve Union Republics, while in the Latvian
and Estonian Republics they have been organized within the
institutes of experimental and clinical departments of oncology. In large Union Republics /the RSFSR and the Ukrainian
SSR/ several oncological and roentgenoradiological institutes
have been created.

The reason for creating larger specialized oncological
centres, apart from the above considerations, is that they
make possible the following:
- to make maximal and most effective use of the expensive
diagnostic and therapeutic equipment for examination and treatment of patients with malignant tumours;
- to carry out organizational measures devoted to a
further improvement of oncological assistance to the population of each Republic;
- their utilization as the permanent basis for scientific
and training purposes and as the basis for improving the
qualifications of physicians specializing in oncology as well
as for the middle-level medical personnel.

In the light of the above, the following objectives pertain to the program of work of the Oncological Centre:

I. Questions Relating to the Organization of Cancer Control

I.1. The study of the incidence of, morbidity, mortality from, and the efficiency of treatment of malignant neoplasms with due consideration to epidemiological features. Creation of a cancer registry on the basis of the Centre with wide-scale program to investigate the above questions.

I.2. Elaboration of effective methods of early detection and diagnosis of tumourous and pretumourous diseases on the basis of mass examinations of the population.

I.2.1. Methods of mass screening of the population /with due consideration of the local conditions/.

I.2.2. Performance of tests with high resolution capacity, which are suitable for mass screening.

I.2.3. Methods of formation of high-risk groups of population who are subject to examination and supervision on a priority basis.

I.2.4. The study of the efficiency of the existing, and the development of new, methods of early diagnosis of tumourous and pretumourous diseases which might be suitable for mass examinations of the population.

I.3. Development of prophylactic methods in the field of malignant neoplasms.

I.3.1. The study and prophylaxis of carcinogenic agents in the human environment.

I.4. The study and development of effective forms and methods of public education about cancer.

II. Questions Relating to Clinical Oncology

II.1. Development of methods of comprehensive diagnosis of malignant neoplasms, their relapses and metastases.

II.2. The study of optimal variants and methods of surgical, comprehensive and combined treatment, radiotherapy, chemotherapy, hormonal treatment of various forms of malignant tumours.

II.3. Development of various patterns of comprehensive therapy and assessment of the results of their application from the point of view of duration and persistence of remissions in case of relapses and metastases.

II.4. Carrying out clinical tests and approbation of new diagnostic and theraupetic methods.

II.5. Development of classification and staging of malignant tumours and their assessment.

III. Questions of the Social Rehabilitation of Patients with Malignant Tumours

III.1. Development of general aspects and methods of restorative treatment in the course of the social-labour rehabilitation of patients.

III.2. The study of limits and possibilities of labour rehabilitation of patients in relation to a number of factors /sex, age, localization of tumour, the nature of treatment which can be carried out, occupation of the patient, possibility of his retraining and so on/.

IV. Training of Oncologists in the Centre

IV.1. Development of the organizational structure of facilities in oncological centres devoted to the training of scientific workers, physicians, medical students and middle--level medical personnel.

V. Coordination of Scientific Research in Experimental and Clinical Oncology

V.1. Determination of the main directions of research of malignant neoplasms within the framework of the activities of the Centre.

V.2. The forms of liaison between the oncological centres and the scientific research and treatment institutions.

V.3. The forms in which the progressive methods of diagnosis, treatment and organization of cancer control should be included into the practical activities of the treatment institutions.

To a certain extent, the activities of oncological centres in the Republics coincide with the program stated

above, though it is necessary to point out here that each
Republican oncological centre has its individual lines of
clinical, experimental and organizational research, which considerably depends on local conditions, on the availability of
personnel and the nature of the material-technical base of
each institute. It should be recalled that, irrespective of
the differences in the directions of scientific research work
between the oncological Republican centres, the problem of
scientific foundations for the organization of cancer control
forms an integral part of their work and occupies a considerable place in their research plans. All these determine to a
great extent their role as cancer control centres in their
Republics.

Before listing the Republican oncological centres we wish
to emphasize that the information given below relates exclusively to their activities on the problem of scientific foundations
for the organization of cancer control because the description
of this problem is the only purpose of this monograph.

Concerning the problem of scientific foundations for the
organization of cancer control the main directions of scientific
research of the oncological and roentgenoradiological centres
at the Republican level may be characterized as follows:

Oncological Centres in the USSR

The head institution of the problem is the Research Institute of Oncology named after Professon N.N. Petrov and decorated
with the Order of the Red Banner of Labour /Ministry of Public
Health of the USSR, Leningrad/.

The Institute was organized in the year 1926 and has been
in charge of the scientific-and-methodological guidance over
the Republican oncological and roentgenoradiological institutes
and the activities of the oncological network of the Soviet
Union since 1966.

As far as the problem of the scientific foundations for
the organization of cancer control is concerned, the Institute
works on such questions as incidence of malignant tumours,
morbidity, efficiency of treatment, and mortality from malignant tumours; it exercises a scientific-and-methodological

guidance with regard to the introduction of a centralized system of processing of data on oncological patients with the aid of electronic computers. In the sphere of scientific interests of the Institute one can also find such questions as the improvement of efficiency of mass prophylactic examinations; the formation of high-risk groups, the problems of social, labour and psychological rehabilitation of oncological patients and the methods of prophylaxis of malignant tumours through identification of carcinogenic agents in the environment. The Institute possesses a hospital registry which is unique for its volume and detailed nature and which has made possible to organize the All-Union Centre for the study of efficiency of treatment of oncological patients. This centre analyses the indicators of treatment of patients with malignant neoplasms and its efficiency on the basis of the information provided by the cooperating oncological institutions of the country which are 40 in number. Within the framework of the CMEA, the Research Institute of Oncology named after Professor N.N. Petrov exercises a general supervision over the work on the problem of the scientific foundations for the organization of cancer control.

The Oncological Research Centre of the Academy of Sciences of the USSR /Moscow/

The Institute was organized in 1952 /formerly it was called the Institute of Experimental and Clinical Oncology of the Academy of Sciences of the USSR/.

This Institute is the head institution for basic research on the problem of malignant neoplasms. This oncological research centre serves as the base for the activities of the Scientific Council for the complex problem of "Malignant neoplasms" under the Presidium of the Academy of Sciences of the USSR.

Concerning the scientific foundations for the organization of cancer control, the Oncological Research Centre works on the coordination of the international scientific cooperation, elaborates the ways and possibilities of using electronic computers in the information retrieval systems, determines the criteria for including patients into the high-risk groups, and also deals with the medical and social rehabilitation of oncological patients and the epidemiology of tumours.

The Moscow Oncological Institute named after P.A. Hertzen of the Ministry of Public Health of the RSFSR, /Moscow/

The Institute was organized in 1920. It is the head institution on the problem of malignant neoplasms in the RSFSR and exercises scientific-and-methodological guidance over the oncological network of the RSFSR.

Its research work concerning the problem of the "Scientific Foundations for the Organizations of Cancer Control" is focussed on the study of improvement of indcators of oncological assistance to the population of the Russian Federation /network, morbidity, mortality, personnel, plant and equipment/.

Several research projects are devoted to the questions of diagnosis of malignant neoplasms in the conditions of the polyclinics of the general health service /stages of examination, duration, typical diagnostic errors, analysis of equipment in the polyclinics of the general health service/. In accordance with the major directions of its activities, the Institute participates in the training of physicians specializing in oncology, successfully introduces into practice the programs of specialization and improvement of qualifications of physicians working in oncology and of physicians working in the general health service.

The Research Institute of Oncology of the Ministry of Public Health of the RSFSR /Rostov-on-Don/

The Institute was organized in 1931; it exercises scientific-and-methodological guidance over the oncological network of the Northern Caucasus.

The Institute is working on questions concerning the improvement of forms and methods of mass prophylactic examinations with the use of diagnostic tests suitable for mass screening, analyses and studies the incidence of, and mortality from, malignant tumours, elaborates the problems of

epidemiology of tumours of different localizations, including
that of the cancer of the lung.

It has to be pointed out here that the Institute investigates also the effect of occupational hazards upon the incidence of cancer of the lung among miners in the Rostov Region.

The Research Institute of Roentgenoradiology and Oncology of the Ministry of Public Health of the Ukrainian SSR /Kiev/

The Institute was organized in 1920. It exercises scientific-and-methodological guidance over the oncological network
of the Ukrainian SSR.

The research work of this institute related to the scientific foundations for the organization of cancer control is
focussed on the study of the efficiency of cancer control in
the Ukraininan SSR, on the analysis of data on morbidity,
mortality, efficiency of treatment, and on the number of patients in advanced stages of the disease. The available information provides the basis for elaboration of measures aimed at a
further improvement of oncological assistance. Wide-scale
research is carried out into the effect of carcinogenic agents
in the environment on the incidence of various forms of malignant tumours.

The Research Institute of Oncology and the Medical Radiology of the Ministry of Public Health of the Byelorussian SSR /Minsk/

The Institute was organized in 1960. It exercises scientific-and-methodological guidance over the oncological network
of the Byelorussian Republic. The main directions of the
research concerning the scientific foundations for the organization of cancer control are focussed on the elaboration of a
centralized, automated system of registration of data on morbidity from malignant neoplasms and on the creation of effective
forms and methods of mass prophylactic examinations for the
detection of tumourous and pretumourous diseases.

The Research Institute of Oncology of the Ministry of Public Health of the Lithuanian SSR /Vilnius/

The Institute was organized in 1957. Its main directions
of research in connection to the scientific foundations for

the organization of cancer control are focussed on the study
of morbidity, mortality and spread of malignant neoplasms in
the Lithuanian SSR and also on the system of registration of
malignant tumours.

The Research Institute of Oncology of the Ministry of Public Health of the Moldavian SSR /Kishinev/

The Institute was organized in 1960. It exercises scientific-and-methodological guidance over the oncological network
of the Republic.

Concerning the problem of the "Scientific Foundations for
the Organization of Cancer Control", the Institute's main effort is directed towards studying the criteria for formation
of high-risk groups, the elaboration of methods of early diagnosis of malignant neoplasms, elaboration of methods of assistance to patients in advanced stages of the disease.

The Azerbaijan Research Institute of Roentgenology, Radiology and Oncology of the Ministry of Public Health of the Azerbaijan SSR /Baku/

The Institute was organized in 1941. It exercises scientific-and-methodological guidance over the oncological network
of the Republic.

The Institute works on the problems of the incidence of,
and mortality from, malignant tumours /including the incidence
and epidemiology of tumours in female genital organs/, the
organization forms of mass prophylactic examinations with the
utilization of the large-frame photoroentgenography for detection of tumours in the gastrointestinal tract.

The Armenian Research Institute of Roentgenology and Oncology of the Ministry of Public Health of the Armenian SSR /Yerevan/

The Institute was organized in 1946. It exercises scientific-and-methodological guidance over the oncological network
of the Republic. With regard to the scientific foundations for
the organization of cancer control, the Institute focusses its
efforts on the study of efficiency of treatment of patients
with malignant tumours, of the indicators of oncological assistance to the population and of the epidemiological

peculiarities of the incidence of tumours in the Armenian SSR.

The Research Institute of Oncology of the Ministry of Public Health of the Georgian SSR /Tbilisi/

The Institute was organized in 1958. It exercises scientific-and-methodological guidance over the oncological network of the Republic. As regards the elaboration of the scientific foundations for the organization of cancer control, the Institute focusses its efforts on the study of the criteria for determination of high-risk groups of patients stricken with cancer of the female genital organs, of the forms of organization of mass prohylactic examinations of the female population, and on the effect of pollution on the incidence of cancer among the population of the Georgian SSR, in its large industrial areas and in the countryside.

The Research Institute of Oncology and Radiology of the Ministry of Public Health of the Kirghiz SSR /Frunze/

The Institute was organized in 1959. It exercises guidance over the oncological network of the Republic. Concerning the elaboration of the scientific foundations for the organization of cancer control the Institute has for a number of years been studying the incidence, epidemiology, morbidity of, and mortality from malignant tumours.

The Institute has made a significant contribution to the elaboration of the principles of the field survey of the population with the purpose to detect tumourous and pretumourous diseases as well as to the study of the effect of the carcinogenic agents on the incidence of cancer of different localizations among certain contingents of the population.

The Research Institute of Oncology of the Ministry of Public Health of the Turkmen SSR /Ashkhabad/

The Institute was organized in 1963. It exercises scientific-and-methodological guidance over the oncological network of the Republic. Its research work in relation to the scientific foundations for the organization of cancer control is focussed on the study of the structure, epidemiology and the indicators of the incidence of, and mortality from, malignant tumours, and, in particular, on the study of the indicators of cancer incidence on the oesophagus which occupies the first place in morbidity in the Republic. The Institute elaborates forms and methods of mass prophylactic examinations of the population /adapting them to local conditions/ and methods of health education of the population.

The Research Institute of Oncology and Radiology of the Ministry of Public Health of the Uzbek SSR /Tashkent/

The Institute was organized in 1958. It exercises scientific-and-methodological guidance over the oncological network.

With regard to the scientific foundations for the organization of cancer control, the Institute focusses its efforts on the assessment of the indicators of medical assistance to oncological patients in the institutions of the general medical service, on the elaboration of methods of the field survey conducted for the detection of tumourous and pretumourous diseases, on the study of the incidence of tumours of certain localizations /e.g. cancer of the oesophagus/ in the Uzbek SSR and on the elaboration of criteria for the inclusion of patients in high-risk groups.

The Research Institute of Oncology and Radiology of the Ministry of Public Health of the Kazakh SSR /Alma-Ata/

The Institute was organized in 1960. It exercises scientific-and-methodological guidance over the oncological network of the Republic. Concerning scientific foundations for the organization of cancer control it focusses its efforts on the development of new forms of mass prophylactic examinations of the population /including the survey method/, on the study of peculiarities of the incidence of some forms of malignant tumours and the study of the indicators of oncological assistance to the population.

Department of Oncology of the Latvian Research Institute of Experimental and Clinical Medicine /Riga/

The Department was organized in 1956. It elaborates first of all the theoretical aspects of malignant neoplasms /morphology of tumours, chemistry of the cancer cell, immunoreactivity of malignant tumours, diagnosis of tumours/. Among the areas of work mentioned above, the laboratory diagnosis of cancer is directly connected to the problem of the scientific foundations for the organization of cancer control, where the successful elaboration and implementation of automatic equipment for the diagnosis of cytological smears in the course of mass examinations of women is going on.

Department of Oncology of the Research Institute of Experimental Medicine of the Ministry of Public Health of the Estonian SSR /Tallin/

The Department was organized in 1947. It elaborates mainly the problems of carcinogenesis and epidemiology of tumours and has made a significant contribution to the study of the problem of the scientific foundations for the organization of cancer control.

The analysis of the main directions of research on the problem of the "Scientific Foundations for the Organization of Cancer Control" carried out in the Republican oncological institutes makes one to arrive to the conclusion that the coordination of scientific research has effectively promoted the concentration of efforts of the institutes in the elaboration of the major tasks arising in connection with the above-mentioned problem.

PERSPECTIVES OF THE IMPROVEMENT OF ONCOLOGICAL
ASSISTANCE TO THE POPULATION
V.P. Demidov and N.P. Napalkov

In considering the possible aspects of the improvement of oncological assistance to the population one should bear in mind that in solving this complicated problem the organization of cancer control occupies a dominant position.

It is obvious that in improving the system of organization of cancer control it is necessary, in the first place, to select the key directions where reorganization should be effected. Such an approach should make it possible to focus attention on their elaboration already in the years to come.

Cancer control consists of a whole series of measures in the field of prophylaxis, detection, diagnosis, treatment, follow-up and rehabilitation of oncological patients, i.e. measures which have the objective to reduce the number of new cases, to increase the number of cured patients and lower the invalidity rate caused by this disease. /The definition of cancer control has been evolved by the WHO Committee of Experts which was convened for this purpose in 1964/.

It is necessary to study the above questions because in many respects they determine the system of organization of oncological assistance to the population.

It should be borne in mind, however, that what serves as basis for the development of research into improving oncological assistance to the population is the availability of reliable statistical data on the morbidity and mortality from malignant tumours. The forecast of the incidence of the main forms of malignant tumours compiled for the nex five-year period shows that one can expect a' higher number of cases subject to radical treatment and further follow-up by the oncological network. Thus, the need arises to develop wide-scale research into the levels of real incidence, morbidity and mortality from malignant tumours in the USSR. In this respect an automated system of centralized registration of patients primarily diagnosed as having a malignant neoplasm acquires a great importance. This system has been in operation since January 1, 1977, and it makes it possible not only to approach the values of real incidence but to broaden considerably the program of study of the incidence of, and mortality from malignant tumours; it should also ensure a prompt registration of patients and facilitate management and planning within the oncological network.

One of the indicators of the efficiency of cancer control programs is the number of patients in whom the disease is detected in a stage when radical treatment is still possible.

There can be no doubt that after an adequate treatment for certain types of tumours patients have the chance to live

as long as healthy people do in the same environment. Therefore, it is incorrect to consider that the only treatment for
cancer control is the palliative one and that and early diagnosis can prolong the life of the patients only by several
months or years. The main purpose of early diagnosis is to
detect the disease in a stage when radical treatment is still
possible.

Early diagnosis of malignant tumours, mainly if made in
a precancerous stage, can produce a high rate of recovery in
case of application of modern methods of treatment. And since
in many cases the development of precancerous conditions takes
months and sometimes years before the appearance of a malignant
neoplasm is confirmed by microscopic and clinical tests, the
recovery from precancerous state prevents a subsequent
development of cancer.

Among the potential possibilities of prophylaxis of cancer and precancerous diseases, a special place belongs to the
removal of carcinogenic factors from the environment /those
already known and those not yet identified/ and also the so-
-called "modifying factors" which promote the development of
endogenic tumours /hormonal inbalance, undernourishment, metabolic disorders and so on/.

In planning research into the scientific foundations for
the organization of cancer control, use should be made not only
of the above-mentioned measures /incidence, morbidity, mortal-
ity/, but also of the efficiency of treatment of oncological
patients which in effect determines and sums up the ultimate
effort of the entire system of oncological assistance to the
population, its social importance and economic efficiency.

Thus, the main problems which are subject to research can
be formulated as follows:

1. Elaboration of the main principles of the statistics
of malignant tumours and creation of a standardized form of
registration and follow-up suitable machine processing /by
computers/.

2. Introduction of the new system of registration in the
activities of the oncological institutions, which should make

possible to obtain more realistic values of morbidity and mortality from malignant tumours, and to assess the activities of the oncological as well as of the general medical service concerning the methodology they use for investigations, prophylaxis and diagnosis of malignant neoplasms.

3. The study and establishment of the regularities associated the incidence of tumours at the main localizations /cancer of the stomach, the lung, the breast and the female genital organs/; on the basis of data thus obtained the development of effective organizational measures for the prophylaxis and early detection of tumours at the above localizations.

4. In the prophylaxis of cancer, an ever greater importance is acquired by the questions of organization of mass prophylactic examinations of the population which constitute the first stage in the transition to a solid monitoring of the entire population of the country. At present intensive search is going on for the optimal forms of organization and of mass prophylactic examinations of the population with a view to raise their efficiency. From among the questions the solution of which play a positive role in improving oncological assistance to the population the following two should be mentioned here:

a/ the study of the main criteria for determining high--risk groups and the creation of rational organizational methods of the formation and investigation of these groups;

b/ development of simple, reliable, highly sensitive tests to be used in the course of mass examinations for detect tumourous and pretumourous diseases.

5. Creation of unified methodology for the study of the efficiency of treatment as well as of the methodology of mathematical forecasting of rational schedules of comprehensive treatment of patients for the main forms of malignant tumours.

6. The study of questions related to the rehabilitation of patients who have undergone radical treatment for malignant neoplasms, with due consideration of such factors as age, education, occupation, the nature of the patient's work; on the basis of data thus obtained elaboration of recommendations concerning the social and labour readaptation of such patients.

Considering that the incidence of cancer is constantly increasing and that the complex and combined treatment of patients with malignant tumours becomes ever more complicated, there is a need of repeated hospitalization for administering the courses of palliative therapy and for treatment of relapses and metastases and consequently of expanding the network of oncological institutions intended for specialized treatment of patients with malignant tumours which should, no doubt, result in the improvement of distant results of treatment.

One of the most urgent tasks of the improvement of oncological assistance to the population is the training of oncologists for the oncological network and also the raising the level of oncological training of medical students. The separation of oncology as a discipline in its own right in the medical universities and the creation of a special curriculum for medical students, for physicians who are specializing in oncology and are refreshing their knowledge in this field as well as for the middle-level medical personnel will make possible to exercise an entirely different approach to the solution of a number of organizational tasks aimed at the timely detection and adequate treatment of patients with malignant neoplasms.

7. Apart from the research mentioned above, measures should be taken to continue and considerably broaden the scope of research aimed at detecting carcinogenic agents in the environment /especially those chemical compounds and substances which are used in industry, agriculture and for domestic purposes/. The maximal permissible concentration of these substances should be studied and established.

Special attention should be given to the development of scientifically substantiated measures for preventing carcinogenic influences in the environment for which we ourselves are responsible.

Coordination of efforts on the part of oncologists, organizers of public health, epidemiologists and hygienists of the USSR should provide the basis for an integrated approach to the solution of this problem.

The implementation of the proposed research should result

in a considerable modernization of the system of oncological assistance to the population.

The number of oncological institutions should increase the structure and the nature of their activities should change and the level of curative and prophylactic assistance to the population should rise, which, in its turn, should bring about a better health status of large contingents of the population, a higher efficiency of treatment of patients with malignant tumours and of their labour and social readaptation.

REFERENCES

1./B.V.Petrovsky/ Петровский Б.В.: 60 лет Советского здраво-
охранения /достижения и пути дальнейшего развития/ ж. "Со-
ветское здравоохранение", 1978,7, с. 3-9

2./B.V. Petrovsky/ Петровский Б.В.: Народное здравоохранение
и медицинская наука за 60 лет Советской власти. Вестн.
АМН СССР, 1978,2, с. 3-19

3./A.V. Chaklin, M.I. Glebova, N.M. Barmina/ Чаклин А.В.,
Глебова М.И., Бармина Н.М.: Организация онкологической службы в СССР /библиотека практического врача/, М., Медицина,
1976, 112 с.

4./Edited by N.N. Blokhin and N.P. Napalkov/ Под редакцией
Н.Н. Блохина и Н.П. Напалкова: Развитие советской онкологии в IX пятилетке, М., Медицина, 164 с.

5./Malignant Neoplasia. USSR statistic data/ Злокачественные
новообразования /статистические материалы по СССР/: под
редакцией проф. А.Ф. Серенко и к.м.н. Г.Ф. Церковного. М.,
Медицина, 1974, 188 с.

6./USSR-75 in Figures. Statistic data collection/ СССР в циф-
рах в 1975 г. /краткий статистический сборник/ М., "Статис-
тика", 1976, 240 с.

7./N.P. Napalkov, V.M. Merabishvili, G.F. Tserkovny et. al./
Н.П. Напалков, В.М. Мерабишвили, Г.Ф. Церковный и др.: Со-
стояние и перспективы развития онкологической статистики в
СССР. Вопр. онкологии, 1978, т. 24, 6, с. 38-44

8./N.P. Napalkov, G.F. Tserkovny, V.M. Merabishvili, M.N.Pre-
obrazhenskaya/ Н.П. Напалков,Г.Ф. Церковный,В.М. Мерабишвили,
М.Н. Преображенская:Злокачественные новообразования в СССР
в 1975 году. - Вопр. онкологии, 1978, 24, 6, с. 8-37

INTERNATIONAL SCIENTIFIC RELATIONSHIPS AND RESEARCH WITHIN THE PROGRAM OF TECHNICAL-SCIENTIFIC COOPERATION OF THE CMEA MEMBER-STATES

N. P. Napalkov and S. Eckhardt

During the last decades, cooperation of efforts in solving problems of major importance in the fields of medicine and public health has become one of the well-established directions in the relations between scientists of various countries. Today, not a single scientist in the world would doubt that the possibilities of solving the problem of cancer transcend national boundaries. The enormous toll of human life taken by this disease calls for global efforts in studying it and winning over it an ultimate victory. But what is required for fundamental research is the availability of the most up-to-date and costly equipment, while for clinical research a large number of observations and their analysis, which might ensure the reliability on of experiment within a shortest time. Organization of cancer control, statistics and registration of morbidity and mortality, epidemiological investigations which make possible to establish the geography of cancer and compare environmental conditions and their likely role in its causation require the scales of the continents for comparisons and conclusions to be made. Wide possibilities open up in this respect before the countries of the socialist community.

Guided by the recommendations of the Council of Mutual Economic Assistance, based on the principles of the socialist internationalism, complete equality, respect for sovereignty and national interests, mutual advantage and comradely assistance, giving much importance to the development of research in the

field of oncology, desiring to enhance its efficiency, to a-
chieve results commensurate with the world level of scientific
development, the CMEA member-states have decided to pool their
efforts in the elaboration of one of the most important problems
of the century - oncology. In accordance with this the competent
organs of Bulgaria, Cuba, Czechoslovakia, GDR, Hungary, Mongolia,
Poland and the USSR have signed an Agreement on Scientific-Technical Cooperation on the Complex Problem of "Malignant Neoplasms"
in Moscow on December 3, 1973.

The signing was preceded by a meeting of directors of leading oncological institutions of the socialist countries who discussed the scope of cooperation, singled out 9 problems which
include all the major and most important departments of experimental and clinical oncology taken as the basis for a long-term
program in the field of oncological research.

Oncology is the first problem which has been included in
the complex program of cooperation within the framework of the
CMEA.

More than 9o institutes of the socialist countries are taking part in the realization of the Research Program.

The utilization of the CMEA platform for the integration
of oncologists of the socialist countries is one of the possibilities for establishing closer scientific contacts which represent a qualitatively new form of cooperation. This form provides for the creation of joint laboratories, temporary international scientific research collectives, etc.

Each participating country has been entrusted according to
the program of the Agreement with the elaboration of individual
scientific aspects of the complex problem.

Problem No.I. "Viral carcinogenesis and its molecular-bio-
logical aspects" - Czechoslovakia /the Institute of Experimental
Oncology of the Slovak Academy of Sciences/;

Problem No.2. "Chemical carcinogenesis" - the USSR /the
Oncological Research Centre of the Academy of Sciences of the
USSR/;

Problem No.3. "Immunology of tumours" - the USSR /the
Moscow Oncological Research Institute named after P.A. Herzen,

Ministry of Public Health of the Russian Federation/;

Problem No.4. "Diagnosis of tumours" - the GDR /the Central Institute of Cancer Research of the Academy of Sciences of the GDR/;

Problem No.5. "Pharmacotherapy of tumours" - Hungary /the State Institute of Oncology/;

Problem No.6. "Radiotherapy of tumours" - Poland /the Institute of Oncology named after Sklodowska-Curie/;

Problem No.7. "Epidemiology of tumours" - the USSR /the Oncological Research Centre of the Academy of Sciences of the USSR/;

Problem No.8. The "Scientific Principles for the Organization of Cancer Control" - the USSR /the Scientific Research Institute of Oncology named after N.N. Petrov of the Ministry of Public Health of the USSR/;

Problem No.9. "Surgical and combined treatment of malignant tumours" - Bulgaria /the Oncological Centre of the Medical Academy/.

The cooperation of research has been assigned to the Scientific Oncological Centre of the Academy of Sciences of the USSR which at present is the Coordination Centre and has a staff functioning on its basis.

For settling the main questions concerning the implementation of the Agreement and the program of scientific research, a Council of Plenipotentiaries has been set up in which each member-state has its representative. For the consideration of scientific and technical aspects of the program of cooperation, a Scientific Council has been set up which is a consultative body for the Council of Plenipotentiaries.

During the period that has elapsed since the signing of the Agreement, a considerable amount of work has been accomplished in realizing the plans of cooperation, which has made it possible to embark on the road of practical implementation of the program of the Agreement with respect to the majority of problems. The experts have been convening on meetings for the consideration of each problem and they have determined the thematic scope of research to be done on cooperation lines, rendered the programs of this research concrete, discussed the possibilities of the standardization of research methods and worked out common criteria for assessment of results.

By now, the number of inter-institute contracts has reached 8o in the field of scientific cooperation with regard to individual themes and assignments in accordance with the working plans.

On the meetings of the Council of Plenipotentiaries and the Scientific Council, conducted by the Coordination Centre, the members consider questions of detailing and elucidation of the Program of Work, scientific training and raising qualification of oncologists, the procedures involved in allocating finances for specialists of the CMEA member-states engaged in joint research in accordance with the Program; they also discuss projects in the field of long-term forecasting and sum up the results of the preceding meetings on individual problems. Within this complex problem a considerable place is assigned to creating and strengthening the experimental base for scientific research: making up a catalogue of various strains of animals and cell cultures used in experimental work by the institutes of the CMEA member-states, establishing a central vivarium which would possess standard, genetically pure strains of animals, setting up on a permanent basis the production of foetal sera and biopreparations, standard laboratory plates and dishes necessary for conducting research by the institutes of the CMEA member-states. The realization of the proposal to create a central tumour bank, a bank of carcinogenic substances necessary for conducting scientific research on the problem of "Chemical Carcinogenesis" has started in the USSR. The CMEA member-states consider supplying the cooperating institutes with modern technology and apparatus to be an important part of their activities: in the GDR, the production of photofluorographs and fluoroscopes using IOO mm films has benn started and a semi-automatic apparatus has been designed for the analysis of photofluorographs; in the GDR and Poland apparatus and instruments are produced for conducting lymphoangiographic investigations. In the USSR an automatic apparatus has been designed for cytodiagnosis which hàs been highly appraised by oncologists all over the world.

A considerable amount of work has been accomplished by the Coordination Centre in the field of forecasting scientific research. A project for this prognosis of the problem as a whole has been outlined and work is going on to improve some of its aspects. Measures have been adopted to complete this work on the prognosis and a respective calendar plan has been outlined. The prognosis contains an analysis of the modern status of research and the results achieved in the field of experimental and clinical oncology.

In accordance with the complex program of socialist economic integration, provision has been made for the further strengthening and improvement of cooperation of the CMEA states on the field of training of scientific and scientific-plus-teaching personnel, especially on the basis of joint scientific research.

The efforts of the countries which are signatory to the Agreement are directed towards raising the level of training of the specialists participating in the elaboration of the above-mentioned problems on the basis of the achievements of science and technology in the socialist countries.

In this connection, it is especially important to provide those participating in the elaboration of the above-mentioned problems with information about the results of research in the sphere of their activities.

Considering the increasing urgency of the cancer problem, the Council of Plenipotentiaries and the Scientific Council have recommended to include oncology in the program of medical faculties as a separate discipline and also to publish textbooks for students on this subject. Work in this direction is carried out in the journal "Neoplasma" and it is planned to organize a discussion on the methods of training and teaching of oncologists in each country which is signatory to the Agreement.

The main forms of cooperation of the CMEA member-states in raising the qualification of scientific and scientific-plus-teaching personnel are as follows:

I. Fellowship training of specialists for studying and mastering methods of research and for familiarization with the achievements in a concrete scientific direction /from one month to two years/.

2. Organization of summer and winter courses for increasing the knowledge of young scientific workers of some concrete questions on their field of specialization or allied disciplines of science and technology /from 7 to I2 days/.

3. Organization of seminars, conferences and colloquia on the most important problems of science and technology /from 3 to 5 days/.

4. Organization of short-term and long-term courses either to provide systematically the latest information on limited area of scientific activity for a definite group of scientists or to retrain specialists in a new direction of development and research /from 7 to 90 days/.

5. Organization of lectures on individual results of scientific research and development.

6. Organization of conferences, symposia and congresses on a wide range of questions pertaining to various aspects of science and technology.

This work is organized by the Coordination Centre.

The first international course "Oncologist-76" was organized in the USSR in October I976 with the participation of I39 young oncologists.

The first international seminar on clinical chemotherapy was held in November I976 in Hungary /the State Institute of Oncology, Budapest/. A didactic laboratory on the topic "Individual planning of irradiation with the aid of electronic computers" has been organized in the GDR /the State Institute of Cancer Research of the Academy of Sciences of the GDR/.

In the training of young specialists a great role has been assigned to the international laboratory for lymphography and angiography which will be based on the Institute of Medical Radiology of the Academy of Sciences of the USSR and it will promote a faster and more successful solution of many tasks of practical importance in the field of diagnostics.

Besides, a number of the institutes of the CMEA member-states, have been selected to serve as international centres for improving qualifications of young specialists in the field of oncology.

A school for medical physicists is being set up at the Institute of Oncology named after M. Sklodowska-Curie in Warsaw.

As a result of the organizational work carried out by the Coordination Centre in the realization of the Program with regard to the individual assignments of the labour plans, the results of scientific work have been brought to the stage where they can be introduced into practice.

The introduction of the scientific results into practice is realized in various forms, namely in monographs, articles, methodological instructions which allow an improved diagnosis of malignant neoplasms.

In 1976, a collective monograph compiled by the oncologists of the socialist countries was published on "Prophylaxis of Cancer" /edited by L.M. Shabad, Member of the Academy of Sciences of the USSR and Professor G. Mitrov, Bulgaria/.

A list of carcinogenic substances has been published; it will be expanded by the inclusion of new substances the carcinogenicity of which will be studied.

The "Information Bulletin on Chemotherapy of Tumours" is issued 6 times a year. Its publication is organized by the State Institute of Oncology in Hungary, which acts as the supervisor for the problem of "Chemotherapy of Malignant Tumours".

A book entitled "Treatment of Generalized Forms of Tumour Diseases" /edited by N.N. Blokhin, Member of the Academy of Sciences of the USSR, and Professor S. Eckhardt, Medicina, Moscow 1978/.

A group of scientists from the USSR, Poland and the GDR is working on the monograph "The Methods of Studying Epidemiology of Malignant Tumours in the CMEA Countries".

A review "Epidemiology of Malignant Tumours in the CMEA Countries" together with a bibliography of works on the subject publushed in the last IO years is under preparation.

This monograph will contain a description of the system of organization of oncological assistance to the population in the CMEA countries. The monograph is intended for oncologists and organizers in the field of public health; being, largely, a reference work, it should be indispensable for those working both in research and in the practice on the problem of malignant neoplasms not only in the countries of the socialist camp but in other countries, too.

The work on the methodology of compilation of an "Atlas of Incidence of Malignant Tumours over the Territory of the CMEA Countries" is being completed.

An effective method has been elaborated for detecting benzopyrene, a cancer-producing hydrocarbon, in automobile exhaust gases, products of internal combustion. This method has been submitted for consideration and adoption for the member-states of the European Economic Community.

Significant practical results are expected also from the joint work on detection and lowering the content of carcinogenic hydrocarbons in foodstuffs.

The cooperation on the complex problem of malignant neoplasms within the framework of the CMEA makes possible to include a whole number of urgent problems of modern oncology in this effort. The principle of cooperation in research may be accomplished because the methods of research are unified and standardized. The coordination of research, which is also one of the principles of scientific cooperation, considerably facilitates the task of elaborating new, modern approaches to the solution of different problems of experimental and clinical oncology.

Apart from the exchange of experience, the principle of mutual assistance is also applied, which considerably increases the technical possibilities of conducting experiments while the exchange of apparatus and instruments contributes to the solution of the tasks in the shortest time possible.

PROSPECTS OF COORDINATION OF CANCER CONTROL IN THE CMEA MEMBER-STATES

N. P. Napalkov and S. Eckhardt

It is evident that, in order to make the fight against malignant neoplasms more effective, it is necessary to combine the efforts and to solve a number of scientific, therapeutic and organizational questions in an integrated way. This is necessitated by a constant growth in the incidence of, and mortality from, malignant neoplasms in the last 60 to 70 years, by the complexity of etiology of the disease, the presence of the latent period and the chronic progression of the disease. The large extent of social and economic losses caused by malignant neoplasms is determined by their specific features, their tendency to develop relapses and metastases, the diffuculties necessarily involved in the process of their early detection and diagnosis and also by the need to resort to complex methods of treatment with the subsequent life-long monitoring of patients, their social and labour rehabilitation.

At its 26th Session /May 23, 1973/ the World Health Assembly formulated the main provisions for long-term planning of international cooperation in the field of oncological research based on the need to join the efforts both in national and international public health in view of the great importance of cancer as one of the main causes of mortality and morbidity in many countries, considering that if the efforts of many countries are not concerted, this problem represents a far too complex task and the probability of its solution is generally low. It is obvious that the selection of key questions, the solution of which on a joint basis can be optimally productive represent the basis for joining the efforts in fighting against malignant neoplasms and for modern trends in this direction. In this respect, the coordination of the efforts of the CMEA member-states on the problem of "Scientific foundations for the organization of cancer control" seems to be a measure which is well substantiated and desireable. The socialist countries have accumulated a considerable experience of the state-organized oncological assistance to the population. This provides the general basis for studying many scientific aspects of the organization of cancer control. The differences in the approach to the solution of some problems cannot put obstacles in the way to conducting joint research into the key aspects of this important problem. This view was the basis for the formulation of the general program of the "Scientific foundations of the organization of cancer control", which is included in the agreement on technical-scientific cooperation of the CMEA member-states on the problem of malignant neoplasms. The object of joint research are problems which offer the greatest possibilities for effective and urgent coordination. These are following:

1. The study of various models of organization of cancer control in the CMEA member-states.

2. Development of organizational forms of prophylactic examinations of the population with respect to the early detection of tumours in common sites /cancer of the lung, the breast, the stomach, the uterus/.

3. Organization of the study on the efficiency of treatment of patients with malignant tumours.

The research is carried out in accordance with the proposed programs; the successful implementation of these programs shows that the possibilities of coordination of scientific research in this field are promising and make possible the further integration of efforts of the CMEA member-states. The study of the organizational patterns of cancer control has demonstrated that the main principles of organization of oncological assistance to the population in the CMEA member--states are identical. This applies to such questions of primary importance as registration systems of incidence of, and mortality from, malignant tumours, follow-up of patients, principles of investigation of patients who are suspected of having a malignant tumour, hospitalization of patients for treatment, care of patients in advanced stages of malignant neoplasms. The common principles of approach to the above-mentioned questions open up wide prospects for the further coordination of scientific research and for the optimization of methods of the improvement of oncological assistance to the population. Thus it seems desirable to create a common cancer registry for all CMEA member-states in the future together with the international program for the study of the incidence, mortality, morbidity and spread of malignant neoplasms. The concentration of efforts concerning the statistics and epidemiology of malignant neoplasms might, no doubt, contribute to the development of an extensive study on the numerous factors which determine the indicators of the incidence of malignant neoplasms and might also determine the methods of their prophylaxis.

At the first stage of the coordination of joint research, some valueable data were obtained which made possible to make a detailed study of the different patterns of in-patient assistance to oncological patients. Now the problem is still far from being solved. Practically, no country in the world is in possession of the necessary number of beds for the hospitalization of every patient primarily diagnosed as having malignant neoplasms. At the same time the growing complexity of the methods of combined treatment of patients with malignant neoplasms having not only local but also regional and also general effects upon the organism require not only the concentration of costly therapeutical equipment but also special knowledge which is obtained only if treatment plans are elaborated in a collective and consultative way. It has been established in many studies that the hospitalization of oncological patients in general medical institutions unavoidably reduces the quality of treatment and, respectively, the length of survival of patients, which can be explained not only by the lack of the entire complex of necessary equipment but also by the in-

sufficient training of physicians in the field of clinical oncology.

It should be stressed here that simultaneously with the
problem of hospitalization of patients with malignant tumours,
a real need arises to solve the questions of follow-up patients, which, in the modern conditions, becomes more active
considering that the special methods of treatment /chemo-,
hormonal and radiotherapy/ require a longer time and considering also the possibilities of the therapy of relapses and metastases at several sites.

The joint research on the problem of creating the theoretical and the practical pre requisites for the rehabilitation
of patients with malignant neoplasms seems highly promising.
This problem has not only moral but also a great national
significance. At present, the factors which determine the
possibilities and limits of rehabilitation of oncological patients, the kinds of work which they can be allowed to engage
in and the optimum volume of work load have not yet been
studied adequately enough. In each CMEA member-state, a certain amount of experience has been accumulated not only in
providing social security for patients with malignant neoplasms but also concerning their job, retraining and the correction of anatomo-functional complications which arise in the
process of treatment. This experience has to be studied and
generalized; it is also desirable and feasible to promote
research on the above-mentioned problem in accordance with
the program including its medical, labour, social and psychological aspects.

Radical treatment is provided in the CMEA member-states
annually for as many as 600 thousand patients primarily diagnosed as having a malignant neoplasm. The analysis and generalization of these data is of primary importance for the
elaboration of effective and adequate therapeutical methods
for tumours at various sites. The diversity of treatment methods, their variants and different combinations, the introduction of new drugs and irradiation sources call for the
creation of an apparatus which would compare them and would

select the most rational and optimal ways of treatment. It is beyond any doubt that, within the framework of the CMEA community, the creation of a system for the study of effectivity of treatment of oncological patients holds out a great promise and all efforts in this direction are modern and perfectly justified. The completion of the first stage of the coordination of research in this direction opens up highly fruitful prospects for their further continuation and the creation of common methodological approaches to the treatment of patients, based on a thorough analysis of the factors which determine the condition of the patient, the nature of the tumour and the degree of its dissemination. Since an assessment of the results of treatment /in the form of survival rates/ can be made only after many years of follow-up it is desirable for the CMEA member-states to coordinate their efforts in order to create of a common method for the implementation of follow-up programs.

Beyond doubt it would be especially desirable to establish a further coordination of efforts of the CMEA member-states with respect to mass examination of large parts of the population for the purpose of early detection of tumours and pre-malignant diseases. It is necessary to emphasize here that the conduct of free of charge prophylactic mass examinations of population has become possible only in the conditions of the socialist system of public health. The fact that the conduct of these examinations is ensured by the state-organized public health creates extremely favourable organizational conditions for their implementation. It should also be mentioned that adequate and reliable tests suitable for mass early diagnosis of tumours have not yet been developed in spite of the definite success of the recent years in this field; modern oncology does not yet have reliable criteria for the selection and identification of patients to be included into high-risk groups. At the first stage of the joint research of the CMEA member-states, various methods have been developed and tested for the formation of high-risk groups and the results obtained in this respect show that the theo-

736

retical pre-requisites and their practical realization are of great interest and should be developed further. It should be also emphasized that research on this problem is very important and urgent; possibilities of detecting tumours in the period before their pre clinical manifestation make possible to plan and carry out their treatment on an entirely different basis. While the modern methods of treatment cannot be considered perfect when the process has been allowed to disseminate widely they, nevertheless, ensure a prolonged and consistent recovery of the patient provided the tumour is diagnosed early and the treatment begins promptly. All that has been said above brings us to the conclusion that coordination of research in this direction seems to be most desirable. The general organizational principles of carrying out mass prophylactic examinations make possible for the CMEA member-states to focus their efforts immediately on the elaboration of principles of early detection of tumours and pre-tumourous diseases on a mass scale.

Thus, the prospects of coordination of efforts of the CMEA member-states on the problem of the "Scientific foundations of the organization of cancer control" are very promising, indeed; the experience accumulated in this direction brings us to the conclusion that a further joining of efforts by the countries of the socialist camp for organization of oncological assistance to the population is justified and feasible.

THE WAYS OF INTEGRATION OF THE SYSTEM
OF ONCOLOGICAL SERVICES
IN THE CMEA MEMBER-STATES

N. P. Napalkov and S. Eckhardt

In socialist countries oncological service is a constituent of the state-organized public health service. Up to now
the CMEA member-states have developed a well-coordinated system of specialized oncological service.

The main trends of activity of the oncological service
are based on the dispensary method in the management of cancer
patients; obligatory registration of patients with newly diagnosed tumours; maximal accessibility of specialized oncological
service to the population; prophylaxis of cancer and precancerous lesions over a wide range.

Despite some differences in the structure of oncological
service in the CMEA member-states the basic principles which
determine not only the ways of further development but also
the possibility of cooperation in the near future, are uniform.

The analysis of statistical data revealing the pattern of
activity of oncological service in the CMEA member-states shows
that it is reasonable and well-grounded to direct further improvement and development along the following guidelines:

1. The establishment of a network of large specialized
oncological hospitals, designed for 300 beds and more, provided
with the necessary facilities and equipment to ensure early
detection, qualified treatment, rehabilitation and follow-up
observation for cancer patients.

2. The establishment of a network of outpatient oncological
departments or units. The activities of these institutions including the organization of prophylactic measures, consultation

service to patients, out-patient treatment, sending the patients for clinical examination and treatment to specialized oncological hospitals, follow-up observation for patients with cancer and precancerous lesions as well as the education of the public in the field of oncology could provide maximal accessibility of oncological service to the population.

3. The improvement of all means of prophylaxis of malignant tumours: a, Elaboration of a program for the protection of environment against pollution with carcinogenic agents. b, The search for more effective organizational forms for conducting mass oncological prophylactic screenings aimed to provide diagnoses of malignant tumours in the preclinical stage of growth.

4. The improvement of therapeutic methods of treatment of malignant tumours directed towards obtaining prolonged and stable effect and maximum rehabilitation possible of cancer patients.

5. Development of an extended program for all national cancer registries to provide intensive studies of such characteristics as morbidity, mortality, effectivity of treatment and epidemiology of malignant tumours.

6. Teaching of oncology as a separate discipline at the medical universities; improvement and extension of the system of special training in the main disciplines of clinical oncology and radiology with the aim to provide highly qualified specialists in oncology, radiology and oncological chemotherapy.

7. Elaboration of programs for further research on etiopathogenesis, treatment, diagnosis and organization of cancer control.

8. Further development of coordination of research on the project "Malignant Tumours".

The above-mentioned program and the progress achieved in the oncological service are the result of the existing plans for the perspective development of oncology in the CMEA member-states. It has to be emphasized that the similarity of the main trends in perspective planning has been stipulated by the common principles in the organization of cancer control in the socialist countries.

It is also obvious that in elaborating the program of integration it is of primary importance to select the items which are the main elements in the system of organization of cancer control in each of the CMEA member-states. The following elements may be included:

1. Registration and reporting of morbidity and mortality of malignant tumours on a nation-wide basis.

2. Prophylaxis of tumours and pretumourous lesions by means of organizing mass prophylactic screenings of different groups of population.

3. System of follow-up observation for patients with tumours and pretumourous lesions.

4. Organization of the system of early diagnosis of malignant tumours.

5. Specialized oncological network at every step of its contact with cancer patients.

6. Studies on the effectivity of surgical, complex and combined methods of treatment of malignant tumours.

7. The system of special training of medical students and physicians in oncology.

In accordance with the above-mentioned program the main problems can be formulated and their elaboration should be recommended as the first stage of integration.

As far as statistics of morbidity and mortality of malignant tumours are the basis on which the scientific planning of oncological service is established, the development of common principles of the study is one of the primary tasks in the field of integration. The approach to this problem involves the following aspects:

1. Elaboration of a common protocol of registration of patients with newly diagnosed malignant tumours.

2. Elaboration of a common system of report on patients with newly diagnosed malignant tumours /organizational scheme of sending and concentraiting primary documentation about cancer patients to the corresponding establishments for processing and studying/.

3. Establishment of a joint cancer registry for the

socialist countries where the data on morbidity and mortality of malignant tumours could be concentrated.

4. Elaboration of a joint program of studying the data on morbidity and mortality of malignant tumours which may be presented as follows:

a, Studies of the tendencies in the incidence, prevalence and mortality rates from malignant tumours in the CMEA member--states.

b, Studies of epidemiology of malignant tumours.

c, Studies of the effectivity of treatment of patients with malignant tumours of the main localizations.

5. The present prophylactic mass screenings with the use of instrumental and laboratory methods of examination are a qualitatively new step in the mass diagnostics of tumours and pretumourous lesions in preclinical stage. Their further improvement is of primary importance and should be concentrated on two aspects:

a, Elaboration of the criteria and organizational forms and methods for determining the groups of population to be screened.

b, Development of effective instrumental and clinical diagnostic methods for mass screenings.

6. Taking into account that patients with malignant tumours visit general medical establishment first, the elaboration of the forms, methods and terms of conducting the examination should comply to the actual requirements and be done according to the following program:

a, Development of the effective forms of early diagnosis of malignant tumours.

b, Elaboration of rational and obligatory methods for complex instrumental and laboratory examinations of the patients suspected for cancer at all stages of their contacts with a physician.

7. The complexity of modern methods of diagnosis, and the complex and combined treatment of cancer patients require rather expensive equipment. It is necessary to elaborate the optimal pattern of an oncological dispensary which could allow the most

effective and economical use of all possibilities of providing adequate examination and treatment of cancer patients.

At the same time, the cooperative elaboration of a joint project of the structure and functions of an oncological dispensary makes possible to raise and solve a number of organizational problems connected with all aspects of oncological service to population.

8. Development of common guidelines in the selection of therapeutic methods for patients with tumours at the main localizations. The variety of therapeutic methods, their different types and constantly increasing combinations require scientifically based principles for the selection of the most rational and optimal way of therapy.

For this purpose it is necessary to have uniform methods for the examination, processing and analysis of the results of treatment as well as the primary information on the cancer patient.

9. Elaboration of a joint program and a textbook on oncology for teaching students at the medical universities.

10. Elaboration of common programs of special training and advanced courses for physicians in the main aspects of oncology /clinical oncology, radiotherapy, chemotherapy, organization of cancer control/.

Up to now, each CMEA member-state has accumulated vast experience in training students and physicians in the field of oncology. The generalization experience in training the choice of more adequate forms of teaching, the elaboration of optimal programmes for special training and advanced courses and the publication of the textbook on oncology will create qualitatively new forms which make possible to improve the system of oncological service to the population.